Sports Injuries
of the Hand and
Upper Extremity

The Hand and Upper Extremity
Volume 12

Editorial Advisory Board

Chairman:
Douglas W. Lamb, F.R.C.S.
Princess Margaret Rose Orthopaedic Hospital
Fairmilehead, Edinburgh, U.K.

W. Bruce Conolly, F.R.C.S, F.R.A.C.S., F.A.C.S.
Hand Unit, Sydney Hospital, Sydney,
New South Wales, Australia

Nicholas Barton, F.R.C.S.
Department of Hand Surgery, University Hospital,
Nottingham, U.K.

Paul R. Manske, M.D.
Orthopedic Surgery, Barnes Hospital Plaza,
St. Louis, Missouri, U.S.A.

Simon P. J. Kay
Department of Plastic Surgery, University
Hospital of St James, Leeds, U. K.

Forthcoming Volumes in the Series

Published Volumes in this series

Sports Injuries of the Hand and Upper Extremity

K. M. CHAN, M.B.B.S, F.R.C.S.(Orth), M.Ch. (Orth), F.R.C.S.

Professor and Chairman
Department of Orthopaedics and Traumatology
Faculty of Medicine
The Chinese University of Hong Kong
Chief of Service
Department of Orthopaedics and Traumatology
Prince of Wales Hospital
Shatin, New Territories, Hong Kong

Churchill Livingstone
New York, Edinburgh, London, Melbourne, Tokyo

Library of Congress Cataloging-in-Publication Data

Sports injuries of the hand and upper extremity / [edited by] K.M.
Chan.
    p.   cm. – (The hand and upper extremity ; v. 12)
    Includes bibliographical references and index.
    ISBN 0-443-07780-0
    1. Shoulder–Wounds and injuries. 2. Sports injuries. 3. Arm–
Wounds and injuries. 4. Hand–Wounds and injuries.   I. Chan, K.
M. II. Series.   III. Series: Hand and upper extremity ; v. 12.
    [DNLM: 1. Athletic Injuries. 2. Hand Injuries.   3. Arm Injuries.
W1 HA51B v. 12 1995 / QT 261 S764 1995]
RD557.S66   1995
617.5′72044–dc20
DNLM/DLC
for Library of Congress   95-14345
                                                                              CIP

Distributed in the United Kingdom by Churchill Livingstone, Robert Stevenson
House, 1–3 Baxter's Place, Leith Walk, Edinburgh EH1 3AF, and by associated
companies, branches, and representatives throughout the world.

Accurate indications, adverse reactions, and dosage schedules for drugs are
provided in this book, but it is possible that they may change. The reader is
urged to review the package information data of the manufacturers of the medications mentioned.

The Publishers have made every effort to trace the copyright holders for bor-
rowed material. If they have inadvertently overlooked any, they will be
pleased to make the necessary arrangements at the first opportunity.

Copy Editor: *Dorothy J. Birch*
Production Supervisor: *Laura Mosberg Cohen*
Cover Design: *Paul Moran*

Printed in the United States of America

First published in 1995   7   6   5   4   3   2   1

Contributors

Marnie Allegrucci, M.S., P.T., A.T.C.

Educational Coordinator, Center for Sports Medicine, University of Pennsylvania Medical Center, Pittsburgh, Pennsylvania

James R. Andrews, M.D.

Professor, Department of Orthopaedic Surgery and Sports Medicine, University of Virginia School of Medicine, Charlottesville, Virginia; Medical Director, American Sports Medicine Institute; Orthopaedic Surgeon, Alabama Sports Medicine and Orthopaedic Center, Birmingham, Alabama

Champ L. Baker, Jr., M.D.

Assistant Professor, Department of Orthopaedics, Tulane University School of Medicine, New Orleans, Louisiana; Staff Physician, Auguston Orthopaedic Clinic, Columbus, Georgia

William Beach, M.D.

Director, Orthopedic Research of Virginia, Richmond, Virginia

John A. Bergfeld, M.D.

Head, Section of Sports Medicine, Department of Orthopaedic Surgery, The Cleveland Clinic Foundation, Cleveland, Ohio

Richard Caspari, M.D.

Professor, Department of Surgery, Virginia Commonwealth University, Medical College of Virginia, School of Medicine; Founder and President, Orthopedic Research of Virginia; Orthopaedist, Department of Orthopaedic Surgery, Tuckahoe Medical Center, Richmond, Virginia

K. M. Chan, M.B.B.S, F.R.C.S.(Orth), M.Ch.(Orth), F.R.C.S.

Professor and Chairman, Department of Orthopaedics and Traumatology, Faculty of Medicine, The Chinese University of Hong Kong; Chief of Service, Department of Orthopaedics and Traumatology, Prince of Wales Hospital, Shatin, New Territories, Hong Kong

G. Dautel, M.D.

Assistant Professor, Department of Plastic and Reconstructive Surgery, NANCY Medical School, Nancy, France; Department of Plastic and Reconstructive Surgery, Centre Hospitalier de NANCY, Nancy, France, and Hôpital Jeanne d'Arc, Toul, France

Ian Davey, M.D.

Lecturer, Department of Diagnostic Radiology and Organ Imaging, The Chinese University of Hong Kong, Shatin, New Territories, Hong Kong

Paul A. Dowdy, M.D.

Resident, Division of Orthopaedic Surgery, Department of Surgery, University of Western Ontario Faculty of Medicine, London, Ontario, Canada

Rhodri M. Evans, M.B., B.Ch.., F.R.C.R

Consultant Radiologist, Department of Radiology, Morriston Hospital, Swansea, West Glamorgan, United Kingdom

Edward S. Forman, D.O.

Fellow, Department of Orthopedic Surgery, Boston University School of Medicine, Boston, Massachusetts

G. Foucher, M.D.

Senior Chief of Clinic, Universite de Strasbourg; Head, SOS Mains, Strausbourg, France

Peter J. Fowler, M.D.

Professor, Division of Orthopaedic Surgery, Department of Surgery, Head, Section of Sports Medicine, University of Western Ontario Faculty of Medicine; Orthopaedic Surgeon, University Hospital, London, Ontario, Canada

Freddie H. Fu, M.D.

Executive Vice Chairman and Professor, Department of Orthopedic Surgery, University of Pittsburgh School of Medicine; Medical Director, Center for Sports Medicine, University of Pittsburgh School of Medicine, Pittsburgh, Pennsylvania

Michael Hayes, M.B.B.S., F.R.A.C.S., FA. Orth. A.

Orthopaedic Surgeon, Sportsmed, SA, Stepney, SA, Australia

Elliott B. Hershmann, M.D.

Executive Associate Director, Department of Orthopaedic Surgery, Lenox Hill Hospital; Staff Nicholas Institute of Sports Medicine and Athletic Trauma, New York, New York

James J. Irrgang, M.D.

Assistant Professor, Department of Physical Therapy, University of Pittsburgh School of Health and Rehabilitation; Director, Outpatient Physical Therapy and Sports Medicine, Center for Sports Medicine, University of Pittsburgh Medical Center, Pittsburgh, Pennsylvania

Robert E. Leach, M.D.

Professor, Division of Orthopaedic Surgery, Department of Surgery, Boston University School of Medicine; Boston University Medical Center Hospital, Boston, Massachusetts

Ping-Chung Leung, M.B.B.S., F.R.C.S, F.R.A.C.S., M.S., D.Sc.

Professor, Department of Orthopaedics and Traumatology, The Chinese University of Hong Kong, Shatin, New Territories, Hong Kong

Terry R. Malone, Ed.D., P.T., A.T.C.

Associate Professor and Director, Division of Physical Therapy, Assistant Professor, Department of Surgery, University of Kentucky College of Medicine, Lexington, Kentucky

Patrick J. McMahon, M.D.

Assistant Professor, Department of Orthopaedic Surgery, University of California, Irvine, College of Medicine, Irvine, California; Staff, Long Beach Veterans Affairs Medical Center, Orange, California

M. Merle, M.D.

Professor, Department of Plastic and Reconstructive Surgery, NANCY Medical School; Chief, Department of Plastic and Reconstructive Surgery, Centre Hospitalier Universitaire de NANCY, Nancy, France

Lyle J. Micheli, M.D.

Associate Professor, Department of Orthopaedic Surgery, Harvard Medical School; Director, Division of Sports Medicine, Children's Hospital, Boston, Massachusetts

Anthony Miniaci, M.D.

Associate Professor, Division of Orthopaedic Surgery, Department of Surgery, University of Toronto Faculty of Medicine; Head, Section of Sports Medicine, The Toronto Hospital–Western Division, Toronto, Ontario, Canada

Lars Neumann, M.D.

Professor, Department of Orthopaedic and Accident Surgery, University of Nottingham; Consultant Orthopaedic Surgeon, King's Mill Hospital and Nottingham Shoulder and Elbow Unit, City Hospital, Nottingham, United Kingdom

Claude E. Nichols III, M.D.

Assistant Professor, Department of Orthopedics and Rehabilitation, McClure Musculoskeletal Research Center, University of Vermont College of Medicine, Burlington, Vermont

Stuart Patterson, M.B.Ch.B, F.R.C.S.C

Assistant Professor, Division of Orthopaedic Surgery, Department of Surgery, University of Western Ontario Faculty of Medicine; Consultant, Hand and Upper Limb Centre, London, Ontario, Canada

Dave Pezzullo, M.S., P.T., A.T.C

Adjunct Assistant Professor, Department of Physical Therapy, University of Pittsburgh School of Health and Rehabilitation Sciences; Physical Therapist IV, Center for Sports Medicine, University of Pennsylvania Medical Center, Pittsburgh, Pennsylvania

Per A. F. H. Renström, M.D., Ph.D.

Professor, Department of Orthopedics and Rehabilitation, McClure Musculoskeletal Research Center, University of Vermont College of Medicine, Burlington, Vermont

Robert S. Richards, M.D., F.R.C.S.C.

Assistant Professor, Division of Plastic and Reconstructive Surgery, Department of Surgery, University of Western Ontario Faculty of Medicine; Attending Staff, Hand and Upper Limb Centre, St. Joseph's Hospital, London, Ontario, Canada

James H. Roth, M.D., F.R.C.S.C, F.A.C.S

Professor, Division of Orthopaedics, Department of Surgery, University of Western Ontario Faculty of Medicine; Director, Hand and Upper Limb Centre, St. Joseph's Hospital, London, Ontario, Canada

John E. Samani, M.D.

Orthopaedic Surgery Resident, Department of Orthopedics and Rehabilitation, McClure Musculoskeletal Research Center, University of Vermont College of Medicine, Burlington, Vermont

Laura A. Timmerman, M.D.

Assistant Professor, Sports Medicine, Department of Orthopaedic Surgery, University of California, Davis, School of Medicine; Sacramento, California

Nathaniel L. Tindel, M.D.

Chief Resident, Department of Orthopaedic Surgery, Lenox Hill Hospital, New York, New York

Hing-Chuen Tseng, M.B.B.S, F.R.C.S.

Lecturer, Department of Orthopaedics and Traumatology, The Chinese University of Hong Kong; Orthopaedic Surgeon, Baptist Hospital, Shatin, New Territories, Hong Kong

W. Angus Wallace, F.R.C.S.Ed.

Professor, Department of Orthopaedic and Accident Surgery, University of Nottingham; Head, Department of Orthopaedic and Accident Surgery, Consultant Orthopaedic Surgeon, University Hospital Queen's Medical Centre and Shoulder and Elbow Unit, City Hospital, Nottingham, United Kingdom

Kevin E. Wilk, P.T.

National Director, Research and Clinical Education, HEALTHSOUTH Sports Medicine and Rehabilitation; Director, American Sports Medicine Institute, Birmingham, Alabama

Susan Zecher, B.S.

Graduate Student, Division of Orthopaedic Surgery, Department of Surgery, Boston University School of Medicine, Boston, Massachusetts

Foreword

One of the most dramatic, important, and rapid advancements in the field of medicine in recent years has been the development of "sports medicine." Until recently, lower extremity injuries have been the most emphasized, despite the frequency of upper extremity injuries threatening the careers of professional athletes and debilitating the amateur athelete as well.

A considerable development in the management of extremity injuries has been a proliferation of sports injury clinics staffed by medical and paramedical experts, including physical therapists, occupational therapists, hand therapists, sports psychologists, and counselors. There is no doubt that sports injury clinics, by examining the physical and psychological aspects of injuries and their victims, have improved the outcome of treatment and therapy of upper extremity injuries. Therefore, it is an opportune time for this book, *Sports Injuries of the Hand and Upper Extremity* to be published. It was not difficult to select Professor K. M. Chan, a distinguished orthopaedic surgeon and professor at The Chinese University of Hong Kong, to be editor. He has done a substantial amount of research and written many impressive papers on the subject. Professor Chan has chosen a most stimulating and experienced team of contributors, mainly from North America, who have played an important part in the development of this subspecialty. There are also many contributors from other parts of the world, who have given of their own experience and expertise.

I know this book will provide much needed information on the management of sports injuries of the upper extremity.

Douglas W. Lamb, M.B., F.R.C.S.E.
Past President, I.F.S.S.H.
Chairman, Editorial Board,
Hand and Upper Extremity Series
Churchill Livingstone

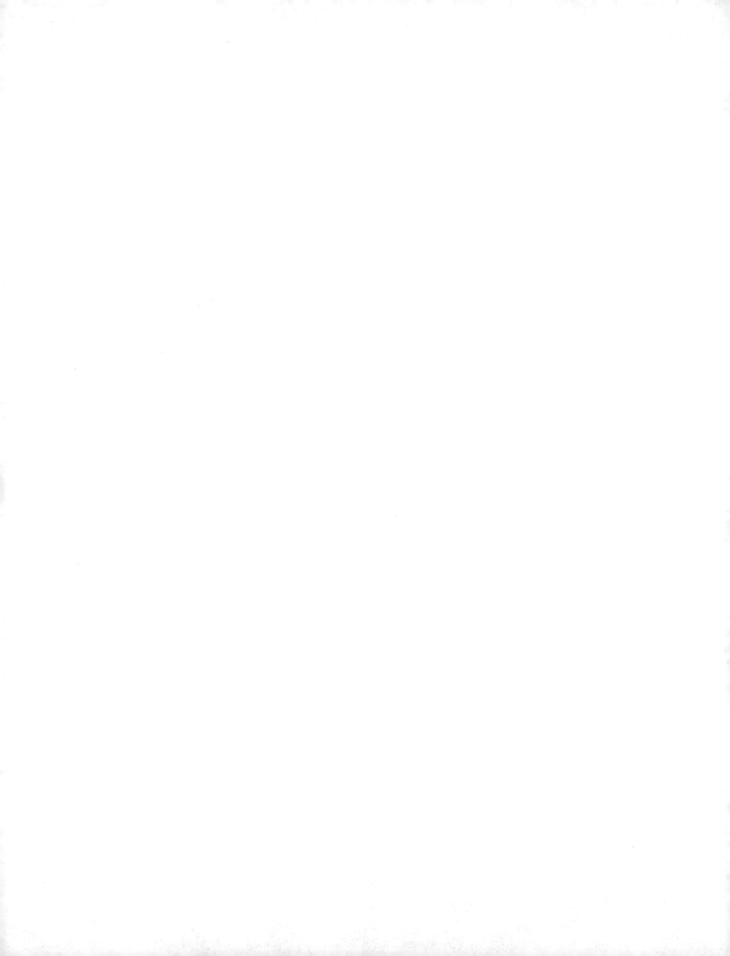

Preface

With the promotion of recreational sports across communities and emphasis on elite athletic training, there is a growing awareness of injuries to the upper extremity caused by tremendous stress in throwing sports or games that require repeated overhead use of the hand and upper extremity. Compared with the lower extremity, there are few books devoted to this important subject.

Sports Injuries of the Hand and Upper Extremity presents a comprehensive view of sports injuries of the upper extremity with sections devoted to the shoulder, elbow, and wrist and hand. Highlights of these sections include a basic understanding of the functional anatomy and applied biomechanics in relation to various sports actions and a practical guide to clinical assessment with clear illustration of relevant physical examination techniques. Recent advances in diagnostic imaging and investigative procedures will assist the surgeon in decision making before embarking on operative procedures. Surgical management of various sports injuries is highlighted with emphasis on recent advances in new techniques, particularly minimal invasive procedures that help return athletes to previous athletic performance within the shortest possible time.

The last section discusses the coordinated effort of the rehabilitation team: the physiotherapist, athletic trainer, and coach. Special consideration is also given to sports injuries of the upper extremity in children and adolescents. There are also specific chapters dealing with brachial plexus injuries related to sports injuries and neurovascular syndrome, some of which may be hidden from the diagnostic arena of sports physicians.

This book is intended for sports physicians and specialists who are interested in the care of athletic injuries of the upper extremity. It is a good reference for all sports medicine clinicians and provides the most updated information and references on the subject.

K. M. Chan, M.B.B.S., F.R.C.S.(Orth), M.Ch. (Orth), F.R.C.S.

Contents

1

Functional Anatomy and Applied Biomechanics of the Shoulder

PATRICK J. MCMAHON
FREDDIE H. FU

INTRODUCTION

An enormous range of mobility is essential at the shoulder to enable the prehensile hand to be placed in all the positions required in everyday life. As a consequence, less bony stability exists at the shoulder in comparison with other diarthrodial joints; however, mechanisms also must exist to guide and limit motion. In this chapter the biomechanics and anatomy of the shoulder are described with reference to specific joints. The kinematics of each joint are described. Attention then centers on stability and mobility of the glenohumeral joint, since this joint is the most frequently injured in sporting activities and has been the center of investigation. Lastly, the clinical conditions that result from glenohumeral pathology are briefly discussed.

Definitions

Even though the term *shoulder* is often used to refer to the glenohumeral joint, normal function of the shoulder requires the coordinated function of four joints: the sternoclavicular, the acromioclavicular, the glenohumeral, and the scapulothoracic.[28] Furthermore, the shoulder is composed of approximately 30 muscles and three bones (humerus, clavicle, and scapula) in addition to the upper thorax (Fig. 1-1). In this chapter, shoulder motion refers to the complex interaction of all these structures.

The actions (either translations or rotations) between the humerus and the glenoid are described as follows. Small linear movements that take place be-

tween the articular surfaces of the humeral head and the glenoid are termed *translations.* When large, these translations are seen clinically as glenohumeral joint instability. Large angular rotations also occur between the humerus and the scapula. In normal shoulders, motion is composed of large angular rotations and small glenohumeral translations.[27,54] For clarity, we define the three possible translations as anterior/posterior, superior/inferior, and medial/lateral. The three rotations are internal/external, adduction/abduction in the scapular plane, and adduction/abduction in the horizontal plane. The importance of this concept is manifest in the problem we call Codman's paradox.

Codman's Paradox

Codman's paradox (Fig. 1-2) can easily be explained by starting with the upper extremity at the side and (1) abducting the shoulder in the scapular plane, then (2) adducting in the horizontal plane, and lastly (3) extending the shoulder until the upper extremity is back at the side. When the extremity returns to the side it is not in the same position as the start. *A rotation has occurred.*

A simple explanation for this phenomenon requires a clearer understanding of the motions we call flexion and extension. All positions of the shoulder can be described with the three rotations described above. We consider that the rotations described as flexion/extension are simply combinations of the other three axial rotations. For example, flexion is a combination of scapular plane abduction, horizontal plane adduction,

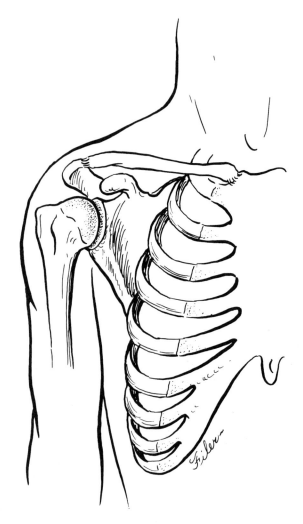

Fig. 1-1. Bones of the shoulder. The bones of the shoulder include the humerus, scapula, clavicle, and upper thorax.

and external rotation. This is much the same concept as circumduction of the thumb, which is a combination of flexion and internal rotation. Thus flexion and extension are not necessary to describe shoulder motion.

To return to Codman's paradox, if we stop after any sequence of shoulder motion and reverse the sequence we return to the original position. In addition, if we eliminate the rotation that occurs outside the three axes described above (because combinations of rotations occur as in flexion or extension), we also return to the original position. As clinicians and researchers we can understand shoulder motion when motion is limited to three planes. In this way Codman's paradox is no longer a problem.

NORMAL SHOULDER ANATOMY AND MOTION
Glenohumeral Anatomy and Motion

The basic structures of the glenohumeral joint are the osteoarticular surfaces, the glenohumeral ligaments (GHLs) and capsule, the labrum, and the glenohumeral muscles.

Osteoarticular Surfaces

The humeral head represents approximately one-third of a sphere. Testut[69] found the average vertical diameter of the humerus to be 48 mm and the average horizontal diameter to be 45 mm. The glenoid, on the other hand, had a 35-mm vertical diameter and only a 25-mm horizontal diameter. The radius of curvature was reported only for the humeral head (25 mm).[69] These findings have been supported more recently by others.[8,13,39,52]

The proximal humerus is generally separated anatomically into four parts: the articular surface, the greater tuberosity, the lesser tuberosity, and the diaphyseal shaft. The lesser tuberosity is the site of insertion of the subscapularis muscle. The remainder of the rotator cuff muscles (the supraspinatus, the infraspinatus, and the teres minor) insert on the greater tuberosity. Between the two tuberosities is the intertubercular groove, in which the tendon of the long head of the biceps brachii muscle lies. This tendon is held in place by the coracohumeral ligament and the transverse humeral ligament.[20,53] With abduction and adduction of the glenohumeral joint, the proximal humerus slides on the tendon of the long head of the biceps brachii much as a tram moves on a monorail track.

In a radiographic study of 20 shoulders, Saha[63] reported three relationships between the humeral head and the glenoid. In the first two, the glenoid and the humeral head did not fit congruently. Either the radius of curvature of the humeral head is larger than that of the glenoid or the reverse is true. In the last circumstance, the two bones are congruent and have the same radius of curvature.

Flatow and co-workers used stereophotogrammetry to demonstrate that the radius of curvature of the humeral head and the glenoid are not statistically different. Additionally, they showed that both surfaces approximated the surface of a sphere. However, this point is controversial and other investigators believe the sur-

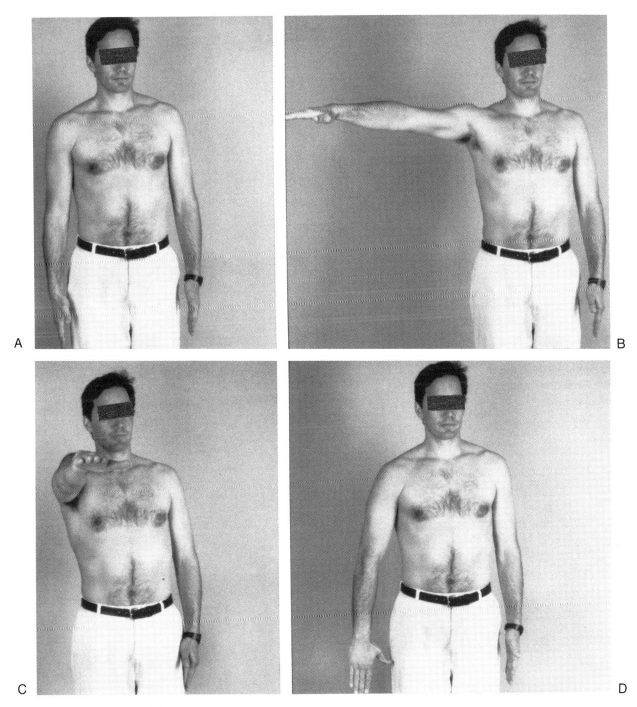

Fig. 1-2. Codman's paradox. Starting with the shoulder at the side, scapular plane abduction, then horizontal plane adduction and lastly shoulder extension result in a new position because internal rotation has occurred.

faces are not conforming and that the contact between them is variable.[5]

Capsuloligamentous Anatomy and Labrum

Although originally disputed, several authors have now agreed that the GHLs are consistently present. (Fig. 1-3)[7,44,70] Variations in the attachments of these ligaments have been described elsewhere.[14,44,50,70] The superior glenohumeral ligament (SGHL) arises near the origin of the long head of the biceps brachii (Figs. 1-4, 1-5). If the glenoid had the markings of a clock, with the 12 o'clock position superiorly and the 3 o'clock anteriorly, the origin of the SGHL would correspond to the area from the 12 o'clock to the 2 o'clock positions. The SGHL runs inferiorly and laterally to insert on the humerus, superior to the lesser tuberosity. The middle (M)GHL usually arises from the glenoid labrum just inferior to the origin of the SGHL or from the adjacent neck of the glenoid and inserts into the humerus just medial to the lesser tuberosity. The presence of the MGHL is the most variable.[14]

The inferior glenohumeral ligament (IGHL) is a complex structure. Originally the IGHL was separated into a superior band, an anterior axillary pouch, and

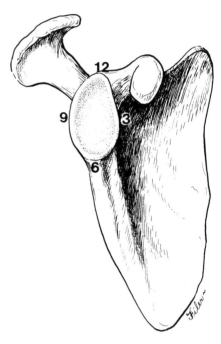

Fig. 1-4. The right glenoid. If markings of a clock were applied to the glenoid, the 3 o'clock position would be anterior. As one moved from 3 to 12 o'clock the motion would be in a clockwise direction.

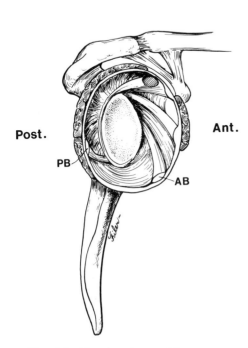

Fig. 1-3. The glenohumeral ligaments.

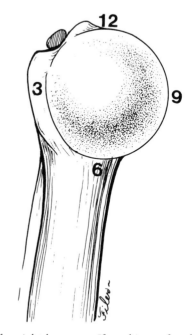

Fig. 1-5. The right humerus. If markings of a clock were applied to the humeral head, the 3 o'clock position would be anterior to match the glenoid. As one moved from 3 to 12 o'clock the motion would be in a counterclockwise direction.

a posterior axillary pouch.[70] More recently, the IGHL has been described as having an anterior and a posterior band, with an axillary pouch between the two bands.[50] Both authors were probably describing the same capsular anatomy: the appearance varies depending on the glenohumeral position. With abduction and external rotation, the anterior band fans out and the posterior band becomes cord-like. Likewise, with internal rotation the posterior band fans out and the anterior band appears cord-like.[50] The anterior band of the IGHL arises from various areas corresponding to the 2 o'clock to 4 o'clock positions on the glenoid, and the posterior band originates at the 7 o'clock to 9 o'clock positions. With the arm at the side, both hands pass through a 90-degree arc and insert on the humerus.[50]

The separation of the rotator cuff tendons from the upper one-half of the capsule is difficult by gross dissection. The lower one-half of the capsule is covered by muscle fibers since the myotendinous junctions of the lower subscapularis and the teres minor muscles are lateral compared with the remainder of the rotator cuff muscles. The inferior capsule has no muscular attachments except for a few fibers from the long head of the triceps muscle.

Based on a study of 45 human embryos and 75 cadaver joints, Moseley and Overguard[44] considered the labrum to be composed of dense fibrous connective tissue devoid of fibrocartilage except at the attachment of the osseous glenoid rim.

Glenohumeral Muscles

Four muscles compose the rotator cuff: the supraspinatus, subscapularis, infraspinatus, and teres minor (Fig. 1-6). The supraspinatus has its origin on the posterior/superior scapula, superior to the scapular spine. It passes under the acromion, through the supraspinatus fossa, and inserts on the greater tuberosity. The supraspinatus is active during the entire arc of scapular plane abduction; paralysis of the suprascapular nerve results in an approximately 50 percent loss of abduction torque.[11] The supraspinatus muscle is capable of abducting the joint without the deltoid muscle action.[11,40]

The infraspinatus and the teres minor muscles originate on the posterior scapula, inferior to the scapular spine, and insert on the posterior aspect of the greater tuberosity. Their tendinous insertions are not separate from each other or the supraspinatus tendon. These

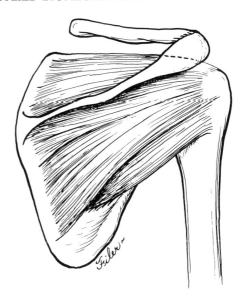

Fig. 1-6. Posterior glenohumeral view. The supraspinatus muscle is above the scapular spine and the infraspinatus and teres minor are below the scapular spine.

muscles function together to externally rotate and extend the humerus.

The subscapularis muscle arises from the anterior scapula and is the only muscle to insert on the lesser tuberosity. The subscapularis is the sole component of the anterior rotator cuff and functions to rotate internally and flex the humerus. The tendinous insertion of the subscapularis is continuous with the anterior capsule; therefore these two structures have been considered responsible for providing anterior glenohumeral stability.[68,70]

The deltoid is the largest of the glenohumeral muscles and covers the proximal humerus on a path from its tripennate origin at the clavicle, acromion, and scapular spine to its insertion midway down the humerus at the deltoid tubercle. The three sections of the deltoid have three separate functions. The anterior portion is primarily a forward flexor of the glenohumeral joint; the middle portion is an abductor; and the posterior portion extends the joint. The deltoid is active throughout the entire arc of glenohumeral abduction; paralysis of the axillary nerve results in a 50 percent loss of abduction torque.[11] The deltoid muscle can fully abduct the glenohumeral joint with the supraspinatus muscle inactive.[11]

Although primarily considered elbow muscles, both heads of the biceps brachii muscle have their origin on the scapula. The long head of the biceps has its origin just superior to the articular margin of the glenoid and is probably a depressor of the humeral head, especially with external rotation of the humerus. In this position, the tendon lies directly over the top of the humeral head. Lucas and Hill[38] reported a 20 percent loss of elevation strength in external rotation with rupture of the long head of the biceps tendon.

The triceps muscle is often forgotten as a shoulder muscle. However, much as the biceps originates above the glenoid, the triceps has its origin on the inferior labrum and glenoid. It is the only muscle on the inferior side of the glenohumeral joint, and fibers of the tendon adjacent to the capsule probably reinforce the inferior capsule.

Glenohumeral Motion

In the glenohumeral joint, three actions are possible: spinning, sliding, and rolling (Fig. 1-7). Spinning occurs when the contact point on the glenoid remains the same while the humeral head contact point is changing. Sliding is pure translation of the humeral head on the articular surface of the glenoid. At the extremes of motion, and certainly in unstable joints, glenohumeral translations occur. In this circumstance, the contact point on the glenoid is moving, while that for the humerus remains the same. The third type of action, rolling, may also occur at the glenohumeral joint. Rolling is a combination of translation and spinning humerus with respect to the glenoid, and the contact point changes on both the glenoid and the humeral head.[43] Some authors believe that all three motions take place at the glenohumeral joint.[43] We discuss glenohumeral motion in more detail later in the chapter.

Scapulothoracic Anatomy and Motion

The scapulothoracic muscles include the trapezius, rhomboid, levator scapulae, serratus anterior, and pectoralis minor. They all act to position the scapula in the proper orientation on the thoracic cage for a given shoulder motion. The trapezius and rhomboid retract the scapula, while the levator scapulae and serratus anterior protract the scapula. Upward rotation of the scapula is accomplished with the trapezius and serratus anterior; the pectoralis minor and levator scapulae are responsible for downward rotation of the scapula. The rhomboid can also elevate the scapula.

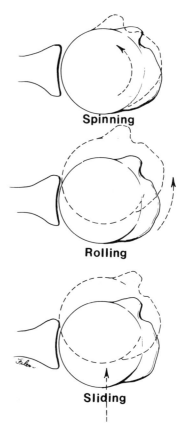

Fig. 1-7. Glenohumeral actions. Three actions are possible at the glenohumeral joint. Spinning is pure rotation. Rolling of the humeral head on the glenoid is much the same as a ball rolling on the floor. Sliding is pure translation.

These muscles position the scapula to provide maximum stability at the glenohumeral joint while maintaining a large range of motion. The glenoid moves with the joint reaction force generated at the interface between the humerus and glenoid so that the force is always directed toward itself.

The relative motion between the scapulothoracic and the glenohumeral joints, during abduction, is the shoulder motion, which has been the most extensively studied.[15,17,28,48,54] This relative motion has also been called the scapulothoracic rhythm, but reports in the literature have often been unclear as to whether abduction was examined in the scapular or the coronal plane. For the first 30 degrees of abduction, glenohumeral motion is much greater than scapulothoracic motion. This ratio has been reported to range from 4 : 1 to 7 : 1.[54,15] Thereafter, both joints move approximately the same amount. Poppen and Walker[54] reported a ratio of 5:4, while Doody and co-workers[15] reported an equal motion for the two joints from 90 to 150 degrees of abduction. In summary, over the entire arc of abduction, the glenohumeral joint moves more than the scapulothoracic joint; however, the difference is greatest at the beginning of abduction and is minimal at the end.

In the resting position, the superior edge of the scapular spine is rotated anteriorly from the frontal plane a mean of 31 degrees.[35] With the initiation of abduction, the scapula can translate medially or laterally, or in rare instances oscillate on the chest wall.[28] As the shoulder abducts, the scapula rotates not only in the plane of abduction, but also in a plane perpendicular to it. The superior edge of the scapula first rotates anteriorly about 6 degrees with the first 90 degrees of shoulder abduction. Past 90 degrees, 16 degrees of posterior scapular rotation occurs.[9]

Abnormalities in the complex motion between the scapula and the thorax can result in pathology. A common history is of a throwing athlete who has a long history of achy shoulder pain during the cocking phase of throwing. The suprascapular nerve originates from the superior trunk of the brachial plexus to innervate the supraspinatus and infraspinatus muscles. Along its path, it can be tethered and compressed in two areas of the scapula: the suprascapular notch and the neck of the spine (spinoglenoid notch).[57] Ringel and co-workers[57] have shown that either the infraspinatus is involved alone, or both muscles are involved, depending on the location of the compression, which is demonstrated on physical examination by muscle atrophy in most cases. The trapezius overlies the supraspinatus muscle, but atrophy of this muscle can be appreciated as a depression over the supraspinatus fossa of the shoulder. Atrophy of the infraspinatus is easy to appreciate as a depression over the lower half of the scapula. Compression results in pain and weakness. Symptoms may preclude pitching more than one or two innings. In the chronic situation, the correct diagnosis can be elusive because the disease has an insidious onset and vague symptoms. Muscle pain and diminished endurance are the important presenting symptoms, but eventually weakness of external rotation and sometimes of abduction appears, depending on the location of the compression.

In summary, the motion that takes place at the glenohumeral and scapulothoracic joints is extremely complex. Athletic endeavors require precise action of these joints, and small alterations in these motions can result in pathology.

Acromioclavicular and Sternoclavicular Anatomy and Motion

The sternoclavicular joint (Fig. 1-8) is stabilized by four ligaments and the intra-articular disc.[24] The interclavicular ligament provides restraint to superior joint motion and is taut when the shoulder is at the side.[58] Anterior and posterior motion is prevented by the anterior and posterior capsular structures, the anterior being the stronger of the two.[1] Inferiorly, the joint is stabilized by the costoclavicular ligaments, which run obliquely and laterally from the first rib to the clavicle. The anterior structures resist superior motion and the posterior structures resist downward motion of the medial clavicle.[1]

The acromioclavicular joint (Fig. 1-9) is stabilized to superior motion by the coricoclavicular ligaments: the conoid and the trapazoid. The acromioclavicular capsule is the primary restraint to anterior and posterior motion, and the acromioclavicular ligament is a superior thickening of the capsule.

The clavicle also moves, the lateral edge rotating approximately 30 degrees superiorly in the coronal plane, during shoulder abduction. The lateral edge also rotates anteriorly approximately 10 degrees with the first 40 degrees of shoulder abduction. No additional anterior rotation of the lateral edge occurs until

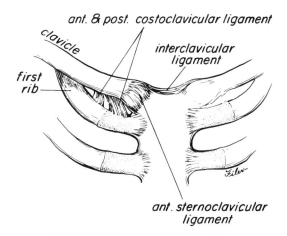

Fig. 1-8. The sternoclavicular joint.

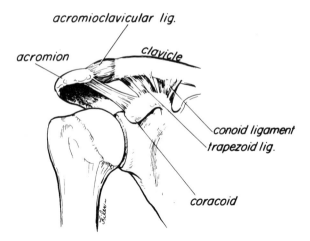

Fig. 1-9. The acromioclavicular joint.

130 degrees of shoulder abduction; then 15 degrees of anterior clavicle rotation occurs until the end of shoulder abduction.[28]

The large axial rotations initially reported by Inman et al.[28] have been questioned recently. By placing pins in the clavicle and the acromion, Rockwood and Green[58] have shown that the clavicle rotates axially less than 10 degrees over the entire arc of shoulder abduction. This finding is supported by the clinical observation that fixing the clavicle to the scapula does not significantly limit shoulder motion. Interruption of normal motion between the clavicle and the thorax can cause thoracic outlet syndrome (TOS). This refers to compression of the nerves and vessels of the upper extremity as they pass under the clavicle and between the scalene muscles over the first rib.[16,61,62] Symptoms are usually vague, making the diagnosis difficult. Typically, a long period of time intervenes from the onset of symptoms until the diagnosis is made. Usually a history exists of paresthesia and pain that radiates down the lateral side of the neck, then moves into the shoulder and the medial side of the arm, and finally continues into the ring and little fingers. Physical findings are usually subtle. Although it is not specific for TOS, Adson's test is positive if the radial pulse diminishes when the arm is abducted, the head is rotated toward the involved side, and a deep breath is held. TOS is also suggested if the patient experiences numbness and tingling when the hands are rapidly opened and closed with the upper extremities elevated.

ROLE OF THE RESTRAINT MECHANISMS IN GLENOHUMERAL TRANSLATIONS

Normal glenohumeral kinematics depend on a normal relationship between the articular surfaces of the glenoid and the humeral head. If the joint is unstable, the kinematics of the joint will undoubtedly change compared with normal. Therefore, the joint restraint mechanisms have three main roles. In the normal joint, these mechanisms (1) guide the joint motion to maintain normal joint kinematics and (2) limit the range of motion, by acting as either a checkrein or a barrier. In other joints, such as the hip, many of these functions are provided by bone. The large range of motion at the shoulder is possible because of the absence of bony restraints, but this has also resulted in increased demands on other shoulder restraints. In their last role the restraint mechanisms are essential to limit abnormal translations. For example, in the individual with anterior glenohumeral subluxation, the restraint mechanisms prevent the joint from dislocating.

The glenohumeral joint is stabilized by a combination of static and dynamic restraints. The static restraints include the geometry of the articular surfaces, the glenohumeral ligaments, the joint capsule, intra-articular pressure, and the labrum, while the dynamic restraints are the muscles that cross the joint. Study of the contribution of static restraints in pathologic joint stability has been extensively studied. Little is known about the manner in which the restraint mechanisms position the humeral head and limit the range of motion of the shoulder, since these concepts are relatively new compared with the role of the restraint mechanisms in pathologic motion.

Defining normal and abnormal glenohumeral translations is difficult due to the inherent laxity of the glenohumeral joint. For example, shoulder laxity tests have shown mean translations as large as 11 mm in normal subjects,[65] yet it is known that during normal shoulder motion glenoid translations are small. Poppen and Walker[54] measured glenohumeral translations in the coronal plane. From 0 to 30 degrees of shoulder abduction, the translation was approximately 3 mm superiorly; thereafter, the translation was minimal (1 to 2 mm inferiorly or superiorly throughout the arc of abduction). Howell and coworkers[27] measured glenohumeral translations in the transverse plane with a similar radiographic technique. In normal subjects, the humeral head translated posteriorly about 4 mm with extension and external rotation of the joint. During other shoulder motions, the translations were minimal (less than 1 mm).

Cadaveric studies to quantify glenohumeral translations have centered on the passive restraints, since it is hard to simulate accurately the dynamic restraints *in vitro*. Harryman and co-workers[26] examined the amount of glenohumeral translation that occurred with specific glenohumeral motion using an electromagnetic sensor to measure the translation and rotation at the joint. They found that significant translations occurred in an anterior direction (4 ± 4 mm) with glenohumeral flexion. The humeral head translated posteriorly (5 ± 3 mm) with glenohumeral extension. Posterior translation (2 ± 2 mm) also occurred with external rotation. Bowen and co-workers[4] examined the effects of internal and external rotation on glenohumeral translation. They found the anterior translation to be about 5 mm with internal rotation and the posterior to be about 5 mm with external rotation. Interestingly, the amount of translation that occurred with the shoulder abducted was significantly diminished when the IGHL was sectioned.

Instability

Anterior Instability

When translations become large, instability results. Anterior dislocation of the shoulder joint usually occurs secondary to a single traumatic event. Subluxation is incomplete dislocation of the joint while contact between the joint surfaces remains. Subluxation is much more common in the throwing athlete secondary to chronic overuse. These patients may not have a history of an acute traumatic event. They have a negative impingement sign, a positive apprehension test, and relief of pain with the relocation test, as described Chapter 2. Proper diagnosis permits the problem to be addressed with physical therapy. Many athletes gain relief of symptoms with rotator cuff strengthening exercises if started early in the course of the disease. Continued instability indicates significant ligament damage, which may require surgical intervention.

Some patients have hyperlaxity of muscle joints and secondary instability. Sometimes impingement is also present. These patients have a positive impingement sign, a positive apprehension test, and relief of pain on the relocation test. However, they also exhibit generalized hyperlaxity, as demonstrated by hyperextension of the elbows, knees, and matacarpophalangeal joints of the hand. Hyperabduction of the thumb to the radius and the ability to touch the palms to the floor without bending the knees are also present.[23] Examination under anesthesia reveals anterior instability of both shoulders, although the involved shoulder may be worse. Computed tomography (CT) arthrogram and arthroscopy usually show anterior labral fraying and may demonstrate increased capsular volume. Initial treatment includes rehabilitation of the rotator cuff and scapular rotator muscles. If the patient remains symptomatic, a capsular shift procedure may be the only option for attaining a successful outcome. Acromioplasty alone, in this setting, has not been successful in our hands.

Posterior Instability

Posterior shoulder instability often goes unrecognized, especially in throwing athletes. Pure dislocation of the joint is rare, but subluxation is not. Two different mechanisms can result in posterior instability. In the first situation, improper pitching technique causes repetitive microtrauma to the posterior capsule. The follow-through phase of the throwing motion is characterized by intense contraction of the shoulder muscles to decelerate the upper extremity. At this time, the shoulder is in the vulnerable position of flexion, adduction, and internal rotation. This creates high stresses in the posterior capsule. Repeated microtrauma resulting from poor pitching technique causes posterior capsule weakness and eventual humeral head subluxation. In the second situation, a single traumatic event initiates the instability. For example, a player falls on the outstretched throwing arm and has immediate posterior shoulder pain. After the pain subsides, throwing velocity and endurance decrease, accompanied by pain during the follow-through. Through either mechanism, the posterior capsule can become attenuated. Complete tears of the capsule from the glenoid, which commonly occur anteriorly, are less common posteriorly.

Patients with posterior shoulder instability complain

of pain in the posterior shoulder, sometimes radiating along the scapula. However, anterior shoulder pain is not unheard of in these patients. A careful physical examination demonstrates the true pathology. Usually the patient has pain with forward flexion, adduction, and internal rotation, and it may be possible to sublux the shoulder posteriorly in this position. The best way to feel the subluxation is to place the patient on the examination table in a supine position. The examiner's hand is placed over the humeral head and the shoulder positioned as described above. A posteriorly directed force applied to the humeral head results in a palpable instability. Radiographic examination may reveal a posterior glenoid spur.[34] However, this lesion is extracapsular and of questionable significance.[39]

Some patients can voluntarily sublux their shoulders, and often these individuals have simply reached the last stage in the spectrum of instability patterns. They should be treated like any other patient with posterior instability, in constrast to the patient with voluntary shoulder dislocation, an associated psychological component, and drug-seeking behavior.

Rehabilitation results in symptomatic improvement in two-thirds of the cases.[41] The external rotators should be strengthened, as well as the posterior deltoid. This exercise program should be well supervised and should last for 6 months. Throwing technique should also be examined to eliminate any activity that may be placing additional stress on the posterior capsule.

Multidirectional Instability

While posterior instability can occur in isolation, it can also be associated with inferior instability and therefore be multidirectional.[36] These patients may complain of a looseness in the shoulder or pain with activities that cause an inferior directed force in the shoulder, such as lifting a heavy suitcase. However, most will present with far more nonspecific symptoms, such as generalized shoulder pain. Only a careful history and physical examination will reveal the multidirectional component of the instability. When anterior instability is also a component of the problem, we suggest an aggressive physical therapy program aimed at strengthening the rotator cuff. In our experience, extensive surgery requiring both an anterior and a posterior approach is required when rehabilitation fails; such surgery should be avoided if possible.

Effects of Intra-articular Pressure

The contribution of atmospheric pressure to shoulder stability is mentioned in *Gray's Anatomy*[25]: "the looseness of the capsule is so great that the arm will fall about an inch from the scapula when the muscles are dissected and a hole is made in it to remove the atmospheric pressure." Other investigators have qualitatively substantiated this finding.[34,60] Anatomic studies, surgical findings, and magnetic resonance studies all confirm that a layer of synovial fluid less than 1 mm thick can be found in the normal glenohumeral joint.[41] Because the joint volume is finite, distraction of the joint surfaces increases volume and results in decreasing intra-articular pressure. A slightly negative intra-articular pressure exists in the normal shoulder that may aid in centering the humeral head and may provide a restraint to pathologic translations.[36,66]

Gibb and co-workers[21] attempted to quantify the role of intra-articular pressure and found that the force required to translate the humeral head from the center of the glenoid to the edge of the glenoid fossa was significantly less in shoulders with the capsule vented to the atmosphere. Ten to 20-N less force was required to translate the humeral head anteriorly, posteriorly, or inferiorly. Qualitative studies are not available on the role of intra-articular pressure in limiting glenohumeral range of motion, or guiding the humeral head in the normal joint.

Effects of the Glenohumeral Ligaments

Role in Guiding the Humeral Head During Normal Motion

Investigators have examined the role of the GHLs in guiding the humeral head during normal motions. Terry and co-workers[68] placed mercury-filled strain gauges on the GHLs, the posterior capsule, and the coracohumeral ligament. They examined the strain values while attempting to maintain normal joint kinematics. In other words, sectioning of restraint structures was not done, and external forces were not applied to the humeral head. With pure flexion, they found that the coracohumeral ligament supported two-thirds of the total tension of the passive restraints. With abduction, the inferior and posterior capsule supported most of the total tension, but with the addition of external rotation the tension increased in the SGHL, MGHL, and

IGHL. In summary, these authors felt that ligament tension is one factor that guides the humeral head as the joint moves to a new position. These glenohumeral motion studies also demonstrate that the GHLs limit the range of motion of the joint. Due to the complexity of the glenohumeral motions produced by their device, Terry and co-workers[68] were unable to correlate strains in the GHLs with the specific position along the arc of motion.

O'Connell and co-workers[51] used intact cadaveric shoulders with Hall-effect strain gauges to examine the strain in the GHLs at three positions of abduction (0, 45, and 90 degrees). At the lower angles of abduction, the SGHL and the MGHL seemed to be most important in guiding the humeral head. However, only the strain in the IGHL was significantly greater at 90 degrees of abduction. It should be noted that considerable variation in strain was seen from shoulder to shoulder.

Role in Limiting Range of Motion

Terry and co-workers[68] found that at the extremes of normal glenohumeral motion, parts of the capsule are under tension while other parts of the capsule are lax. For example, in the flexed position the strain was greatest in the coracohumeral ligament and the midportion of the posterior capsule. When external rotation was added, the strain increased in the anterior GHLs and decreased in the posterior capsule. In these static positions, portions of the capsule become taut to limit motion in one range of motion, while in another position other parts of the capsule become taut to limit another range of motion.

Role in Limiting Pathologic Motion

The role of the GHLs in limiting pathologic translations has been the most intensively studied of all the restraint mechanisms. Turkel and co-workers examined the role of the anterior joint structures in limiting anterior translations.[70] The subcapularis muscle and the three GHLs were sectioned in different sequences and the joint was then externally rotated. As the GHLs were serially sectioned, the joint became more mobile until the range of motion had increased to such a degree that the joint finally dislocated. In other words, they recognized two roles of the restraint mechanisms: limiting pathologic translations and limiting normal glenohumeral range of motion. Results showed that the subcapularis muscle prevents anterior dislocation at 0 degrees of

glenohumeral abduction. At 45 degrees of glenohumeral abduction the subscapularis muscle, the MGHL, and the anterior fibers of the IGHL act as barriers to dislocation. The IGHL alone prevents anterior dislocation of the glenohumeral joint at 90 degrees of abduction.

O'Brien et al.[49] arthroscopically labeled the GHLs in cadaveric shoulders. With an anterior-to-posterior force applied to the glenohumeral joint in 90 degrees of abduction and neutral rotation, selective cutting of the capsular structures was performed. The anterior superior band of the IGHL was the primary capsular restraint to anterior translation at −30, 0, and 30 degrees of horizontal flexion. The MGHL was a secondary barrier, and only minor contributions were made by the SGHL and the posterior capsule. After sectioning all three of the GHLs and the associated capsule, Galinat and Howell[19] reported that the articular glenoid, the fibrous labrum, and the glenohumeral capsule-ligament complex function to limit anterior instability.

The role of the GHLs in limiting inferior translation has also been examined.[3,72] With a 50-N superior-to-inferior force applied to the proximal humerus, the structure-limiting inferior instability was dependent on joint position. In all positions of abduction the IGHL plays a role in limiting inferior translation; however, with the joint in 0 degrees of abduction the SGHL also is significant. These selective ligament cutting studies emphasize the important role of the passive restraints in limiting large glenohumeral translations. However, it is known that large glenohumeral translations are abnormal.[27,54]

Effects of Joint Geometry/Bone

Cyprien and co-workers[13] used plain radiographs to measure a number of glenohumeral relationships in both normal shoulders and shoulders with anterior instability. No difference was found in humeral retroversion, glenoid inclination, dimension of the glenoid, or width of the humeral head. In the patients with recurrent anterior dislocation, significant differences were found between contralateral sides for the diameter of the humeral head and the contact index (the ratio of the diameter of the glenoid to the diameter of the humeral head). It is unclear if the significantly smaller sizes are responsible for, or secondary to, recurrent anterior dislocation. Randelli and Gambrioli[55] used CT to quantify similar glenohumeral relationships. They also found no significant difference in the relationships of normal and unstable shoulders, but believed that erosions or fractures affect the joint congruity in unstable shoulders.

Itoi and co-workers[29] examined the influence of scapular inclination of inferior instability in a cadaveric study. With the shoulder fully adducted and the scapula inclined −15, 0, 15, or 30 degrees, an inferior load was applied to the humeral head (sulcus test). Increased inclination of the scapula prevented dislocation of the joint. With the joint abducted 90 degrees and an inferior load applied to the humeral head (Feagin's test), increased scapular inclination resulted in greater displacement of the humeral head. Note that in the Feagin's test the humerus became less abducted relative to the scapula as the scapular inclination increased. Thus the capsular structures responsible for preventing inferior translation probably changed with the scapular inclination.

Lippett and co-workers[37] examined the stabilizing effect of compressing the humeral head into the glenoid. Using 50 and 100 N of compressive load, they found that the humeral head resisted tangential forces of up to 56 N. The effect was lessened when the labrum was removed. Thus concavity-compression may be important in providing stability when large compressive loads occur during normal muscle action.

Effects of Dynamic Restraints

The rotator cuff muscles and the biceps tendon have a role in stabilizing the glenohumeral joint[30,59] but it is likely that other muscles that cross the glenohumeral joint[41] or position the scapula also aid in this function. In addition to their large number, the dynamic restraints can be difficult to study because they have a dual function. First, they act as primary movers of the joint and second, they provide stability.

Role in Guiding the Humeral Head During Normal Motion

Glousman and co-workers[22] examined the electromyographic (EMG) activity of various shoulder muscles in normal throwers and those with anterior glenohumeral instability. They found a significant difference in the EMG activity of all the muscles tested except for the middle deltoid. The biceps and the supraspinatus muscles had increased activity in the unstable shoul-

ders. This was felt to be a compensatory mechanism to "help stabilize the humeral head against the glenoid fossa." In addition, other muscles, such as the infraspinatus, showed increased activity during certain phases of the pitching motion (specifically the late cocking phase) in patients with instability. Assuming that the rotator cuff muscles act to guide the humeral head, this pattern of activity could actually add to the anterior instability of the joint. Whether or not abnormal kinematics occurred during the throwing motion in these patients is not known.

In a cadaveric study of glenohumeral abduction in the scapular plane, McMahon and co-workers[42] found that minimal translation of the humeral head occurred. Three different muscle force combinations were used in the supraspinatus and the middle deltoid, with the subscapularis and teres minor/infraspinatus muscle forces being constant for each abduction angle tested. Many different muscle forces result in the same amount of glenohumeral rotation; this study indicates that the force required to move the glenohumeral joint also acts to provide stability. This hypothesis is supported by Kelar and coworkers, who also found minimal translations of the joint with scapular plane abduction.[33]

Role in Limiting Range of Motion

The ability of the dynamic restraints to limit motion is demonstrated in a study by Rodosky and coworkers.[59] With the rotator cuff muscles simulated, the load to the long head of the biceps tendon was varied. Using a cadaveric model, the glenohumeral joint was abducted to 90 degrees and the torque required to rotate the humerus externally was determined. The maximum torque required to rotate the humerus externally was significantly increased as the load applied to the long head of the biceps tendon was increased. The authors conclude that "for a given external torque, the long head of the biceps tendon is able to reduce the amount of external rotation."

Role in Limiting Pathologic Motion

Matsen and co-workers[41] have described how the dynamic restraints can act as barriers to pathologic motion. When a patient is relaxed, the humeral head can be translated on the glenoid, as is done in stability testing. If the patient then contracts the muscles "the anterior-posterior excursion can be virtually eliminated."[41] These and other authors have shown that selective contraction of the rotator cuff muscles can counteract displacement forces on the humeral head.[41, 44, 67] It has been demonstrated that activities such as swimming, which enhances the coordinated activity of the dynamic restraints, can reduce symptoms of instability.[31]

Blasier and co-workers[2] found that a load in any of the cuff tendons resulted in a measurable and statistically significant contribution to anterior joint stability. In addition, the long head of the biceps brachii plays a role in limiting glenohumeral translations.[30] Using a magnetic tracking device to record the position of the humeral head, a load was applied to the long head of the biceps brachii and a force was applied to the humeral head in various directions in an attempt to translate it on the glenoid. No load was applied to any other tendons about the shoulder. Loading of the long head of the biceps tendon significantly decreased posterior translation and anterior translation (with the humeral head in neutral or external rotation). Thus the long head of the biceps tendon was shown to act as a barrier to pathologic glenohumeral translations.

Rotator cuff disease provides an excellent example of the importance of the dynamic restraints. Rotator cuff disease has extrinsic and intrinsic etiologies.[18] The extrinsic causes are forces acting outside the rotator cuff that cause injury to the tendons. Impingement syndrome, which Neer[45] implicated in 95 percent of rotator cuff tears, is an example of extrinsic rotator cuff disease.

The most common injuries that occur in the shoulder from throwing result from the constant irritation of anterior shoulder structures.[12] Impingement is defined as compromise of the space between the coracoacromial arch and the proximal humerus. The coracoacromial arch includes the coracoid, the coracoacromial ligament, the acromioclavicular joint, the acromion, and the subacromial bursa. These structures make up the roof over the anterior glenohumeral joint. The supraspinatus tendon and the tendon of the long head of the biceps brachii are the most commonly compressed structures. When the humerus is flexed and internally rotated, the insertion of the supraspinatus tendon is brought under the coracoacromial arch and constant irritation can ensue. This is especially true when the space between the acromion and the humerus is further compromised by anterior acromial osteophytes. Patients complain of anterior shoulder pain, especially with overhead activities. The athlete initially complains of pain in the anterior shoulder during the acceleration phase or sometimes during the follow-through phase. Initially the pain resolves after a short period of rest. However, the condition relentlessly progresses if the offending activity is not stopped. With time, the pain becomes more intense, especially with forward flexion and internal rotation (impingement sign). Physical examination reveals tenderness on palpation of the anterior acromion and a positive impingement sign and test.

Extrinsic causes of rotator cuff disease also include instability of the glenohumeral joint. Jobe and co-workers[32] have shown that muscle activity becomes abnormal about the shoulder as it begins to sublux. In an attempt to stabilize the shoulder girdle, the scapula becomes fixed. The rotator cuff muscles attempt to subsitute for the lost scapulothoracic motion. Muscle overuse and muscle fatigue occur. If this condition persists, spasm and pain result. Muscle fatigue leads to abnormal shoulder kinematics and contributes to instability. A downward spiral then ensues. Eventually, instability causes the humeral head to impinge on the coracoacromial arch. This situation is very different from that of pure impingement, and a careful evaluation for shoulder instability is required. These patients occasionally report that their shoulder feels as though it is moving anteriorly. However, anterior shoulder pain is usually the only complaint. Careful physical examination reveals the subtle anterior instability. CT arthrogram may show an avulsion of the anterior-inferior labrum from the glenoid (Bankart lesion). In addition to demonstrating the Bankart lesion, arthroscopy can show anterior labral fraying (the only lesion in some cases). A small posterior-lateral humeral head compression fracture (Hill-Sachs lesion) may also be present.

Intrinsic causes of rotator cuff disease include traction injuries and primary cuff degeneration not related to impingement syndrome. A critical zone of hypovascularity exists at the insertion of the supraspinatus tendon.[10,56] Most rotator cuff pathology occurs in this area. Uhthoff and co-workers[71] showed that most tears of the rotator cuff begin on the articular side of the tendon, which supports a role for intrinsic etiologies of rotator cuff disease. Nirschl[47] wrote of angiofibroblastic changes occurring in the tendon with secondary development of rotator cuff calcification, erosion, and impingement. Undoubtedly both extrinsic and intrinsic factors play a role in rotator cuff pathology.

Motion of all four joints (sternoclavicular, acromioclavicular, scapulothoracic, and glenohumeral) is essential to normal shoulder kinematics. This can be assessed both actively and passively. Differences between active and passive motion can be due to neuromuscular deficiency such as a rotator cuff tear. Motion should always be compared with the contralateral shoulder. Brown and co-workers[6] found that major league pitchers have different ranges of motion between shoulders. In the pitching arm, with the shoulder in abduction, 11 degrees less extension, 15 degrees less internal rotation, and 9 degrees more external rotation are seen. Therefore, comparison with the contralateral arm should be done with this variance in mind.

Throwing a baseball subjects the rotator cuff to many insults (impingement, traction, and contusion) that can result in failure of the tendon fibers. Repeated, small episodes of partial rotator cuff tearing can occur. The incidence of partial rotator cuff tears rises with age. In a series of 233 patients with rotator cuff tears, Neer and co-workers[46] found that 97 percent occurred in individuals over the age of 40 years. These patients commonly present with a long history of intermittent shoulder tendonitis that likely represents tendon fiber failure. Most full-thickness rotator cuff tears occur in a tendon that is already weakened by earlier pathology. Eventually the patients experience increasing shoulder pain that may wake them up at night, especially when sleeping on the affected shoulder. Elevation of the arm in the scapular plane against resistance becomes increasingly difficult partly because of the tear and partly because of disuse atrophy. Samuilson and Binder[64] found that the most common symptoms of complete rotator cuff tears were pain, weakness in shoulder elevation, and subacromial crepitus. Partial rotator cuff tears are characterized by less severe symptoms.

REFERENCES

1. Bearn J: Direct observation of the function of the capsule of the sternoclavicular joint in clavicular support. J Anat 101:159–170, 1967
2. Blasier R, Guldberg R, Rothman E: Anterior shoulder stability: contributions of rotator cuff forces and the capsular ligaments in a cadaveric model. J Shoulder Elbow Surg 1:140–150, 1992
3. Bowen M et al: Role of the inferior glenohumeral ligament complex in limiting inferior translation of the glenohumeral joint. Trans Orthop Res Soc 17:497, 1992
4. Bowen M, Deng XH, Warner JP et al: Kinematics of the glenohumeral joint: Coupled translation with rotation. Personal communication, 1992
5. Bowen M, Deng XH, Hannafin JA et al: An analysis of the patterns of glenohumeral joint contact and their relationship to the glenoid "bare area." Trans Orthop Res Soc 17:496, 1992
6. Brown L, Niehues SL, Harrah P et al: Upper extremity range of motion and isokinetic strength of the internal and external rotators in major league baseball players. Am J Sports Med 16:577–578, 1988
7. Warner JSP, Caborn DNM, Berger R et al: Dynamic capsuloligamentous anatomy of the glenohumoral joint. J Shoulder Elbow Surg 2:115–133, 1993
8. Clark I, Gruen T, Hoy A et al: Problems in glenohumeral surface replacements—real or imagined? Eng Med 8:161–175, 1979
9. Cleland FRS: Notes on raising the arm. J Anat Physiol 18:275, 1884
10. Codman E: Rupture of the supraspinatus tendon and other lesions about the subacromial bursa. In: The Shoulder. Thomas Todd, Boston, 1934
11. Colachis S Jr, Strohm B: Effect of suprascapular and axillary nerve blocks on muscle force in upper extremity. Arch Phys Med Rehab 52:22–29, 1971
12. Collins H, Lund D: Baseball injuries. p. 64. In Schneider R, Kennedy J, Plant M (eds): Sports Injuries: Mechanisms, Prevention, and Treatment. Williams & Wilkins, Baltimore, 1986
13. Cyprien J et al: Humeral retrotorsion and glenohumeral relationship in the normal shoulder and in recurrent dislocation (scapulometry). Clin Orthop 175:8–17, 1983
14. DePalma A, Callery G, Bennett G: Shoulder joint: variational anatomy and degenerative lesions of the shoulder joint. AAOS Instructional Course Lectures, 6:255–281, 1949
15. Doody S, Freedman L, Waterland J: Shoulder movements during abduction in the scapular plane. Arch Phys Med Rehab 51:595–604, 1970
16. Falconer M, Li F: Resection of the first rib in costoclavicular compression of the brachial plexus. Lancet 1:59, 1962
16a. Flatow E, Soslowsky L, Ateshian G et al: Shoulder joint anatomy and the effect of sublaxations and size mismatch on patterns of glenohumeral contact. Orthop Trans 15:803–804, 1991
17. Freedman L, Munro R: Abduction of the arm in the scapular plane. J Bone Joint Surg [Am] 48A:1503–1510, 1966
18. Fu F, Harner C, Klein A: Shoulder impingement syndrome: a critical review. Clin Orthop 269:162–173, 1991
19. Galinat B, Howell S: The glenohumeral ligament. Orthop Trans, 12:143, 1988
20. Gerber C, Terrier F, Zehnder R et al: The subcoracid space: an anatomic study. Clin Orthop 215:132–138, 1987
21. Gibb T, Sidles J, Harryman D et al: The effect of capsular

venting on glenohumeral laxity. Clin Orthop 268:120–127, 1991

22. Glousman R, Jobe F, Tibone J et al: Dynamic electromyographic analysis of the throwing shoulder with glenohumeral instability. J Bone Joint Surg [Am] 70A:220–226, 1988

23. Grana W, Moretz J: Ligamentous laxity in secondary school athletes. JAMA 240:1975–1976, 1978

24. Grant J: Method of Anatomy. 7th Ed. Williams & Wilkins, Baltimore. 1965

25. Gray H: The shoulder joint. p. 253. In Pick TP, Howden R (eds): Gray's Anatomy, Crown, New York, 1977

26. Harryman D, Sidles J, Clark J et al: Translation of the humeral head on the glenoid with passive glenohumeral motion. J Bone Joint Surg [Am] 72A:1334–1343, 1990

27. Howell S, Galinat B, Renzi A et al: Normal and abnormal mechanics of the glenohumeral joint in the horizontal plane. J Bone Joint Surg [Am] 70A:227–232, 1988

28. Inman V, Saunders J, Abbott L: Observations on function of the shoulder joint. J Bone Joint Surg 26:1–30, 1944

29. Itoi E, Motzkin N, Morrey B et al: Scapular inclination and inferior instability of the shoulder. Trans Orthop Res Soc 17:288, 1992

30. Itoi E, Motzkin N, Morrey B, An K-N: Stabilizing function of the long head of the biceps in the hanging position. J Shoulder Elbow Surg 3:135–142, 1994

31. Jobe F: Unstable shoulders in the athlete. AAOS Instr Course Lec 34:228–231, 1985

32. Jobe F, Tibone JE, Jobe CM et al: The shoulder in sports. In p. 961: Rockwood C, Matsen F (eds): The Shoulder. WB Saunders, Philadelphia, 1990

33. Kelkar R, Newton P, Armengol J et al: 3-Dimensional kinematics of the GH joint during abduction in the scapular plane. Trans Orthop Res Soc 18:136, 1993

34. Kumar V, Balasubramanian P: The role of atmospheric pressure in stabilizing the shoulder. J Bone Joint Surg [Br] 67B:719–721, 1985

35. Laumann U: Kinesiology of the shoulder joint, p. 23. In Kolbel R (ed): Shoulder Replacement. Springer-Verlag, Berlin, 1985

36. Levick J: Joint pressure-volume studies: their importance, design and interpretation. J Rheum 10:353–357, 1983

37. Lippett S, Vanderhooft J, Harris S et al: Glenohumeral stability from concavity-compression: a quantitative analysis. J Shoulder Elbow Surg 2:27–34, 1993

38. Lucas L, Hill J: Humerus varus following birth injury to the proximal humerus. J Bone Joint Surg 29:367–369, 1947

39. Maki S, Gruen T: Anthropometric studies of the glenohumeral joint. Trans Orthop Res Soc 13:162, 1988

40. Markhede G, Monastyrski J, Stener B: Shoulder function after deltoid muscle removal. Acta Orthop Scand 56:242–244, 1985

41. Matsen FI, Thomas S, Rockwood CJ: Anterior glenohumeral instability. p. 526. In Rockwood CJ, Matsen FI (eds): The Shoulder. WB Saunders, Philadelphia, 1990

42. Deleski R, McMahon P, Thompson W et al: A new dynamic testing apparatus to study glenohumeral motion. J Biomech, 1994 (in press)

43. Morrey B, An K-N: Biomechanics of the shoulder. p. 216. In Rockwood CJ, Matsen FI (eds): The Shoulder. WB Saunders, Philadelphia, 1990

44. Moseley H, Overgaard B: The anterior capsular mechanism in recurrent anterior dislocation of the shoulder. J Bone Joint Surg, [Br] 44B:913–927, 1962

45. Neer C: Impingement lesions. Clin Orthop 173:70–77, 1983

46. Neer C, Flatow E, Leach O: Tears of the rotator cuff: long term results of anterior acromioplasty and repair. In: 4th Meeting of the American Shoulder and Elbow Surgeons, Atlanta, 1988

47. Nirschl R: Rotator Cuff Tendonitis: Basic Concepts of Pathoetiology. AAOS Instructional Course Lectures, Park Ridge, IL, 1989

48. Nobuhara K: The Shoulder: Its Function and Clinical Aspects. Igaku-Shoin, Tokyo, 1987

49. O'Brien S, Schwartz R, Warren R et al: Capsular restraints to anterior/posterior motion of the shoulder. Orthop Trans. 12:143, 1988

50. O'Brien S, Arnoczsky S, Warren R, Rozbruch S: Developmental anatomy of the shoulder and anatomy of the glenohumeral joint. p. 1–33. In Rockwood CJ, Matsen FI (eds): The Shoulder. WB Saunders, Philadelphia, 1990

51. O'Connell P, Nuber G, Mileski R et al: The contributions of the glenohumeral ligaments to anterior stability of the shoulder joint. Am J Sports Med 18:579–584, 1990

52. Perry J: Biomechanics of the shoulder. In Rowe C (ed): The Shoulder. Churchill Livingstone, New York, 1988

53. Petersson C: Spontaneous medial dislocation of the tendon of the long biceps brachii. An anatomic study of prevalence and pathomechanics. Clin Orthop 211:224–227, 1986

54. Poppen N, Walker P: Normal and abnormal shoulder motion. J Bone Joint Surg [Am] 58A:195–201, 1976

55. Randelli M, Gambrioli P: Glenohumeral osteometry by computed tomography in normal and unstable shoulders. Clin Orthop 208:151–156, 1986

56. Rathman R, McNab I: The microvascular pattern of the rotator cuff. J Bone Joint Surg [Br] 52B:540–553, 1970

57. Ringel S et al: Suprascapular neuropathy in pitchers. Am J Sports Med 18:80–86, 1990

58. Rockwood C Jr, Green D: Fractures in Adults. 2nd Ed. JB Lippincott, Philadelphia, 1984

59. Rodosky MW, Rudert MJ, Harner CH et al: Significance of a superior labral lesion of the shoulder: A biomechanical study. Trans Orthop Res Soc 15:276, 1990

60. Romanes G: Upper and lower limbs. p. 75. In: Cunningham's Manual of Practical Anatomy. Oxford University Press, London, 1966

61. Roos D: Transaxillary approach to the first rib to relieve thoracic outlet syndrome. Ann Surg 163:354–358, 1966

62. Roos D: Congenital anomalies associated with thoracic outlet syndrome. Anatomy, symptoms, diagnosis and treatment. Am J Surg 132:771–778, 1976

63. Saha A: Theory of Shoulder Mechanism: Descriptive and Applied. p. 11. Charles C Thomas, Springfield, 1961

64. Samuilson R, Binder W: Symptomatic full thickness tears of the rotator cuff: an analysis of 292 shoulders in 276 patients. Orthop Clin North Am 6:449–466, 1975

65. Sidles J, Harryman II D, Harris S et al: In vivo quantification of glenohumeral stability. Trans Orthop Res Soc 16:646, 1991

66. Simkin P: Structure and function of joints. In Schumacher H (ed): Primer on the Rheumatic Diseases. Arthritis Foundation, Atlanta, 1988

67. Symeonides P: The significance of the subscapularis muscle in the pathogenesis of recurrent anterior dislocation of the shoulder. J Bone Joint Surg [Br] 54B:476–483, 1972

68. Terry G, Hammon D, France P et al: The stabilizing function of passive shoulder restraints. Am J Sports Med 19:26–34, 1991

69. Testut L: Traité d'Anatomie Humaine. Tome I. Osteologie, Arthrologie, Myologie. p. 504. Doin, Paris, 1921

70. Turkel S, Panio M, Marshall J et al: Stabilizing mechanisms preventing anterior dislocation of the glenohumeral joint. J Bone Joint Surg [Am] 63A:1208–1217, 1981

71. Uhtoff H, Loehr J, Sarkar K: The pathogenesis of rotator cuff tears. p. 211. In The Shoulder. Takagishi N (eds): Tokyo Professional Postgraduate Services, Tokyo, 1987

72. Warner J et al: Static capsuloligamentous restraints to superior-inferior translation of the glenohumeral joint. Trans Orthop Res Soc 16:210, 1991

2

Clinical Assessment of Shoulder Injuries

ANTHONY MINIACI
PAUL A. DOWDY
PETER J. FOWLER

INTRODUCTION

Shoulder injuries in sports are very common and lead to significant morbidity and cost. At least 10 percent of competitive swimmers have shoulder pain significant enough to interfere with activities.[22] Shoulder problems, most notably pain, are extremely common in competitive tennis players[18] and throwing athletes.[15,16] These problems also occur not infrequently with athletes of all calibers in swimming, golf, volleyball, and hockey, as well as many other sporting activities.[14,20]

In order to treat shoulder injuries properly, an accurate diagnosis must be made, beginning with a complete history, and physical examination not only of the shoulder, but of the complete musculoskeletal system and the body in general. The importance of clinical skills in the evaluation of shoulder injuries has been emphasized in the literature.[7,11,21,30]

HISTORY

An accurate history is essential for a proper diagnosis in the athletic shoulder. The initial patient profile should be obtained, including age, occupation, hand dominance, sports participated in, and activity level. Taking the history allows the doctor to develop a relationship with the athlete and also gives initial impressions as to the magnitude of the injury and the patient's expectations. The most common presenting symptom is pain. Evaluation of its onset, duration, location, pre-

cipitating and relieving factors, quality, and degree of interference with sport or work activity of the pain are essential. The presence of pain at rest or pain at night often signifies significant pathology.[15,16] Shoulder, arm, and hand position at the time of symptoms and the relationship of the onset of the pain to the specific portion or phase of the activity that precipitates it may elucidate its etiology.[23] For example, anterior shoulder pain that occurs in the late cocking phase of pitching may signify anterior glenohumeral subluxation.[15,16]

Other common presenting symptoms include instability, deformity, or associated symptoms from neurovascular compression or disruption. A patient with instability symptoms may complain that the shoulder dislocates or feels as if it is coming out of joint. Alternatively, pain or an uncomfortable sensation may only be experienced when the arm is positioned in a potentially unstable position. A high index of suspicion is required. A patient with recurrent subluxation can experience "dead arm syndrome" (episodic pain and the sensation that the arm has gone numb).[35]

In thoracic outlet syndrome, the athlete experiences pain in the shoulder radiating down the arm, with overhead activity; it may be associated with extremity blanching and temporary ischemic changes. Leffert and Gumley[17] have noted the coexistence of anterior glenohumeral subluxation and thoracic outlet syndrome.

Any treatment prior to the assessment (including medications) is important, not only for diagnostic impressions but also for determining other treatment options. An assessment of any significant associated medical conditions as well as a history of previous similar shoulder problems can aid in diagnostic and therapeutic decision making. Although not common in most athletes, systemic diseases such as diabetes mellitus or systemic lupus erythematosus indicate higher risk of complications after surgery, such as wound-healing problems or adhesive capsulitis. Janda and Hawkins[13] have recently presented a series of patients with adhesive capsulitis in whom diabetes was the underlying predisposition to the condition.

A positive family history of shoulder problems is important and should be documented. Patients with such a history have been shown to have a higher postoperative recurrence rate[25] and a higher rate of bilateral instability and postoperative subluxations.[3]

Medications the patient may be taking that can affect the musculoskeletal system (e.g., corticosteroids, nonsteroidal anti-inflammatory drugs) should be determined and taken into account for treatment. A judicious but delicate search for drug, alcohol, and anabolic steroid use should be made. A systematic review of symptoms in other anatomic areas of the musculoskeletal system is made, looking for either a systemic arthropathy or other sports-related injuries to prevent or treat.

A complete history will give a good idea of the diagnosis. The injuries can be broken down into acute and chronic:

1. Acute injuries
   a. Fractures
      i. Clavicle
      ii. Scapula
      iii. Humerus
   b. Dislocation
      i. Sternoclavicular joint
      ii. Acromioclavicular joint
      iii. Glenohumeral joint
   c. Rotator cuff tears
2. Chronic injuries
   a. Rotator cuff tendinopathy
   b. Acromioclavicular arthrosis
   c. Recurrent glenohumeral instability
   d. Chronic pain syndromes
      i. Referred pain (cervical spondylosis)
      ii. Thoracic outlet syndrome
      iii. Suprascapular nerve entrapment
      iv. Quadrangular space syndrome

PHYSICAL EXAMINATION

A detailed history can lead to the most likely diagnosis(es) and the physician can focus the examination accordingly. However, the importance of a general examination, especially examination of the cervical spine, cannot be overemphasized.[12]

Many of the physical findings in athletes with shoulder injuries are subtle, so a consistent approach to the evaluation to these problems is required. When the shoulder is being examined, one should remember that the shoulder actually consists of five areas of articulation; the sternoclavicular, acromioclavicular, scapulothoracic, and glenohumeral joint as well as the subacromial articulation. Sports-related injuries can occur at any of these articulations.

General examination of the athlete's shoulder begins with inspection and palpation of the entire shoulder, both active and passive range of motion (ROM), and neuromuscular testing. Special tests for impingement, instability, and bicipital tendinitis as well as thoracic outlet syndrome are performed. Injection techniques can then be utilized in the shoulder area, as needed, for both diagnostic and therapeutic purposes.

Inspection

Inspection begins with noting the general attitude of the patient and contour of the shoulder. The patient with pain in the shoulder may hold that shoulder higher and may support it with the contralateral hand. Careful inspection of the shoulder anteriorly, laterally, and posteriorly will reveal muscle wasting. For example, with supraspinatus wasting the scapular spine is prominent and normal muscle bulk above it is lost. The skin is inspected for swelling, erythema, scars, or deformities. Swelling and erythema may reflect the acuteness of the injury or may indicate an impending reflex sympathetic dystrophy. The presence of deformities may help to localize the diagnosis. Anterior prominence of the sternoclavicular joint or cephalad prominence of the distal clavicle may represent disruption of these joints. Winging of the scapula may be due to traumatic injury of the long thoracic nerve[19,37] or to muscular imbalance, with a relative deficiency of serratus anterior function.[23]

Palpation

We palpate the patient's shoulder by moving systematically from the sternoclavicular region, out laterally along the clavicle, and on to the acromion, greater tuberosity region, bicipital groove, and body of the scapula. Any tenderness, crepitus, or instability is noted and correlated with the patient's symptoms.

Range of Motion

Both active and passive ROM is measured for forward elevation, external rotation of 0 degree abduction (Fig. 2-1), external rotation at 90 degrees abduction (Fig. 2-2), and internal rotation (measured as the highest point that the thumb reaches (Fig. 2-3). In shoulder impingement and rotator cuff tears active forward elevation may be decreased. In shoulders with degenerative changes after a repair for recurrent shoulder instability either decreased external rotation[9,34,36] or internal rotation may be seen.[2,9] Decreased active ROM

with maintained passive ROM is of muscular etiology, while decrease in both active and passive ROM is due to physical limitations either intrinsic or extrinsic to the joint.

Neuromuscular Testing

A detailed neurologic examination is performed, if indicated, including testing the tone and reflexes of the upper extremities, as well as muscular strength (Fig. 2-4) and sensation (light touch, pinprick, two-point discrimination). A complete examination of the cervical spine is required to rule out a neuromuscular cause of the patient's symptoms.[12]

Impingement

The impingement sign is elicited by forcibly taking the arm from the side to maximal elevation.[8,26] The test is positive when this motion causes significant anterior

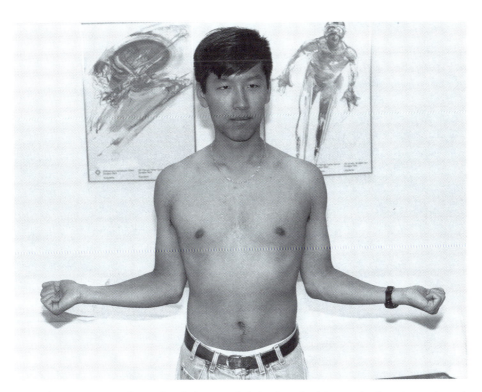

Fig. 2-1. External rotation is performed at 0-degree of abduction. In this way, both active and passive external rotation can be measured.

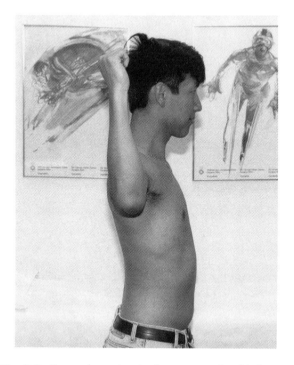

Fig. 2-2. External rotation is also measured at 90 degrees of abduction. This is an especially important motion to measure in the athlete who participates in overhead sports.

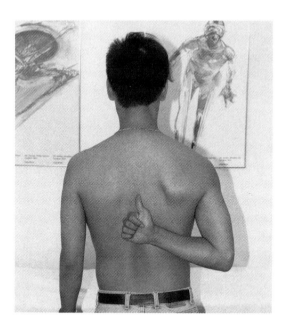

Fig. 2-3. Internal rotation is measured as the highest anatomic structure that the thumb reaches. In this case, the subject is internally rotating to T7.

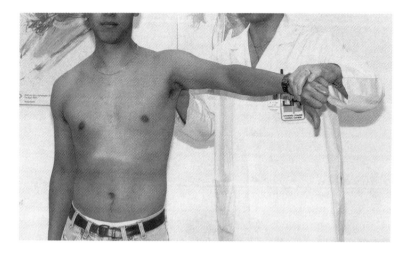

Fig. 2-4. Resisted abduction with the arm at 90-degrees of abduction, 30-degrees forward elevation, and full internal rotation (thumbs pointing to the floor) measures supraspinatus strength.

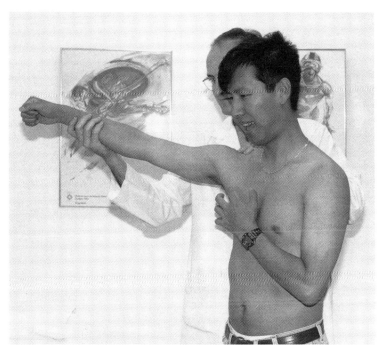

Fig. 2-5. The impingement sign is elicited by stressing the arm into full elevation. A positive sign is noted when the patient suddenly feels pain as the supraspinatus tendon impinges on the anteroinferior acromion.

shoulder pain (Fig. 2-5). This causes the distal bursal surface of the supraspinatus tendon to impinge on the rigid coracoacromial arch, which elicits the pain. Another impingement sign is performed by flexing the elbow 90 degrees, elevating the arm 90 degrees, and internally rotating the arm[7] (Fig. 2-6). This maneuver also causes pain by impinging on the insertion of the supraspinatus tendon and greater tuberosity against the anteroinferior acromion and the coracoacromial ligament.

Instability Testing

When testing for instability it is essential to have a well-relaxed and cooperative patient. In this fashion instability can be tested using apprehension and relocation tests, as well as humeral translation tests. Anterior apprehension is elicited by forcibly externally rotating the 90 degree abducted arm (Fig. 2-7). Apprehension that the shoulder is coming out of joint marks a positive test. Sometimes patients complain of pain with this maneuver. In these patients, the disappearance of the

pain with a posteriorly directed force on the humeral head suggests underlying instability as the cause of the pain. This is the relocation test (Fig. 2-8). The positive anterior apprehension test signifies anterior glenohumeral instability. Posterior apprehension is elicited by maximally internally rotating the 90 degree abducted arm while applying a posterior force on the humeral head (Fig. 2-9). In a positive test the patient feels as if the shoulder is about to dislocate. O'Driscoll[29] has found this test to be highly sensitive and specific for posterior shoulder instability. Another test that the authors have found to be particularly useful in assessing for the presence of posterior instability is the flexion-pivot test. In this test the patient's arm is positioned in 90 degrees abduction and neutral rotation with the elbow flexed 90 degrees. The examiner holds the patient's elbow with one hand and places the opposite hand on the patient's ipsilateral anterior axillary fold, while stabilizing the acromion and clavicle (Fig. 2-10A). The examiner then forward flexes and adducts the patient's arm while exerting a posteriorly directed force on the humeral head (Fig. 2-10B). In a positive

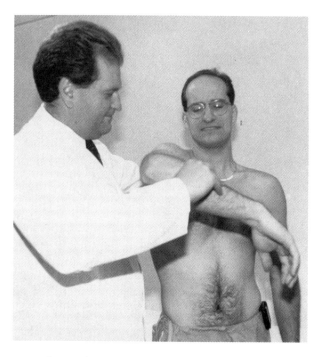

Fig. 2-6. An alternative to the classical impingement sign. The arm is elevated 90 degrees and stressed into maximal internal rotation. This produces pain as the supraspinatus tendon impinges on the corocoacromial ligament.

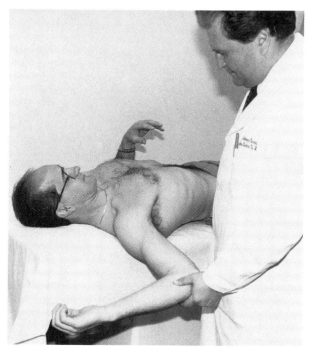

Fig. 2-7. The anterior apprehension sign. Although shown here supine, it is also done sitting. The most important point is complete relaxation of the patient prior to testing.

test the glenohumeral joint subluxes posteriorly, reproducing the patients symptoms and occasionally producing a palpable "clunk."

When examining a shoulder for glenohumeral translation it is imperative that the joint be concentrically reduced prior to forcing translation. For example, if the joint is already posteriorly subluxed, a posterior force applied to the humeral head may not produce any more translation, thereby giving a falsely negative test.

The anteroposterior (AP) translation or load-and-shift tests are performed by grasping the humeral head with one hand and performing a concentric reduction. Anterior and posterior loads are applied to the humeral head, in an attempt to translate it out of the joint (Fig. 2-11). This test is graded 0 to 3 for the amount of translation (Table 2-1). The sulcus sign is evaluated by asking the patient to sit comfortably with hands at the sides while one of the examiner's hands concentrically reduces the shoulder joint. The examiner's other hand produces a downward force, in line with the long axis

of the humerus, trying to translate the humeral head inferiorly (Fig. 2-12). This test is similarly graded 0 to 3 (Table 2-1). It is important to remember when performing these tests that normal shoulders can translate significantly.[5,6] Bilateral examination is crucial in assessing pathology, assuming that only one side is affected.

Table 2-1. Translation of Humeral Head out of Glenohumeral Joint[a]

Grade	Instability
0	None
1	Mild (0–1-cm translation)
2	Moderate (1–2-cm translation or to glenoid rim)
3	Severe (>2 cm translation or over glenoid rim)

[a] Degree of translation is graded 0–3, according to the magnitude of the translation and whether the humeral head is translated completely out of joint or not.

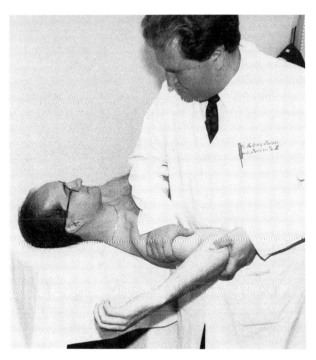

Fig. 2-8. The relocation test relieves the patient's apprehension symptoms. This is done simply by applying a posteriorly directed force to the humeral head in a patient in whom the anterior apprehension sign is positive.

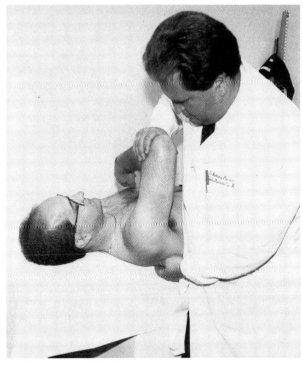

Fig. 2-9. The posterior apprehension sign is performed by placing a posterior force on the humeral head when the arm is at 90 degrees of abduction and full internal rotation. The sign is positive if the patient feels apprehensive that the shoulder is about to dislocate. Pain is not a positive test.

Acute Injuries

Clavicle Fracture

Athletes with clavicle fractures present with a definite history of either direct or indirect shoulder trauma followed by shoulder pain and deformity overlying the clavicle. Examination reveals ecchymosis and swelling of the skin surrounding the fracture site. The skin may be tented, but open injuries are unusual. The affected shoulder appears lower and droops inferomedially. The patient's neck may be bent laterally toward the injury and rotated toward the opposite side, to try and overcome the effects of the trapezius and sternocleidomastoid muscles. A prominence may be present at the fracture site because of pull on the proximal fragment by the sternocleidomastoid muscle and pull on the distal fragment by the pectoralis muscles. Bony crepitus is palpable at the fracture site, which is easily accessible because of its subcutaneous location. Any movement of the shoulder joint produces pain at the fracture site.

A thorough neurovascular examination as well as a chest examination is performed, looking for complications of this fracture.

Proximal Humerus Fracture

An athlete rarely suffers a proximal humerus fracture in sports. However, with severe direct or indirect trauma or through pathologic bone, this can happen. The athlete presents with sudden onset of severe pain in the shoulder and arm area accompanied by inability to use the extremity. The patient may complain of paresthesias in the involved extremity. The shoulder area is swollen, red, and bruised. Normal shoulder contour may be lost from fracture displacement. A fracture-dislocation must be suspected. A detailed neurovascular examination must be performed since injury to these structures is fairly common. The diagnosis of proximal humeral fracture is suspected clinically but is confirmed with appropriate radiology, including

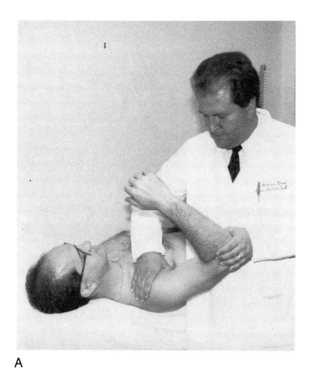
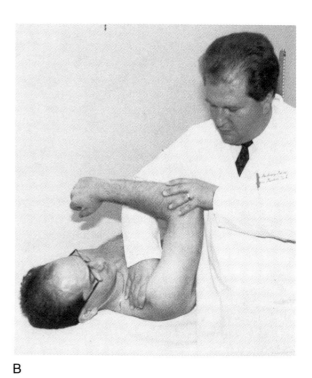

A

B

Fig. 2-10. **(A, B)** The flexion-pivot test for posterior instability is performed by flexing and adducting the patient's arm from the 90-degree abducted position and applying a posteriorly directed force on the humeral head. In a positive test the humeral head translates out of the glenohumeral joint.

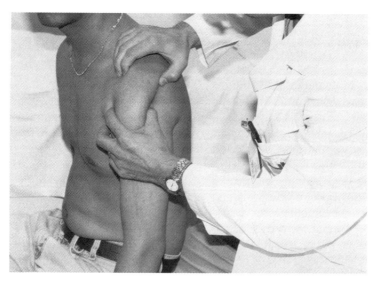

Fig. 2-11. The AP translation or load-and-shift test is performed by holding the humeral head into concentric reduction and then applying anterior and posterior forces to translate the humeral head on the glenoid cavity.

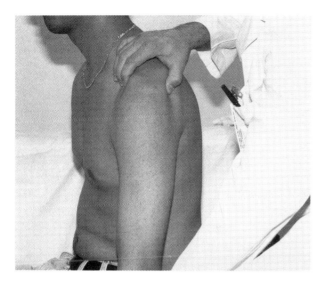

Fig. 2-12. The sulcus test is performed to assess inferior translation of the humeral head.

AP in the scapular plane, Y-lateral, and axillary radiographs.

Scapula Fracture

Scapular fractures can occur as isolated fractures of the glenoid, coracoid process, and acromion or as fractures of the scapular neck or body, often with associated life-threatening injuries. The latter fractures are extremely uncommon in athletic activity, being more commonly seen after major trauma. Glenoid rim fractures after acute shoulder dislocations are the most common scapular fractures occurring in sports. Patients with scapular fractures present with their arm held tightly adducted to their chest. Any ROM, especially abduction, causes severe pain. Crepitus may be present with passive arm movement. A detailed neurovascular and chest examination needs to be performed to rule out associated injuries such as axillary artery disruption, brachial plexus injury, pneumothorax, or pulmonary contusion. Appropriate radiographic examination is required to make the diagnosis of scapular fracture.

Glenohumeral Instability

Shoulder instability is extremely common in overhead sporting activity. Instability is classified by direction (anterior, posterior, or multidirectional) and timing (acute, chronic, recurrent).[10] Examination of an athlete

with an acute glenohumeral dislocation will reveal loss of the normal shoulder contour. Any motion will exacerbate the extreme pain. There may be a fullness either anteriorly or posteriorly, depending on the direction of dislocation. A complete neurovascular examination of the upper limb must be performed. Particular attention is paid to the status of the axillary nerve, since this is the most frequent nerve damaged after anterior shoulder dislocation. The axillary nerve is assessed by testing pinprick sensation over the deltoid and ability of the deltoid muscle to contract voluntarily.

In our experience, chronic unreduced shoulder dislocations are rarely seen in the athletic population and thus are not discussed here.

The clinical assessment of athletes with recurrent glenohumeral instability is of utmost importance for the proper management of these difficult problems. Patients with recurrent shoulder instability give a history of recurrent pain or numbness, a feeling that the shoulder is coming out of joint, or frank dislocations with provocative activity. Athletes with anterior instability usually experience their symptoms with the arm above the horizontal plane. By contrast, athletes with posterior instability usually experience symptoms with the arm below the horizontal plane. In athletes with recurrent anterior instability, the anterior apprehension sign is positive if they have had recurrent dislocations. With recurrent subluxations, the relocation test is positive. Speer and colleagues[38] have recently emphasized the importance of calling the relocation positive only if instability symptoms are reproduced with the test. If reproduction of pain during the relocation test is counted as a positive test, they suggest that this reduces the sensitivity and specificity of the test. In these patients, increased anterior translation of the glenohumeral joint can be demonstrated. In recurrent posterior instability, posterior apprehension may be demonstrated.[29] These patients show increased posterior glenohumeral translation on the flexion-pivot and load-and-shift tests. Athletes with multidirectional instability will have a positive sulcus test. They will also show evidence of anterior or posterior (or both) shoulder instability on examination.

Acromioclavicular Joint Disorders

Acute Conditions

Acromioclavicular joint disruption is a common sports injury. Most commonly, it is the result of the direct force produced by a fall on the tip of the shoulder with the arm adducted to the side. Less commonly, it results from a fall on the outstretched hand and is classified as types I to VI.[32] In type I the acromioclavicular ligament is sprained and all other ligaments are intact. In type II the acromioclavicular ligament is disrupted and the coracoclavicular ligaments are sprained. Subluxation of the acromioclavicular joint may be present. In type III both the acromioclavicular and coracoclavicular ligaments are completely disrupted. In type IV the distal clavicle is dislocated posteriorly, buttonholing itself through the trapezius. In type V the acromioclavicular joint is dislocated and the distal clavicle is grossly elevated above the scapula. In type VI the clavicle is dislocated inferiorly, below the coracoid.

Athletes with acromioclavicular joint disruption all have pain localized to this joint. Swelling and mild erythema of the skin and soft tissues around the joint may be present. In types I and II this is all that may be seen clinically. In type III injuries the distal clavicle is prominent superiorly; in type V injuries this is marked. In type IV injuries the distal clavicle may be palpated as a prominence posteriorly in the trapezius muscle. In type VI injuries (extremely rare) the acromion is prominent superiorly, and the coracoid process is palpated by directly stepping down from the acromion. In all types of injury, the acromioclavicular joint is tender to palpation. Decreased shoulder ROM is observed, secondary to pain at the joint.

Chronic Conditions

Chronic acromioclavicular joint symptomatology in athletes is usually related to the presence of arthritis in this joint after previous conservative or surgically managed sprains or dislocations of the same joint. These patients present with pain, usually worse with activity, localized to the joint. Examination may reveal superior prominence of the distal clavicle from previous acromioclavicular joint dislocation. Tenderness along the joint is present. The acromioclavicular arthrosis may lead to crowding of the subacromial space, which may cause mechanical impingement and subsequent rotator cuff tendinitis. Translation of the clavicle inferiorly, anteriorly, and posteriorly may be possible. Crepitus may be palpable. Radiographs will often show degenerative changes of the joint.

Sternoclavicular Joint Disorders

Sternoclavicular joint injuries are a rare, but important, cause of shoulder complaints. Sporting injuries are the second most common setting in the etiology of injury to this joint. Injuries can occur from anteriorly or posteriorly directed forces on the shoulder joint, producing posterior or anterior sternoclavicular joint subluxation or dislocation. Lateral compressive forces can also cause sternoclavicular joint disruption, with the direction of disruption depending on whether anterolateral or posterolateral compression, is present. These forces produce anterior or posterior dislocation, respectively. Alternatively, a posterior dislocation can be produced by a direct posteriorly applied force on the medial end of the clavicle. Anterior dislocations of the sternoclavicular joint are far more common than posterior dislocations.

The athlete with sternoclavicular joint disruption presents with pain and swelling localized to this area. The medial clavicle may be prominent anteriorly if the joint is dislocated anteriorly. In posterior dislocations the lateral edge of the sternum is prominent and the normal prominence of the medial clavicle is lost. In patients with posterior sternoclavicular dislocation venous engorgement or ischemia of the ipsilateral upper extremity, shortness of breath, or difficulty in swallowing may be seen, or the patient may be in hypovolemic shock. These latter signs and symptoms in posterior sternoclavicular joint dislocation are caused by compression of the mediastinal structures in close proximity to the sternoclavicular joints. This condition represents a surgical emergency and must be dealt with promptly in the operating room.

Rotator Cuff Tendinopathy

Rotator cuff tendinopathy or "*impingement syndrome*" in athletes (see Ch. 5) occurs most commonly in overhead sports. Tendinosis can result from rotator cuff and scapular rotator imbalance and subsequent stretching of static constraints, which can lead to anterior shoulder instability and secondary impingement.[15,16] These patients present with anterior shoulder pain upon overhead activities. Pain at rest may signify a rotator cuff tear. Examination reveals the presence of anterior apprehension and a positive relocation test. The impingement sign is negative initially but may be positive with prolonged symptomatology.

Acute Rotator Cuff Tears

Acute rotator cuff tears can occur in the setting of proximal humerus fractures or fracture-dislocations,[4] acute anterior glenohumeral dislocations,[27,28] or, less commonly, with supraphysiologic eccentric rotator cuff contractions. After their acute injuries have settled patients present with a painful arc of motion, supraspinatus muscle weakness, and inability to elevate their arm above 90 degrees. A drop-arm test may be positive. In this test the examiner passively elevates the patient's arm and asks the patient to hold the arm in that position. In a positive test the patient is unable to hold the arm against gravity, and it simply drops.

Bicipital Tendinitis

Bicipital tendinitis is best evaluated clinically by testing for the presence of tenderness in the bicipital groove using Yergason's and Speed's tests. In Yergason's[41] test the patient's arm is at the side, flexed 90 degrees at the elbow, fully pronated, while the examiner instructs the patient to supinate actively against resistance. In Speed's test, the arm is extended at the elbow, placed at the side, fully supinated, and the patient elevates the arm against the examiner's resistance. In both Yergason's and Speed's tests a positive response occurs when the test elicits pain localized to the bicipital groove.

Thoracic Outlet Syndrome

Thoracic outlet syndrome causes shoulder pain and can occur in athletes. It can be evaluated with Wright's hyperabduction test and Adson's maneuver. In the hyperabduction test, bilateral radial pulses are palpated, both with the patient resting the arms comfortably at the sides and with the arms hyperabducted.[40] Decrease or disappearance of the radial pulse, usually unilaterally, with the reproduction of symptoms constitutes a positive test. In Adson's[1] maneuver the arm of the affected side is placed on the sitting patient's thigh. With the forearm supinated, the patient turns the head to the affected side and extends the neck while holding the breath. In a positive test the radial pulse will diminish or disappear and the symptoms will be reproduced. The importance of symptom reproduction with these tests cannot be overemphasized since approximately 20% of the normal population will have decreased radial pulses with these maneuvers.[39]

Suprascapular Nerve Entrapment

Patients with suprascapular nerve entrapment present with vague dull shoulder aching and no sensory deficits. Examination reveals wasting of both supra- and infraspinatus muscles, as well as weakness of external rotation. Occasionally only the infraspinatus will be affected. Fully adducting the extended arm stretches the nerve and may exacerbate the pain.[31] Definitive diagnosis is difficult. Electromyography and nerve conduction tests are helpful in detecting the pathology.

Quadrangular Space Syndrome

Quadrangular space syndrome involves compression of the posterior humeral circumflex artery and axillary nerve in the quadrangular space. It typically presents as poorly localized pain and paresthesias in the posterior shoulder region. It generally occurs in the dominant extremity of young active individuals. Examination usually reveals diffuse tenderness on the anterolateral aspect of the shoulder, but point tenderness over the area of the quadrangular space is present. Symptoms can be reproduced by maintaining the shoulder abducted and externally rotated for approximately 1 minute.[24]

Cervical Spondylosis

The cervical spine must always be considered in the differential diagnosis of shoulder pain, especially in older individuals. The cervical spine is examined by first inspecting how the patient is holding the neck. A patient who keeps the head slightly laterally bent may have cervical spine muscle spasm. Having the patient fully flex, extend, and laterally bend the neck can reproduce pain from the cervical spine and also give the examiner an idea of cervical spine ROM. Complete muscular strength testing as well as sensory and reflex examination is required to evaluate whether the cervical spine is the cause of a patient's shoulder pain. If the examiner is still in doubt, then relief of pain with manual in-line cervical spine traction and reproduction of symptoms with manual cervical compression is highly suggestive that the cervical spine is the origin of the patient's shoulder pain.

INJECTION TECHNIQUES

Assessment of shoulder injuries would be incomplete without a discussion of techniques of injecting local anesthetic with or without corticosteroids around the shoulder girdle. These techniques are used both diagnostically and therapeutically. In subacromial injection, we prefer to enter anteriorly, with the patient supine. The injection consists of 2–5 ml of 2 percent lidocaine with or without a long-acting corticosteroid. If rotator cuff tendinitis is the cause of the patient's symptoms, then this injection should relieve them swiftly and completely. The impingement sign should become negative after the injection (positive impingement test).

Normally the bicipital groove is facing 10 to 20 degrees laterally with the arm in the anatomic position. Local anesthetic with or without corticosteroid is injected here in the evaluation and management of bicipital tendinitis. In suprascapular nerve entrapment, local infiltration of anesthetic around the suprascapular notch may relieve the patient's symptoms and also help to differentiate nerve entrapment from rotator cuff impingement and cervical spine pathology.[31,33] In acromioclavicular joint arthrosis, injection of anesthetic with or without corticosteroid is done by pointing the needle 15 degrees external to the sagittal plane and directly infiltrating the joint.

CONCLUSION

A thorough and consistent clinical assessment of athletes with shoulder injuries is a good start for optimal management of these demanding clinical problems. A complete history and physical examination augmented by the use of various injection techniques (when indicated), along with the judicious use of basic and special radiologic studies (see Ch. 3), will allow an appropriate diagnosis in the vast majority of cases.

REFERENCES

1. Adson AW: Surgical treatment for symptoms produced by cervical ribs and the scalenus anticus muscle. Surg Gynecol Obstet 85:687–700, 1947
2. Dowdy PA, O'Driscoll SW: Osteoarthritis following stabilization for recurrent anterior shoulder instability. Am J Sports Med 1993
3. Dowdy PA, O'Driscoll SW: Shoulder instability. An analysis of family history. J Bone Joint Surg [Br] 75B:782–784, 1993
4. Flatow EL, Cuomo F, Maday MG et al: Open reduction and internal fixation of two-part displaced fractures of the greater tuberosity of the proximal part of the humerus. J Bone Joint Surg [Am] 73A:1213–1218, 1991
5. Harryman DTI, Sidles JA, Clark JM et al: Translation of the humeral head on the glenoid with passive glenohumeral motion. J Bone Joint Surg [Am] 72A:1334–1343, 1990
6. Harryman DTI, Sidles JA, Harris SL, Matsen FAI: Laxity of the normal glenohumeral joint: a quantitative in-vivo assessment. J Shoulder Elbow Surg 1:66–76, 1992
7. Hawkins RH, Hawkins RJ: Failed anterior reconstruction for shoulder instability. J Bone Joint Surg [Br] 67B:709–714, 1985
8. Hawkins RJ, Kennedy JC: Impingement syndrome in athletes. Am J Sports Med 8:151–158, 1980
9. Hawkins RJ, Angelo RL: Glenohumeral osteoarthrosis. A late complication of the Putti-Platt repair. J Bone Joint Surg [Am] 72A:1193–1197, 1990
10. Hawkins RJ, Mohtadi NG: Clinical evaluation of shoulder instability. Clin J Sports Med 1:59–64, 1991
11. Hawkins RJ, Chris T, Bokor D, Kieter G: Failed anterior acromioplasty. A review of 51 cases. Clin Orthop 243:106–111, 1988
12. Hawkins RJ, Bilco T, Bonutti P: Cervical spine and shoulder pain. Clin Orthop 258:142–146, 1990
13. Janda DH, Hawkins RJ: Shoulder manipulation in patients with adhesive capsulitis and diabetes mellitus: a clinical note. J Shoulder Elbow Surg 2:36–38, 1993
14. Jarvinen M: Epidemiology of tendon injuries in sports. Clin Sports Med 11:493–504, 1992
15. Jobe FW, Kvitne RS: Shoulder pain in the overhead throwing athlete. The relationship of anterior instability and rotator cuff impingement. Orthop Rev 18:963–975, 1989
16. Kvitne RS, Jobe FW: The diagnosis and treatment of anterior instability in the throwing athlete. Clin Orthop 291:107–123, 1993
17. Leffert RD, Gumley G: The relationship between dead arm syndrome and thoracic outlet syndrome. Clin Orthop 223:20–31, 1987
18. Lehman RC: Shoulder pain in the competitive tennis player. Clin Sports Med 7:309–327, 1988
19. Mah JY, Otsuka NY: Scapular winging in young athletes. J Paediatr Orthop 12:245–247, 1992
20. Maylack FH: Epidemiology of tennis, squash, and racquetball injuries. Clin Sports Med 7:233–243, 1988
21. McAuliffe TB, Pangayatselvan T, Bayley I: Failed surgery for recurrent anterior dislocation of the shoulder. Causes and management. J Bone Joint Surg [Br] 70B:798–801, 1988

22. McMaster WC, Troup J: A survey of interfering shoulder pain in United States competitive swimmers. Am J Sports Med 21:67–70, 1993

23. Miniaci A, Fowler PJ: Impingement in the athlete. Clin Sports Med 12:91–109, 1993

24. Miniaci A, Tibone JE: Uncommon surgical approaches to the shoulder. In p. 103. Paulos E, Tibone JE (eds): Operative Techniques in Shoulder Surgery. Aspen, Gaithersburg, 1991

25. Morrey BF, Janes JM: Recurrent anterior dislocation of the shoulder. Long term follow-up of the Putti-Platt and Bankart procedures. J Bone Joint Surg [Am] 58A:252–256, 1976

26. Neer CSI, Welsh RP: The shoulder in sports. Orthop Clin North Am 8:583–591, 1977

27. Neviaser RJ, Neviaser TJ, Neviaser JS: Concurrent rupture of the rotator cuff and anterior dislocation of the shoulder in the older patient. J Bone Joint Surg [Am] 70A:1308–1311, 1988

28. Neviaser RJ, Neviaser TJ, Neviaser JS: Anterior dislocation of the shoulder and rotator cuff rupture. Clin Orthop 291:103–106, 1993

29. O'Driscoll SW: A reliable and simple test for posterior instability of the shoulder. J Bone Joint Surg [Br] suppl. 1. 73B:50, 1991

30. Ogilvie-Harris DJ, Wiley AM, Sattarian J: Failed acromioplasty for impingement syndrome. J Bone Joint Surg [Br] 72B:1070–1072, 1990

31. Post M, Mayer J: Suprascapular nerve entrapment. Clin Orthop 223:126–136, 1987

32. Rockwood CAJ, Young DC: Disorders of the acromioclavicular joint. p. 422. In Rockwood CAJ, Matsen FAI (eds): The Shoulder. WB Saunders, Philadelphia, 1990

33. Rose DL, Kelly CK: Shoulder pain. Suprascapular nerve block in shoulder pain. J Kansas Med Soc 70:135–136, 1969

34. Rosenberg BN, Richmond JC, Levine WN: Long-term follow-up of Bankart reconstruction: incidence of late glenohumeral arthrosis. p. 37. In: AOSSM, 19th Annual Meeting, Sun Valley, Idaho. American Orthopaedic Society for Sports Medicine, San Diego, 1993

35. Rowe CR, Zarins B: Recurrent transient subluxation of the shoulder. J Bone Joint Surg [Am] 63A:863–872, 1981

36. Samilson RL, Prieto V: Dislocation arthropathy of the shoulder. J Bone Joint Surg [Am] 65A:456–60, 1983

37. Schultz JS, Leonard JA: Long thoracic neuropathy from athletic activity. Arch Phys Med Rehab 73:87–90, 1992

38. Speer KP, Hannafin JA, Altchek DW, Warren RF: An evaluation of the shoulder relocation test. p. 32. In: AOSSM 18th Annual Meeting. American Orthopaedic Society for Sports Medicine, San Diego, 1992

39. Stallworth JM, Horne JB: Diagnosis and management of thoracic outlet syndrome. Arch Surg 119:1149–1151, 1984

40. Wright IS: The neurovascular syndrome produced by hyperabduction of the arms. Am Heart J 29:1–19, 1945

41. Yergason RM: Supination sign. J Bone Joint Surg 13:160, 1931

3

Diagnostic Imaging Techniques of Shoulder Injuries

RHODRI M. EVANS
K.M. CHAN
IAN DAVEY

INTRODUCTION

The shoulder is an anatomically and biomechanically complex joint composed of five functional articulations: glenohumeral, subacromial, acromioclavicular, sternoclavicular, and scapulothoracic. The selection of diagnostic imaging techniques in various kinds of shoulder injuries depends on the anatomic site. It is therefore important to have a thorough understanding of the functional anatomy of the various articulations as well as the relevant biomechanical implications. In this chapter, the various diagnostic imaging techniques are discussed in the light of specific injuries, and the relative merits and limitations are presented.

PLAIN RADIOGRAPHY

Plain radiographs are usually the initial radiologic investigation in the assessment of shoulder trauma. With the advent of newer imaging modalities such as computed tomography (CT), arthrography, and magnetic resonance imaging (MRI), the subtleties of plain film diagnosis are becoming more frequently overlooked, and plain film diagnosis appears to be assuming a minor role. This is not necessarily cost-effective.

Which views to choose? At times the plethora of radiographic views available for the shoulder is perplexing. The basic concept, as in all trauma, is to obtain two films of the region of interest at right angles to one another. Tailoring the patient's position and appro-

priate angulation of the central beam according to the region of interest should yield the greatest information.

Clavicle and Acromioclavicular Joint

When assessing the clavicle, the beam should be angulated 10 to 15 degrees in a cephalic direction. In order to assess the medial third of the clavicle, greater cephalic angulation is needed, approximately 35 to 40 degrees. Optimal visualization of the acromioclavicular joint can be achieved by 10 to 15 degrees cephalic angulation. Stress views are of questionable value.

A clinical and radiologic classification exists for acromioclavicular injuries.[66] However, the appearance of the normal joint varies considerably.[32] Many individuals with wide or "malaligned" acromioclavicular joints are asymptomatic. As always, close correlation of radiographic findings to the clinical situation is needed when assessing this joint. As a rule of thumb, if, in the anteroposterior (AP) projection, the inferior cortical margin of the acromion and the inferior aspect of the distal clavicle form a continuous arc, an acromioclavicular separation can be excluded (Fig. 3-1).[27] If the inferior aspect of the clavicle is displaced superiorly to align with the superior margin of the acromion, disruption of the acromioclavicular ligaments (Rockwood type III injury) is generally implied (Fig. 3-2). Disruption of the coracoclavicular ligament complex is signified by an increase of 5 mm or more in the distance between the undersurface of the clavicle and the superior surface of the coracoid of the injured side compared with the normal side (normal range, 11 to 13

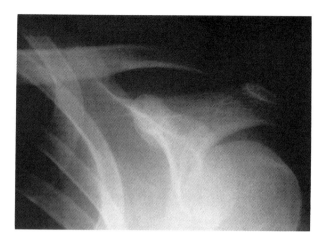

Fig. 3-1. AP view. Normal acromioclavicular joint.

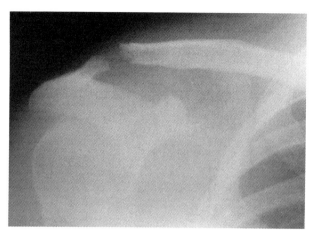

Fig. 3-3. AP view. Post-traumatic osteolysis of outer end of clavicle.

mm) (Fig. 3-2).[23] Post-traumatic osteolysis may follow acromioclavicular separation (Fig. 3-3).

In the assessment of impingement syndrome, conventional AP radiographs of the acromioclavicular joint may underscore the incidence of subacromial bony proliferation. Early diagnosis of bony spurring or an abnormally long anterior acromial process may initiate early surgical intervention for impingement syndrome. Many radiographic views have been proposed. Cone et al.[9] initially described an erect AP radiograph with 30-degree caudal angulation of the tube (Fig. 3-4). The use of the supraspinatus "outlet" view has also been emphasized in order to assess the incidence of subacromial spurs, but this view is undoubtedly more

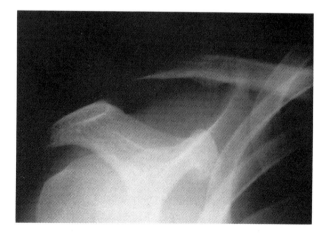

Fig. 3-2. AP view. Acromioclavicular separation and widening of coracoclavicular distance.

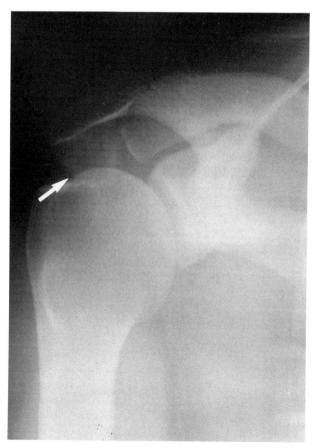

Fig. 3-4. AP view plus 30-degree caudal angulation. The anterior acromial process is well seen (*arrow*).

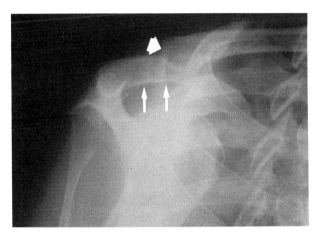

Fig. 3-5. Supraspinatus outlet view. The undersurface of the acromion can be seen (*thin arrows*), as well as the lateral end of the clavicle (*thick arrow*).

difficult to perform (Fig. 3-5).[35] Some authors[59] have proposed that the degree of angulation should be assessed fluoroscopically to attain the optimal angulation for assessing the acromioclavicular joint, pointing out that the degree of acromial tilt can vary from 13 to 34 degrees.[2] When seeking a cause for impingement syndrome, it should be borne in mind that the incidence of low-lying or anterior acromions and subacromial spurs in the asymptomatic population is not known. Despite the increasing use of complex imaging, we should not forget that radiography is the simplest, cheapest, and most reproducible method of demonstrating a low-lying or bulbous acromion, or a subacromial spur formation.[23]

Dislocation/Instability

Considerable controversy exists as to the optimal initial film series in suspected shoulder trauma or instability. For a comprehensive review the reader is directed to Raffi's[65] text. While American authors favor two AP views of the shoulder (in internal and external rotation) as standard, in the United Kingdom a more conservative approach is used with a single AP view in external rotation (Fig. 3-6) combined with an axillary view, if possible. The Y view or anterior oblique view of the scapula is underutilized in shoulder trauma (Figs. 3-7 and 3-8). No shoulder movement is required, and therefore it is better tolerated by the trauma patient

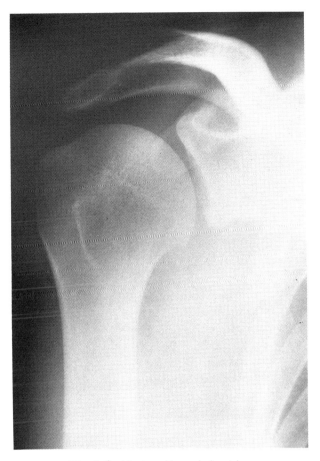

Fig. 3-6. AP view. Normal shoulder.

than the traditional axillary view. The shoulder being studied is rotated anteriorly 60 degrees, allowing a tangential view of the scapula. The acromion forms the posterior limb of the Y, the coracoid forms the anterior limb, and the normal head sits within the glenoid at the junction of the body of the scapula. Its use in suspected dislocation should become more widespread.

Posterior glenohumeral dislocation (approximately 5 percent of all dislocations) is still a commonly missed diagnosis on AP radiographs (Figs. 3-9 to 3-11). Emphasis of the radiographic signs is warranted:

1. "Light bulb" appearance of the humeral head
2. Glenohumeral joint space wider than 6 mm
3. Loss of parallelism of the glenoid and the humeral head

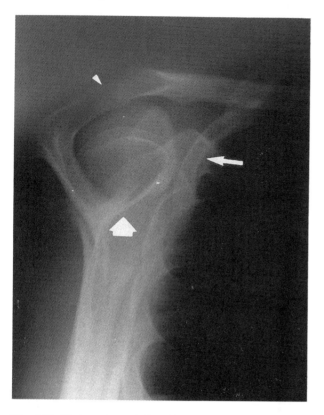

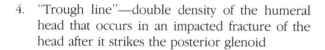

Fig. 3-7. Y view. Normal shoulder, showing acromion (*arrowhead*), coracoid process (*thin arrow*), and humeral head overlying glenoid cavity (*thick arrow*).

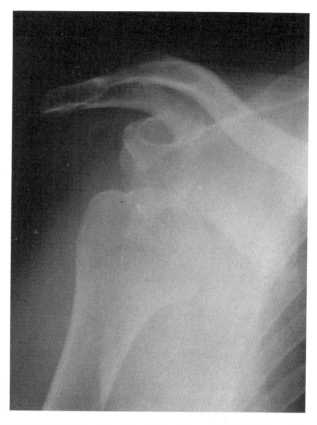

Fig. 3-8. AP view. Anterior dislocation of the shoulder. Inferior displacement of the humeral head is well seen.

4. "Trough line"—double density of the humeral head that occurs in an impacted fracture of the head after it strikes the posterior glenoid

When looking for signs of previous dislocation or instability (i.e., Hill-Sachs deformity of the humeral head or the Bankart lesion), it is important to tailor the radiographic series accordingly. More than 50 percent of anterior dislocations are associated with a Hill-Sachs defect, the compression fracture of the posterolateral surface of the humeral head that occurs in anterior dislocation.[29] Gold and Bassett[23] state that the AP view with the arm in 70 to 90 degrees of internal rotation is the best view for identifying a Hill-Sachs defect (Figs 3-12 and 3-13). However, Rozing et al.[69] state that the Stryker view is the best.

The Bankart lesion,[3] an avulsion fracture of the anterior-inferior glenoid rim, is now regarded as pathognomic of anterior instability (Fig. 3-14).[4] The Bankart lesion is best seen on axillary (Fig. 3-15) or modified axillary views (e.g., Westpoint view). Pavlov et al.[60] have shown that the maximal yield in diagnosing the lesions of anterior instability (i.e., the Bankart lesion and the Hill-Sachs defect) is obtained when a combination of three views are obtained: AP in internal rotation, Stryker notch view (tangential view of posterosuperior aspect of humeral head), and either Westpoint or Didiee views (modified axillary views).

When the examiner is searching for ectopic calcification around the shoulder joint, the humeral head must be rotated to allow depiction of the insertions of the component muscles of the rotator cuff. Supraspinatus calcification is best seen capping the greater tuberosity when the arm is in external rotation. The next most frequently calcified tendon is the infraspinatous tendon. As this inserts more posteriorly and inferiorly onto the greater tuberosity, an AP view with the arm in internal rotation is optimal, since this projects the calcification laterally. Calcification in the teres minor is similarly detected, whereas calcification in the sub-

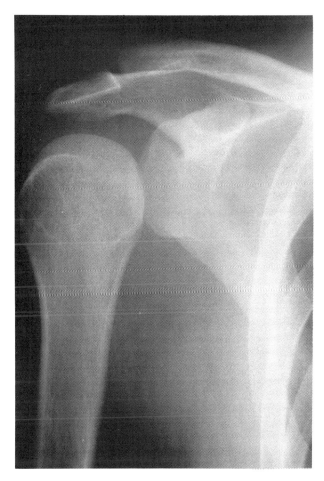

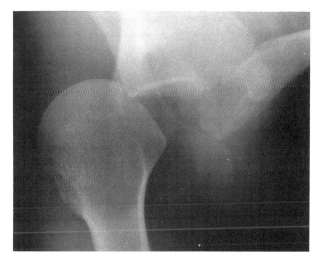

Fig. 3-10. Axillary view. Posterior dislocation of the shoulder. Humeral head is displaced posteriorly from the glenoid.

Fig. 3-9. AP view. Posterior dislocation of the shoulder. The humeral head has a "light bulb" appearance, and the glenohumeral joint space is widened.

scapularis tendon is best depicted on an axillary view to demonstrate the lesser tuberosity origin. Bursal calcification can be contused with tendinous calcification, however, bursal calcification tends to be denser and usually possesses a lobular configuration (Fig. 3-16).

ULTRASONOGRAPHY

The possible use of ultrasonography in diagnosis of rotator cuff pathology was suggested in 1977.[45] By the early to mid-eighties, several groups had published their techniques for evaluation of the rotator cuff.[11,42,48,50,72] As with many new techniques, the initial research into the use of ultrasonography as a noninva-

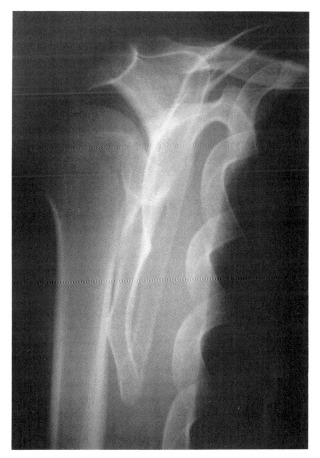

Fig. 3-11. Y view. Posterior dislocation of the shoulder. Posterior displacement of the humeral head is well depicted.

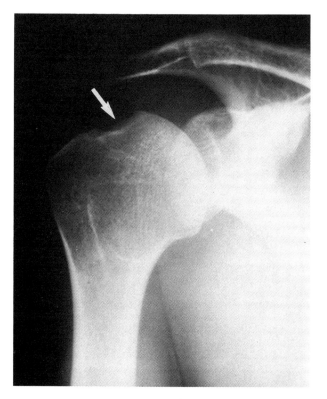

Fig. 3-12. AP view. A large Hill-Sachs deformity is seen related to the superior surface of the humerus (*arrow*).

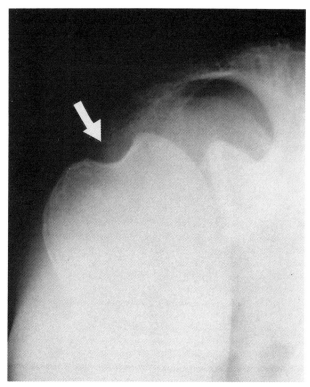

Fig. 3-13. Modified axillary view. Hill-Sachs deformity of shoulder instability (*arrow*).

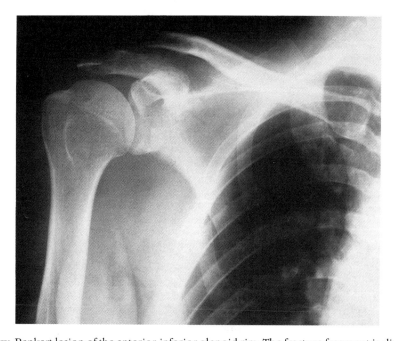

Fig. 3-14. AP view. Bankart lesion of the anterior-inferior glenoid rim. The fracture fragment is displaced medially.

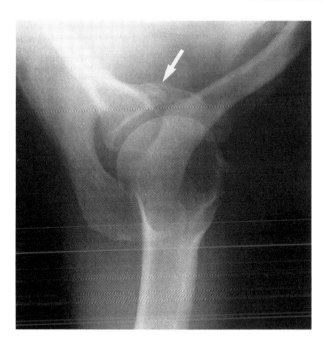

Fig. 3-15. Axillary view. Bankart lesion of the glenoid rim (*arrow*).

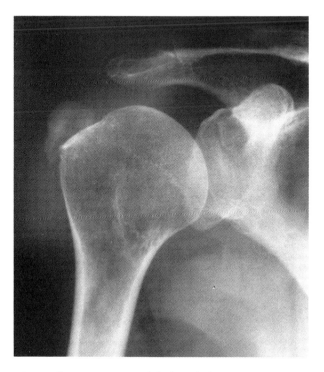

Fig. 3-16. AP view. Dense lobular calcification in the subdeltoid bursa.

sive, safe means of imaging the shoulder was positive and encouraging. As more and more centers have evaluated ultrasonography, less positive reports have emerged.

Brandt and his colleagues[5] stated in 1989 that ultrasonography has a limited role in assessment of rotator cuff injury. They found a sensitivity of 57 percent and a specificity of 76 percent for detection of a rotator cuff tear when compared with surgery, yet positive reports continue to emerge. Soble et al.[74] quoted a sensitivity of 93 percent and specificity of 73 percent for detection of a tear. Hodler et al.[30] in their prospective comparative trial found that ultrasonography demonstrated 14 of 15 tears, whereas MRI imaged only 10 of 15. They concluded that with regard to cost and patient compliance ultrasonography should be the initial examination for rotator cuff tears. However, other studies suggest otherwise; Misamore and Woodward[53] compared ultrasonography and arthrography in 32 patients. They found an accuracy of only 37 percent for ultrasonography compared with 87 percent for arthrography.

Why does such disparity exist in the current literature? As with any ultrasonographic examination, the skill of the operator is paramount. Middleton[47] states that rotator cuff sonography rivals carotid sonography as the most difficult sonographic examination to master. In addition to a thorough understanding of the anatomy of the shoulder, a detailed understanding of the basic principles of sound interaction with acoustic interfaces is needed.

Any budding shoulder ultrasonologist is advised to read the research of Crass et al.[12] on tendon echogenicity. They showed that the echogenicity of a tendon was quite angle dependent, a tendon characteristic known as anisotropy. Normal tendon is composed of parallel bundles of collagen with a scanty stroma, which act as specular reflectors. When the collagen bundles are parallel to the axis of the transducer, a reflective (bright) image results (Fig. 3-17). If the transducer is tilted relative to the long axis of the tendon or vice versa, a decrease in the returning echos results in a hypoechoic (black) region. Thus if the transducer head is curved or a linear array transducer is used to assess a curved tendon (e.g., supraspinatus tendon), hyperechoic and hypoechoic areas will be seen within a normal tendon. Some of the earlier reports of false-positive and false-negative ultrasonographic findings in assessing the rotator cuff have certainly failed to realize the concept of anisotropy.

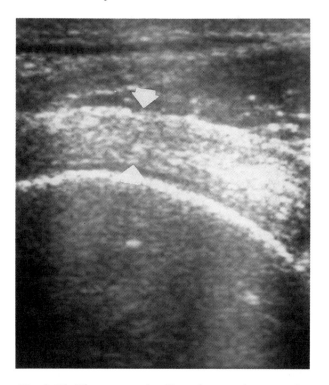

Fig. 3-17. Ultrasonography. Normal supraspinatus tendon, seen as a uniformly echogenic band (*arrows*).

cuff tear are: (1) nonvisualization of the cuff, which results from large tears, as the deep surface of the deltoid directly opposes the humeral head; nonvisualization should have a 100 percent predictive value for a complete tear[43,50]; (2) focal thinning the cuff; focal thinning due to a tear is abrupt and should be sharply demarcated from normal rotator cuff tissue[49]; and (3) discontinuity of the tendon fibers; when clearly asymetric, this is an unequivocal sign of a tear (Fig. 3-18).[47]

In addition to these three major criteria, two other minor criteria may be helpful in diagnosing rotator cuff tears. The visualization of a small subdeltoid bursal effusion, especially when intra-articular fluid is detected, may be the only finding in a small tear.[50] The probability of detecting fluid is increased by scanning the region above the greater tuberosity with the arm held in extension and internal rotation.[48] The bright echoes of the subdeltoid bursa normally form a convex upward curve. In full-thickness tears a concave configuration may be seen.

The use of ultrasonography has been advocated in the postoperative patient.[44] Scanning the postoperative

The basic technique of shoulder ultrasonography is outlined by Mack et al.[43] The first principle is that any tendon should be examined in two orthogonal planes whenever possible. High-frequency (7.5 to 10 MHz) linear array probes are essential. The use of sector or curved array transducers will lead to error. The technique is an active one; scanning during shoulder movement is essential and will help to identify subtle defects. Hyperextension of the shoulder should always be performed, allowing assessment of the maximum area possible of the supraspinatus tendon. The subacromial portion of the supraspinatus will always be a blind spot for ultrasonography. However, as the vast majority of tears involve the distal portion of the supraspinatus, which is well seen, this is not thought to represent a significant problem.

What ultrasonic criteria should be used for a rotator cuff tear? As the technique has evolved, some earlier criteria (i.e., hyperechoic foci) thought to represent small tears filled with granulation tissue or hypertrophied synovium[19] have been found to be unreliable.[5] The three most reliable ultrasonic features of a rotator

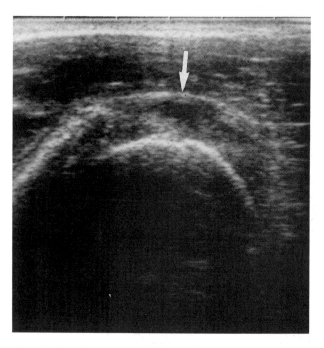

Fig. 3-18. Ultrasonography. Tear of the supraspinatus tendon. The tendon fibers are discontinuous, as indicated by a dark cleft within the tendon (*arrow*).

patient is an infinitely more complex examination. While excellent results have emerged from one major referral center, the results have not yet been duplicated. This reflects the degree of expertise that needs to be achieved in order to interpret postoperative appearances reliably.

Is there a role for ultrasonography in the evaluation of the shoulder? The main proviso has to be an experienced operator. If that exists, it would be reasonable to use this method as the initial investigation in suspected impingement syndrome or rotator cuff tear, especially when MRI access is limited. In younger patients in whom symptoms persist, a negative ultrasonogram should be followed by other imaging modalities.

ARTHROGRAPHY

The use of arthrography in the shoulder to demonstrate rotator cuff tears was first described in 1939.[41] It was not until the late 1970s that double-contrast arthrography became the vogue.[22] The most common indication for arthrography is a suspected rotator cuff tear.[25] Neer[56] stated that his indications for arthrography were unresponsive impingement syndrome (for those older than 40 years), sudden weakness after trauma, bicipital tendon rupture, and glenohumeral instability (for those older than 40 years). Few current authors would now agree with Neer's indications. Pure arthrography is now becoming a historical technique. The prime reason for using shoulder arthrography these days is to perform a CT arthrogram.

Is the dwindling usage of shoulder arthrography totally justified? Mink et al.[52] showed a greater than 99 percent accuracy in the detection of surgically proven full-thickness tears. The easiest diagnosis to make on arthrography is a "complete" rupture of the cuff, since frank extravasation of contrast exists from the glenohumeral joint into the subacromial bursa (Fig. 3-19). A "complete" tear is a full-thickness tear resulting in abnormal communication between joint and bursa. Soble and his colleagues,[74] in comparing sonography with arthrography in 30 patients with rotator cuff tears who subsequently underwent surgery, describe a sensitivity for sonographic detection of a tear of 93 percent with a specificity of 73 percent, while for arthrography sensitivity was 87 percent and specificity was 100 percent. Which is the superior technique?

Arthrography can detect "complete" tears of the rotator cuff or incomplete tears that involve the inferior (articular) surface of the cuff. It cannot, however, detect partial tears of the superior surface or intrasubstance

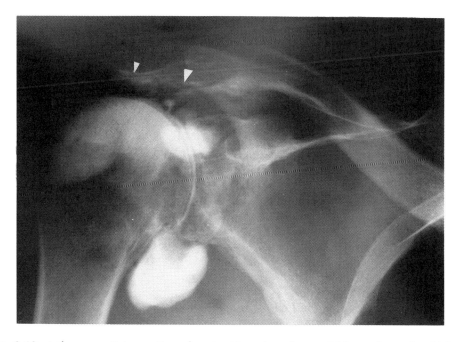

Fig. 3-19. Arthrogram. Extravasation of contrast into the subacromial bursa (*arrowheads*) is seen.

tears. The management of such partial tears is controversial.[36] It could be argued that a didactic approach is warranted (i.e., all acute traumatic complete tears or chronic tears that are unresponsive to conservative management should be repaired).[46] If such management of acute complete tears is to be pursued, then perhaps the declining use of arthrography is unwarranted. Yes, arthrography is invasive, but this argument is facile in the light of recent literature extolling the virtues of MR arthrography.[20,31] When Hodler et al.[30] prospectively evaluated MRI and ultrasonography, they used arthrography as the "gold standard."

Noninvasive and nonionizing investigations (i.e., MRI) will ultimately ensure that arthrography is a truly historic technique, but when MRI is not available, a strong case can still be made for its continued use, both as standard arthrography and in conjunction with CT (i.e., computed arthrotomography).

While the results of arthrography for detection of full-thickness rotator cuff tears are excellent, false-positive and false-negative results can occur. False-positive arthrograms usually result from the misinterpretation of normal structures[24]; the biceps tendon sheath filled with contrast can mimic a tear with the shoulder in external rotation, as can the superior extension of the capsule in the region of the glenoid. Occasionally the normal fat line outlining the subacromial subdeltoid bursa can be mistaken for air. False-negative studies are usually the result of inadequate postexercise films. Complete and partial tears can be missed or complete tears misdiagnosed as partial tears.

COMPUTED ARTHROTOMOGRAPHY

Combining CT with double-contrast shoulder arthrography was first suggested in 1987.[73] Since then, numerous authors have described their techniques. The main value and use of computed arthrotomography is in the assessment of shoulder instability and in demonstrating the labral and capsular abnormalities associated with instability. The technique is basically that of a standard double-contrast arthrogram followed by CT with axial sections taken through the shoulder. For a detailed review of the technique, the reader is directed to El-Khoury's text.[16]

What plain films should be taken prior to the study? As a high association is known to exist between the presence of a Hill-Sach's lesion and glenoid margin fractures with labral tears, any plain films taken prior to the study should be directed at demonstrating these bony abnormalities.[77] An AP view, an axillary view, and a view with a high sensitivity for the Hill-Sachs deformity (e.g., Stryker or Didiee views) are recommended. CT arthrography is allegedly less sensitive in the detection of the Hill-Sachs deformity than plain radiography.[62,73] DeHaven et al.[13] found a sensitivity of only 70 percent. However, Deutsch et al.[15] state that CT arthrography is highly sensitive in the detection of the Hill-Sachs deformities and will detect them when plain films have failed to do so. If CT arthrography does fail to detect a Hill-Sachs deformity it is probably of no significance, since it means the lesion will be small and will probably be of no significant clinical consequence; if significant instability exists, other features should be present that should allow a positive diagnosis (e.g., labral or capsular abnormalities). If a brief set of appropriate preliminary films is accompanied by CT arthrography, the false-negative incidence for the detection of a Hill-Sachs fracture will be insignificant.

Is it relevant to take postcontrast films prior to CT? Occasionally a rotator cuff tear will be detected on CT arthrography, and although Wilson et al.[77] state that CT arthrography is more sensitive than conventional arthrography in their series, it is often a difficult diagnosis to make on CT arthrography. Since the presence of a rotator cuff tear has management implications, the taking of postcontrast AP radiographs in internal and external rotation is prudent. Postexercise films are not recommended and although this may mean a small incidence of false-negative examinations, it is preferable, since vigorous exercise increases the likelihood of extracapsular extravasation of contrast with a subsequent poor-quality study.

The positioning of the shoulder during CT scanning is critical. Raffi[65] contends that while external rotation allows better visualization of the posterior labrum/capsule complex[61] by relaxing the posterior capsule and allowing air to move posteriorly, it may cause difficulty in the interpretation of the anterior structures. Scanning performed in the neutral position should allow better dispersal of contrast and air around the joint. Extra sections with the hand in external rotation can then be taken if further assessment of the posterior labrum is required.

Labrum

The bony glenoid cavity is surrounded by a triangular fibrous structure called the labrum, which acts as a brace to prevent excessive translational movement of the oversized humeral head within the smaller glenoid cavity. It may also act like the rim of a suction cup, which allows the motion of the humeral head to induce strong negative pressures within the glenoid, thus helping to maintain glenohumeral stability.[28]

On CT arthrography, at the midglenoid level, the labrum has a triangular shape, more pointed anteriorly and more rounded in outline posteriorly (Fig. 3-20). The posterior labrum is usually smaller than the anterior labrum. Unfortunately, while it is usually easy to confirm normality by CT arthrography, difficulty arises in the distinction between normal and abnormal. Wilson et al.[77] define an abnormal labrum as one that is absent, deformed, or fragmented, has irregular margins, or contains contrast media within, on more than one section. No series of asymptomatic individuals have undergone CT arthrography. MRI studies of asymptomatic shoulders confuse the situation by revealing normal variants of labral morphology that were previously regarded as pathologic. In Neumann et al.'s[58] MRI study on asymptomatic shoulders a 6 percent incidence of absent anterior labrum and an 8 percent incidence of absent posterior labrum was found. The definition of an "isolated" labral injury in the light of such variance in normal anatomy will continue to cause diagnostic problems. Despite such difficulties, CT arthrography has excellent sensitivity for identifying labral tears or fractures. In the largest series to date that has surgical correlation an accuracy of 97 percent was obtained.[77] In a smaller, earlier study, a slightly lower accuracy rate (84 percent) was found.[65]

CT arthrography is often used in the assessment of athletes who have "functional instability" (i.e., patients with a clinically stable glenohumeral joint but who have the sensation of an unstable joint).[55] They may complain of pain, clicking, or "catching" in the joint. Raffi[65] states that a frequent finding in throwing athletes with shoulder pain but no clinical instability was detachment of the superior labrum. This is thought to arise from the pull of the biceps tendon on its origin at the superior labrum during the throwing act.[1] However, De Palma[14] believes that this represents a progressive degeneration that starts in the second decade. An

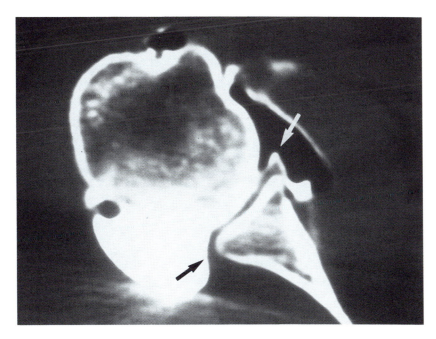

Fig. 3-20. CT arthrography. Normal labrum. The anterior labrum is more pointed (*white arrow*), while the posterior labrum is more rounded (*black arrow*).

incidence of a detached superior labrum greater than 60 percent by the fifth decade is quoted. These changes may progress to a hypertrophy of the superior labrum as synovial tabs and fringes form, particularly anteriorly. This has been reported to be associated with pain in both the stable and unstable shoulder.[1] This complex region is difficult to assess with axial images, and MRI with its multiplanar imaging capability is likely to shed more light.[55] The next most frequently found "isolated" labral tear in the athlete with a stable shoulder is a tear of the middle portion of the anterior labrum.[62] This is thought to arise from impingement of the labrum between the humeral head and subscapularis tendon during the throwing action.

Current literature regarding the appearance of the normal and abnormal labrum is confusing. As more MRI studies are performed on asymptomatic shoulders, we should learn more of the natural morphology of the labrum and how it varies with age. MRI studies may not clarify the situation, however, as illustrated by Garneau's recent work.[21] MRI images of 9 asymptomatic volunteers and 15 patients with surgically documented labral tears were blindly reviewed by two musculoskeletal radiologists. In the 15 symptomatic shoulders (with surgically documented labral tears) the two radiologists had sensitivities of 44 and 77.8 percent with specificities of 66.7 and 66.7 percent, respectively. Clearly, diagnosing labral abnormalities in isolation is fraught with difficulty. When assessing for instability, other signs should be present to reinforce a radiologic diagnosis of instability.

When can we say that the labrum is abnormal on CT arthrography? If air or contrast is clearly seen within the labrum or dissects between the labrum and its attachment to the articular surface of the glenoid, we can regard these as signs of trauma (Fig. 3-21). Similarly, an abrupt amputation of the labrum may be indicative of trauma (Fig. 3-22). This may be associated with an intra-articular loose body [i.e., a free-floating labral fragment (Fig. 3-23)]. If a fracture of the glenoid is present or a periosteal reaction is seen related to the glenoid margin, this usually implies major trauma to the labrum.

Capsule

Because the capsule is distended with air and contrast media, CT arthrography affords better delineation of

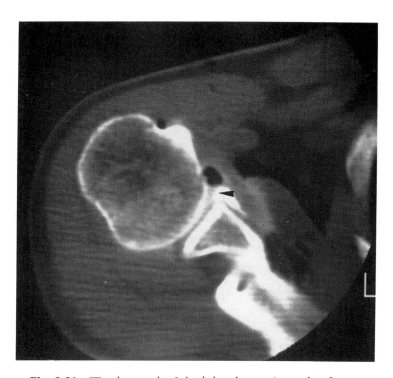

Fig. 3-21. CT arthrography. Labral detachment (*arrowhead*).

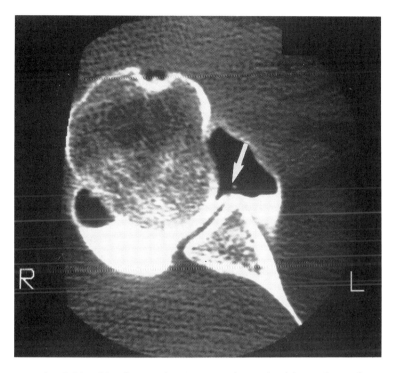

Fig. 3-22. CT arthrography. Amputated anterior labrum (*arrow*).

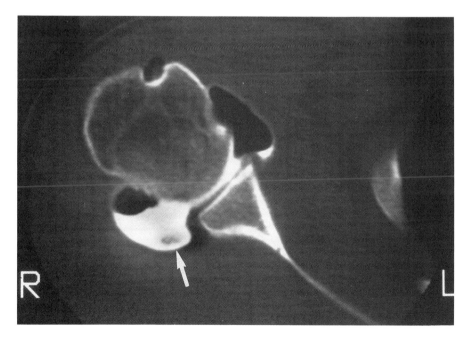

Fig. 3-23. CT arthrography. An anterior labral fragment is seen in the posterior capsular recess (*arrow*).

the capsule and its attachments than MRI. Unless an effusion is present or MR arthrography is performed, the capsule can be difficult to assess on MRI.[78] The normal capsule is thickened anteriorly by the superior, middle, and inferior glenohumeral ligaments. Whether these are clearly demonstrated on CT arthrography is contentious.[16,63] The capsule envelops the glenohumeral joint and is attached to the anatomic humeral neck laterally and the scapula medially.

The scapular insertion of the anterior capsule is a subject of great interest and debate when discussing the unstable shoulder. Wilson et al.[77] give an arbitrary classification of anterior capsular attachments, dividing the scapular neck into three divisions: lateral, middle, and medial. Insertion of the anterior joint capsule beyond the glenoid margin has been called abnormal and was thought to result from stripping of the capsular attachment secondary to trauma (Fig. 3-24).[13,63,65,73] Many authors [68,77,78] believe a medial anterior capsular insertion (i.e., not into the glenoid margin) to be a normal anatomic variant and a poor indicator of shoulder instability. Wilson et al[77] found that the frequency of labral injury increased as the anterior capsular attachment moved medially. Whether the medial insertion of the anterior capsule is a predisposition to insta-

bility or is simply the result of anterior subluxation with capsular stripping is debatable.[63,65] Interestingly, capsular size has been found to have no correlation with labral injury.[77] Occasionally new bone formation can be seen along the capsular margin, confirming that a recent injury with some stripping of the capsular insertion has occurred.

When should we regard a medial capsular insertion as abnormal? Some authors would advocate simply stating the insertion of the anterior capsule and avoiding a definition of normality or abnormality. We find Wilson et al.'s[77] advice the most sensible option: anterior capsular insertion should only be considered abnormal when it inserts into the medial third of the scapular neck. If the insertion is more lateral it may be normal and should be evaluated in connection with other possible findings of instability. If the remainder of the study is normal it is safe to ignore capsular insertions into areas I and II (i.e., lateral and middle divisions).

Just as the clinical diagnosis of instability in the glenohumeral joint is often not clear, the radiologic diagnosis of instability can be problematic. The normal variants of labral and capsular anatomy are diagnostic traps for the unwary, if interpreted in isolation. Al-

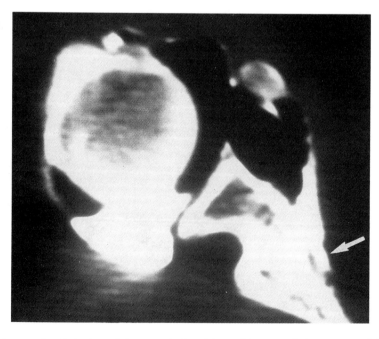

Fig. 3-24. CT Arthrography. Stripping of the capsule is evidenced by a medial insertion of the anterior capsule (*arrow*).

though it is invasive, CT arthrography allows excellent delineation of labral morphology, the joint capsule and its attachments, and any associated bony abnormality that may occur in instability. If these are assessed together, CT arthrography plays a major role in the assessment of shoulder stability.

MAGNETIC RESONANCE IMAGING

MRI, with its superior soft tissue contrast and multiplanar capabilities, is having a large impact on imaging of the shoulder. The fact that it is a nonionizing and noninvasive technique means that its use will become more widespread.

The new technology and its complex associated terminology can often perplex the uninitiated. The vast array of potential imaging techniques and pulse sequences only confuses the situation. The examination must always be tailored to the clinical question being asked, but for most shoulder problems an imaging technique that scans in a coronal oblique plane (i.e., parallel to the supraspinatus tendon) and in an axial plane to delineate the glenoid/labral/capsular complex should allow adequate assessment of the common areas of pathology. Pulse sequences will be individually tailored but proton density or T_1-weighted images should always be obtained.

Impingement Syndrome

A major contribution of MRI to shoulder imaging is in its evaluation of the impingement syndrome and rotator cuff disorders.[7,18,33,38,64,70,79] Its proponents claim that MRI allows precise delineation of the tears that occur in late impingement syndrome, in addition to the spectrum of pathologies associated with impingement syndrome (e.g., tendonitis, subacromial/subdeltoid bursitis, acromial spurs, and acromioclavicular joint arthritis).

Tendonitis is diagnosed on MRI when abnormal intermediate signal intensity is seen within the tendon that does not brighten to fluid intensity on T_2-weighted sequences (Figs. 3-25 and 3-26). An enlarged tendon with an inhomogenous signal pattern and an associated bursitis are strong indications for a symptomatic tendonitis. Raffi[64] provides some histologic correlation for the region of increased signal intensity seen within the supraspinatus tendon. In the cadavers studied, his

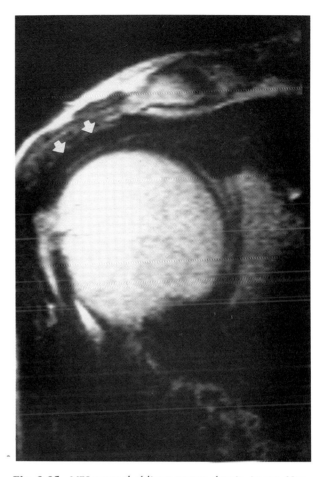

Fig. 3-25. MRI coronal oblique proton density image. Normal supraspinatus tendon, which is homogenously dark (*arrow*).

group found histologic changes of tendon degeneration. Kieft et al.[33] reported myxoid degeneration and inflammation of the supraspinatus tendon in regions of increased signal intensity. Similar conclusions to Raffi et al.[64] have been reached by Kjellin et al.[37] in their evaluation of 13 cadaveric shoulders. They observed that tendons with findings suggestive of tendonitis on MRI failed to demonstrate histologic confirmation of acute inflammation. Indistinctness of the tendon margin correlated with several histologic features including eosinophilic, fibrillary, and mucoid degeneration and scarring. Areas of increased signal intensity on T_2-weighted images were associated with severe degeneration and disruption of the supraspinatous tendon, but again no signs of acute inflammation were seen. They also concurred with prior investigators that

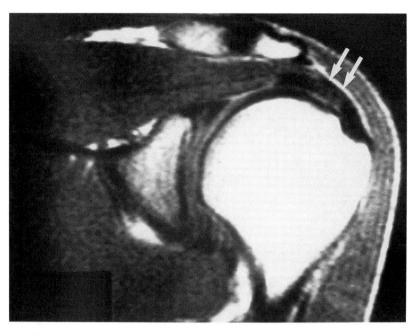

Fig. 3-26. MRI coronal oblique proton density image. Tendonitis is evidenced by increased signal within an intact supraspinatus tendon (*arrows*).

the high signal intensity seen on T_2-weighted images in tears may well represent joint fluid that has penetrated the tendon.

Several authors have noted a relatively high signal region (a signal similar to muscle and less than that of fluid) in the distal supraspinatus tendon that corresponded to the "critical zone."[8,51] The critical zone is a region approximately 1 cm in length situated 1 cm proximal to the insertion of the supraspinatus tendon into the greater tuberosity. It frequently demonstrates increased signal intensity on T_1-weighted images and may be misinterpreted as a tear or tendonitis. This region of higher signal intensity may be related to an inherent hypovascularity of the zone, which may result in early degenerative changes.[68] However, other workers have shown that this region is not less vascular but does represent a watershed zone of anastamoses between osseous and tendinous vessels.[54] Still others have used laser Doppler studies to demonstrate considerable blood flow within the critical zone.[75] Perhaps this "avascular" region is more prone to degenerative change and because of its anatomic position is vulnerable to mechanical trauma by the process of impingement. While these changes may be seen in "asymptomatic" individuals and may simply be part of an aging

process, the chain of events is likely to be accelerated by repetitious shoulder activity or trauma.[6]

Two further points need to be made in the context of supposed abnormal hyperintense areas in asymptomatic shoulders. The assumption that asymptomatic shoulders are normal is not necessarily correct. Repeated microtrauma may well have taken place without symptoms. The second point is the phenomenon of the "magic angle," whereby normal tendon will exhibit focal areas of increased activity on T_1-weighted images when oriented at 55 degrees to the constant magnetic induction field (Bo).[17] In these cases, normal signal intensity was seen on T_2-weighted images, emphasizing the need for T_2-weighted images in evaluating the rotator cuff.

Inflammation and scarring of the subacromial subdeltoid bursa are believed to be secondary to "tendonitis." Neer and Welsh[57] state that a thickened and fibrotic bursa occurs in stage II impingement syndrome. Widening of the peribursal fat on T_1-weighted images[70] and loss of the peribursal fat signal due to fluid accumulation within the bursa[79] have both been described as indicators of bursitis. The fluid may not originate from the glenohumeral joint but from within the bursa itself.[64] The possible causes of impingement should always be sought, and MRI often depicts them. A low-lying acromion is a not infrequent companion of impingement. On coronal oblique images one should be able to draw a relatively straight line under the distal clavicle, the acromioclavicular joint, and the anterior acromion. A low-lying or down-sloping acromion will fall well below this line. Hypertrophy of the acromioclavicular capsule and degenerative spur formation may induce impingement and can be demonstrated by MRI.

MRI is sensitive in the detection of full-thickness tears, the most accurate criterion being a region of intense signal activity seen within the tendon on T_2-weighted images[64] (Fig. 3-27). Changes in tendon morphology, retraction of the musculotendinous junction, and fluid within the subacromial bursa are secondary signs. In Rafii et al.'s[64] series of 31 patients with full-thickness tears a region of intense activity on T_2 weighting was seen in 22 cases. In partial tears this was only seen in just under half of the patients (7 of 16). Farley et al.,[19] in a retrospective trial, found discontinuity of the tendon with a region of water intensity within to be the most accurate criterion for a tear (22 of 31 shoulders; 89 percent). They also were less successful in the detection of partial tears.

While MRI can achieve reasonable accuracy in the detection of full-thickness tears (although not yet as accurate as double-contrast arthrography in some authors' eyes), a poorer accuracy is obtained in diagnosing partial tears.[30] The distinction between the MRI diagnoses of "tendonitis," tendon degeneration, and partial tear is blurred, and more MRI studies with histopathologic correlation are needed to define these diagnoses. However, in management terms, the distinction is probably academic unless an aggressive surgical approach is adopted for the treatment of partial tears.

Glenohumeral Instability and the Glenoid Labrum

Initial experience with MRI in the evaluation of shoulder instability was encouraging. Although the study populations were small, in general the results were good.[51,71] As more centers published their data, slightly less positive results have emerged. In Garneau et al.'s[21] small double-blind trial sensitivities of only 44 and 77.8 percent and specificities of 66.7 percent were obtained.

As in CT arthrography, the variable normal anatomy of the labra causes problems; Neumann et al.'s[58] study of asymptomatic individuals clearly demonstrates the wide range of normality (Fig. 3-28). As experience is

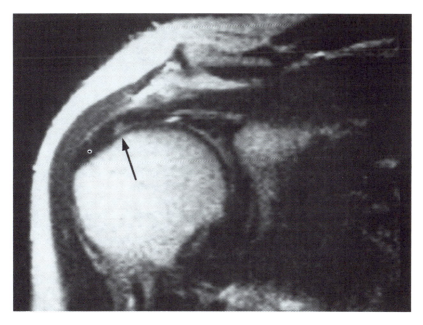

Fig. 3-27. MRI coronal oblique T_2 image. High signal is seen within the supraspinatus tendon, indicating a tear (*arrow*).

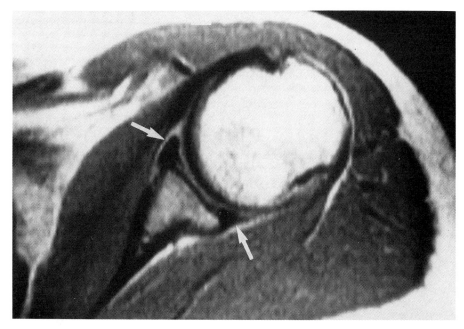

Fig. 3-28. MRI axial proton density image. The normal anterior and posterior labra are seen as dark triangles (*arrows*).

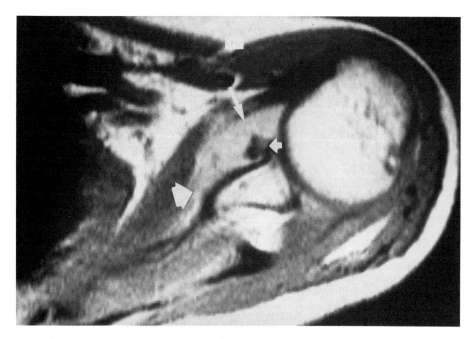

Fig. 3-29. MRI axial proton density image. The capsule is distended by fluid (*thin arrow*), which dissects along the scapular neck (*thick arrow*). A detached labral fragment is also evident (*small arrow*).

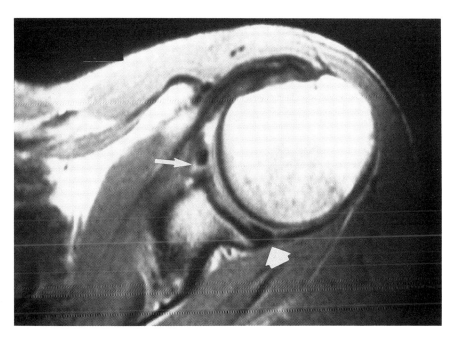

Fig. 3-30. MRI axial proton density image. The anterior labrum is small and lies posterior to a prominent glenohumeral ligament (*thin arrow*). Posterior labrum is normal (*thick arrow*).

gained, many centers are now producing studies showing MRI to be comparable to if not better than CT arthrography in delineation of the labrum. In a series of 39 shoulders with surgical correlation Lannotti and his colleagues[39] produced a sensitivity of 88 percent and specificity of 93 percent in the diagnosis of labral tears. In a young athletic population, Gross et al.[26] performed a retrospective study on 48 shoulders corrected by surgery. Their results included a sensitivity of 90.6 percent. However, MRI correctly identified only 11 of 16 normal labra, resulting in a lower specificity of 68.8 percent. In a more detailed study in which arthroscopic correlation was available for 88 shoulders, Logan et al.[40] showed excellent sensitivities and specificities for anterior labral tears (95 and 86 percent, respectively), as well as slightly less sensitive (75 percent) but highly specific (99 percent) appearances for superior labral tears. However, when assessing posterior labral (77 percent) and inferior (40 percent) tears the sensitivity was poor.

Although isolated labral tears may be seen on MRI (as a line of brighter signal within the normal signal void of the labrum), the more common finding is an avulsion of the labrum from the glenoid associated with a tear in the capsule. Evidence of a capsular tear on MRI is seen by the detection of fluid within the subscapularis tendon or muscle or dissection of fluid along the scapular neck (Fig. 3-29). Just as in CT arthrography, knowledge of the variants of capsular anatomy are essential—the superior delineation of the glenohumeral ligaments on MRI can cause problems in diagnosis. The middle glenohumeral ligament occasionally shows a high attachment, may originate adjacent to the anterior glenoid labrum, and may be confused with a tear (Fig. 3-30).[10] MRI may well be more sensitive than CT arthrography in the detection of the Hill-Sachs lesion, as it may detect changes of marrow edema (i.e., "bone bruising" without frank fracture), thus assisting in the diagnosis of instability.

In summary, MRI is now widely used in the evaluation of the shoulder; provided the examination is tailored to the clinical problem, the accuracy will be as high if not higher than the other imaging modalities.

REFERENCES

1. Andrews JR, Carson WG, McCleod WD: Glenoid labrum tears related to the long head of the biceps. Am J Sports Med 13:337–341, 1985
2. Aoki M, Ishi S, Usui M: The slope of the acromion and

rotator cuff impingement. Presented at the Annual Meeting of the American Shoulder and Elbow Surgeons, New Orleans, LA, February, 1986

3. Bankart AJB: Recurrent or habitual dislocation of the shoulder joint. BMJ 2:1132–1133, 1923

4. Bankart AJB: The pathology and treatment of recurrent dislocation of the shoulder joint. Br J Surg 26:23, 1938

5. Brandt TD, Caslone BW, Grant TH et al: Rotator cuff sonography: a reassessment. Radiology 173:323–327, 1989

6. Brewer BJ: Aging of the rotator cuff. Am J Sports Med 7:102–110, 1979

7. Burk DL, Karasick DK, Kutz AB et al: Rotator cuff tears: prospective comparison of MR imaging with arthrography, sonography and surgery. AJR 153:87–92, 1989

8. Chandnani V, Ho C, Gerharter J et al: MR findings in asymptomatic shoulders: A Blins analysis using symptomatic shoulders as controls. Clin Imaging 16:25–30, 1992

9. Cone RO, Resnick D, Danzing L: Shoulder impingement syndrome: radiologic evaluation. Radiology 150:29–33, 1984

10. Coumas J, Waite RJ, Goss TP, et al: CT and MR evaluation of the labral capsular ligamentous complex of the shoulder. AJR 158:591–597, 1992

11. Crass JR, Craig EV, Thompson RC, Feinberg SB: Ultrasonography of the rotator cuff: surgical correlation. JCU 1984, 12:487–492, 1984

12. Crass JR, Lucy vende Vegte G, Harkary LA: Tendon echogenicity: ex vivo study. Radiology 167:499–501, 1988

13. De Haven JP et al: A prospective comparison study of double contrast CT arthrography and shoulder arthroscopy. Walter Reed Army Medical Center. Paper presented at the AOSS, San Francisco, January, 1987

14. De Palma AF: Surgery of the Shoulder. p. 211–298. 3rd Ed. JB Lippincott, Philadelphia, 1983

15. Deutsch AL et al: Computed and conventional arthrotomography of the glenohumeral joint: normal anatomy and clinical experience. Radiology 153:603, 1984

16. El-Khoury GY, Renfrew DL: Computed arthrotomography of the shoulder. p. 83–95. In Seeger LL (ed): Diagnostic Imaging of the Shoulder. Williams and Wilkins, Philadelphia, 1992

17. Erickson SJ, Cox IH, Hyde JS, et al: Effect of tendon orientation on MR imaging signal intensity: a manifestation of the 'magic angle' phenomenon. Radiology 181:389–392, 1991

18. Evancho AM, Stiles RGT, Rajman WA et al: MR imaging diagnosis of rotator cuff tears. AJR 151:751–754, 1988

19. Farley TE, Neumann CH, Steinbach LS et al: Full thickness tears of the rotator cuff of the shoulder: Diagnosis with MR imaging. AJR 158:347–351, 1992

20. Flannigan B, Kursmogh-Brahme S, Snyder S et al: MR arthrography of the shoulder: comparison with conventional MR Imaging. AJR 155:829–832.

21. Garneau RA, Renfrew DL, Moore TE et al: Glenoid labrum: evaluation with MR imaging. Radiology 179:519–522, 1991

22. Ghelman B, Goldman A: The double contrast shoulder arthrogram: evaluation of rotator cuff tears. Radiology 124:251, 1977

23. Gold RH, Bassett LW: Disorders of the shoulder: plain radiographic diagnosis. p. 13–51. In Seeger LL (ed): Diagnostic Imaging of the Shoulder. Williams and Wilkins. Philadelphia, 1992.

24. Goldman AB: Shoulder arthrography. p. 52–87. In Seeger LL (ed): Diagnostic Imaging of the Shoulder. Williams and Wilkins, Philadelphia, 1992

25. Goldman AB, Ghelman B: The double contrast shoulder arthrogram. Radiology 127:655–663, 1978

26. Gross ML, Seeger LL, Smith JB et al: Magnetic resonance imaging of the glenoid labrum. Am J Sports Med 18:229–234, 1990

27. Harris JH: p. 1251. In Grainger RG, Allinson DJ (eds): Diagnostic Radiology. Churchill Livingstone, New York. 1986

28. Harryman DT, Sidles JA, Clark JM et al: Translation of the humeral head on the glenoid with passive glenohumeral motion. J Bone Joint Surg [Am] 72A:1334–1343, 1990

29. Hill HA, Sachs MD: The grooved defect of the humeral head: a frequently unrecognized complication of dislocation of the shoulder joint. Radiology 35:690–700, 1940

30. Hodler J, Terrier B, Von Schulthess GL, Fuchs WA: MRI and sonography of the shoulder. Clin Radiol 43:323–327, 1991

31. Hodler J, Kursmough-Brahme S, Snyder SJ et al: Rotator cuff disease: assessment with MR arthrography versus standard MR imaging in 36 patients with arthroscopic confirmation. Radiology 182:431–436, 1992

32. Keats PE, Pope TL Jr: The acromioclavicular joint: normal variations and the diagnosis of dislocation. Skeletal Radiol 17:159–162, 1988

33. Kieft GS, Bloem JL, Rozing PM et al: Rotator cuff impingement syndrome: MR imaging. Radiology 166:211–214, 1988

34. Kieft GJ, Bloem JL, Rozing PM, Obermann WR: MR imaging of anterior dislocation of the shoulder: comparison with CT arthrography. AJR 150:1083–1087, 1988

35. Kilcoyne RF, Reddy PK, Lyons F, Rockwood CA Jr: Optimal plain film imaging of the shoulder impingement syndrome. AJR 153:795–797, 1989

36. Killoran PJ, Marcore RC, Freibeger RH: Shoulder arthrography. AJR 103:658, 1968

37. Kjellin L, Ho CP, Cervilla V et al: Alterations in the supraspinatus tendon at MR imaging: correlation with histopathologic findings in cadavers. Radiology 181:837–841, 1991

38. Kneeland BJ, Middleton WD, Carrera GF et al: MR imaging of the shoulder: rotator cuff tears. AJR 149:333–337, 1987

39. Lannotti JP, Zlatkin MB, Estrhai JL et al: Magnetic resonance imaging of the shoulder: sensitivity, specificity and predictive value. J Bone Joint Surg [Am] 73A:17–29, 1991

40. Legan JM, Burkhard TK, Goff WB II et al: Tears of the glenoid labrum: MR imaging of 88 arthroscopically confirmed cases. Radiology 179:241–246, 1991

41. Lindbloom K: Arthrography and roentgenography in ruptures of tendons of the shoulder joints. Acta Radiol, 20:548, 1939

42. Mack LA, Matson FA, Kilcoyne JF et al: Ultrasound evaluation of the rotator cuff. Radiology 157:205–209, 1985

43. Mack LA, Nyberg DA, Masten FA III: Sonographic evaluation of the rotator cuff. Radiol Clin North Am 26:161–177, 1988

44. Mack LA, Nyberg DA, Matsen FR et al: Sonography of the postoperative shoulder. AJR 150:1089–1093, 1988.

45. Mayer V: Ultrasound of rotator cuff letter. J Ultrasound Med 4:608, 1985

46. McLaughlin ML: Rupture of the rotator cuff. J Bone Joint Surg [Am] 41A:978–983, 1963

47. Middleton WD: Status of rotator cuff sonography. Radiology 173:307–309, 1989

48. Middleton WD, Edelsteing G, Reinus WR et al: Ultrasonography of the rotator cuff: technique and normal anatomy. J Ultrasound Med 3:549–551, 1984

49. Middleton WD, Reinus WR, Melson GL et al: Pitfalls of rotator cuff sonography. AJR 146:555–569, 1986

50. Middleton WD, Reinus WR, Totty WG et al: Ultrasonographic evaluation of the rotator cuff and biceps tendon. J Bone Joint Surg [Am] 68:440–450, 1986

51. Microwitz SA: Normal rotator cuff: MR imaging with conventional and fat suppression techniques. Radiology 180:735–740, 1991

52. Mink JH, Harris E, Rappaport M: Rotator cuff tears: evaluation using double contrast shoulder arthrography. Radiology 157:621, 1985

53. Misamore GW, Woodward C: Evaluation of degenerative lesions of the rotator cuff. J Bone Joint Surg [Am] 73:704–706, 1991

54. Moseley HF, Goldie I: The arterial patterns of the rotator cuff of the shoulder. J Bone Joint Surg [Br] 45:780–789, 1963

55. Munk PL, Holt GR, Helms CA, Genard HK: Glenoid labrum: preliminary work with use of a radial sequence MR imaging. Radiology 173:751–753, 1989

56. Neer CS: Impingement lesions. CORR 173:70, 1983

57. Neer CS II, Welsh RP: The shoulder in sports. Orthop Clin North Am 8:583–591, 1977

58. Neumann CH, Peterson SA, Jahnke AH: MR imaging of the labral-capsular complex: normal variations. AJR 157:1015–1021, 1991

59. Newhouse KE, EL Khowy GT, Nepola JV, Montgomery WV: The shoulder impingement view: a fluoroscopic technique for the detection of subacromial spurs. AJR 151:539–541, 1988

60. Pavlov H, Warren RF, Weiss CB, Dines DM: The roentgenographic evaluation of anterior shoulder instability. Clin Orthop 194:153, 1985

61. Pennes DR, Jonsson K, Buckwalter K et al: Computed arthrotomography of the shoulder: comparison of examinations made with internal and external rotation of the humerus. AJR 153:1017–1019, 1989

62. Raffi M, Minkoff J, De Stefano V: In Seeger LL (ed): Diagnostic Imaging of the Shoulder. Williams & Wilkins, Philadelphia, 1992

63. Raffi M, Kroozmia H, Golumba C et al: CT arthrography of the capsular structures of the shoulder. AJR 146:361–367, 1986

64. Rafii M, Zsoozmia H, Sherman O et al: Rotator cuff lesions: signal patterns of MR imaging. Radiology 177:817–823, 1990

65. Raffi M, Firooznia H, Bonamo JJ et al: Athlete shoulder injuries: CT arthrographic findings. Radiology 162:559–564, 1987

66. Rockwood CA Jr, Young DC: Disorders of the acromioclavicular joints. p. 413. In Rockwood CA Jr, Matson FA III (eds): The Shoulder, Vol. 1. WB Saunders, Philadelphia, 1990

67. Rothman RH, Rarke WW: The vascular anatomy of the rotator cuff. Clin Orthop 541:176–186, 1965

68. Rothman RH, Marvel JP, Hapenstall RB: Anatomic considerations in the glenohumeral joint. Orthop Clin North Am 6:341–352, 1975

69. Rozing PM, de Bakker HM, Obermann WR: Radiographic views in recurrent anterior shoulder dislocation. AA Orthop Scand 57:328, 1986

70. Seeger LL, Gold RH, Bassett LW, Ellman H: Shoulder impingement syndrome: MR findings in 53 shoulders. AJR 150:343–347, 1988

71. Seeger LL, Gold RH, Bassett LW: Shoulder instability: evaluation with MR imaging. Radiology 168:695–697, 1988

72. Seltzer SE, Tinberg HJ, Weissman BN: Arthrosonography technique, sonographic anatomy and pathology. Invest Radiol 15:19–28, 1980

73. Singson RD, Feldman F, Bigliami L: CT arthrographic patterns in recurrent glenohumeral instability. AJR 149:749, 1987

74. Soble MG, Kaye AD, Gray RC: Rotator cuff tear: clinical experience with sonographic detection. Radiology 173:319–321, 1989

75. Swiontowski MF, Iannotti JP, Bonlas HJ, Esterhai JL: Intraoperative assessment of rotator assessment of rotator cuff vascularity using laser Doppler flowmetry. p. 208. In Post M, Morrey BF, Hawkins RJ (eds): Surgery of the Shoulder. Mosby Yearbook, St. Louis, 1990

76. Tirman R, Nelson CS, Tirman WS: Arthrography of the shoulder joint: state of the art. CRC Rev Diagn Imaging 17:19–76, 1981

77. Wilson AS, Totty WG, Murphy WA, Hardy DC: Shoulder joint: arthrographic CT and long term follow up with surgical correlation. Radiology 173:329–333, 1989

78. Zlatkin M, Bjorliengren AG, Gylys V et al: Cross sectional imaging of the capsular mechanism of the glenohumeral joint. AJR 150:151–158, 1988

79. Zlatkin MB, Lamnott JP, Roberts MC et al: Rotator cuff tears: diagnostic performance of MR imaging. Radiology 1782:223–229, 1989

4
Shoulder Instability

LARS NEUMANN
W. ANGUS WALLACE

INTRODUCTION

In athletes younger than 40, instability is the most common shoulder disorder, usually after one episode of acute trauma that produces an injury to the joint or after repeated stretching injuries at the extremes of the range of movement (ROM) of the shoulder. In traumatic cases, the initial episode of subluxation or dislocation usually causes a persistent lesion, and a tendency toward recurrence is often seen. This may lead to a severe disablement that not only restricts sports, but also influences daily living.

When diagnosing and treating shoulder instabilities, the aim must be to restore normal shoulder function and to bring patients back to the same level of activity they had before the initial episode. When treating athletic shoulder instability, the authors' aim is to return athletes to their previous level of sports. However, shoulder instability results from a very varied group of pathologies, and in order to select the correct treatment for the individual case and achieve a good result from treatment, an exact diagnosis is necessary. It is important to choose a method of treatment known to produce good results with a low morbidity; in particular, the ROM of the shoulder should not be restricted by the treatment and ideally no long-term secondary effects from the operation such as arthritis should be seen.

The dislocating shoulder is a common problem for the young adult, and a large number of surgeons will have the expertise to treat most of these patients (mainly the traumatic recurrent anterior dislocations) with good results. However, to provide a satisfactory result for athletes involved in throwing sports and for those who take part in overhead activities such as rac-

quet players (who place high demands on their shoulders), a very experienced shoulder surgeon is required: for these athletes, a loss of only a few degrees of external rotation after an operation may lead to the end of their sporting careers. The second difficult group comprises athletes with multidirectional instability, particularly swimmers, who require a highly specialized rehabilitation program.

FUNCTIONAL ANATOMY

The shoulder is susceptible to instability because of the construction of the joint itself. The main shoulder joint (the glenohumeral joint) is not an isolated entity, but one of several components of the mechanically complicated shoulder complex. This complex allows a very large ROM of the arm but at the cost of a joint that is mechanically less stable.

Hard Tissues

The glenohumeral joint is a ball-and-socket type in which the surface area of the socket corresponds to only about 25 to 30 percent of that of the ball, with the result that the bones provide poor stability by themselves. The plane of the transverse axis of the glenoid is normally retroverted about 7 degrees to the blade of the scapula.[64] However, the angle alters measuring from the superior to the inferior pole of the glenoid. The size of the glenoid is approximately 4.5 cm from the superior to the inferior pole. Recent detailed research work has shown that the humeral head is retroverted 21 degrees relative to the transepicondylar plane at the elbow, and that the head is slightly offset posteriorly from the axis of the humeral shaft. The articular surface of the head is close to being a sphere and has a diameter of approximately 50 mm.[59] The curvature of the glenoid articular surface is greater than that of the humeral head, thus reducing the stability produced by the hard tissues.

Soft Tissues

The glenoid surface is made more congruent to the humeral head by the presence of the fibrous glenoid labrum. This structure surrounds the glenoid and is attached to the capsule at its insertion to the glenoid rim. It has been shown that the negative intra-articular pressure of the glenohumeral joint and the suction-cup effect of the labrum are major stabilizers of the glenohumeral joint and that this may account for up to 50 percent of the stability of the joint.[28] Inferior subluxation of the humeral head can often be seen after a traumatic injury partly as a result of the loss of this stabilizing mechanism. Other important stabilizing factors are the surrounding soft tissues; the capsule and ligaments are static, and the muscles and tendons are dynamic.

The joint capsule itself can be very thin, perhaps as a congenital variation. Its reinforcements are often considered to be ligamentous structures. A detailed study by Clark and Harryman[14] concludes that the function of the different ligaments that lie within the joint capsule has not yet been exactly defined. It is clear, however, that these ligamentous structures are of major importance for the day-to-day stability of the joint. The position of these ligaments is shown in Figure 4-1.

Coracohumeral Ligament

The coracohumeral ligament is a capsular reinforcement that originates from the base of the coracoid process and inserts laterally onto the greater and lesser tuberosities. This structure probably helps to prevent inferior subluxation, and it has been shown to become taut in external rotation.[8]

Superior, Middle, and Inferior Glenohumeral Ligaments

The superior glenohumeral ligament (GHL) originates from the glenoid rim just anterior to the insertion of the long head of the biceps and inserts close to the lesser tuberosity. Schwartz et al.[65] have shown that after detachment of the inferior GHL and the capsule, when

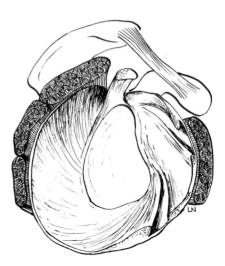

Fig. 4-1. The glenohumeral ligaments. Looking at the glenoid joint surface from a lateral view with the humeral head removed, the glenohumeral ligaments are seen as antero-inferior capsular reinforcements.

this ligament is cut, the humeral head is able to translate posteriorly and inferiorly. Thus its major contribution to stability may be to prevent inferior instability.

The middle GHL originates from the supraglenoid tubercle just medial to the insertion of the superior ligament and also from the anterior/superior labrum. It blends laterally with the subscapularis tendon before inserting on the medial aspect of the lesser tuberosity. It is taut in the critical position of external rotation and abduction of the humerus and is acknowledged to be a major anterior stabilizer of the shoulder.[18,67]

The inferior GHL is not always very clearly defined, and may be considered to consist of most of the capsule originating from the middle and lower part of the glenoid from anteroinferior to posteroinferior; it attaches at the capsular insertion on the humerus inferior to the head.[67] It is slack with the arm in neutral but becomes taut in external rotation and abduction. The ligament becomes detached when an anterior inferior Bankart lesion is present, and most authors now attribute most instabilities to this lesion. Schwartz et al.[65] showed that sectioning this ligament caused anterior and inferior subluxation of the humeral head, especially when the superoposterior capsule was also cut.

Muscles and Tendons

The dynamic stabilizers of the shoulder joint are the four muscles of the rotator cuff: the subscapularis, the supraspinatus, the infraspinatus, and the teres minor.

They also act as passive stabilizers, as has been shown by Ovesen and Nielsen[51] in cadaveric studies. When these muscles, especially the subscapularis, were cut, increased anterior and posterior translation was made possible. Their active contribution is to stabilize the shoulder by centering and compressing the humeral head onto the glenoid and thus assisting the previously mentioned suction-cup effect of the joint. They also tense the ligaments during movement, as is seen when the supraspinatus muscle acts as an external rotator during elevation and tightens the inferior ligaments of the joint.[17] When the muscles are contracted, they act as slings, preventing translation of the humeral head.

The sequence in which the different muscles act during movement of the arm and the relative force yielded by each muscle are important factors in keeping the shoulder in joint during motion. If imbalance develops, or if an individual adapts an unusual motion pattern, instability may result. Only when normal muscle strength and movement patterns are restored can the stability of the shoulder be assessed. In general one should consider all these many stabilizers as one entity, working together during the dynamics of the shoulder movement, rather than looking at them one by one.

DEFINITIONS OF DIAGNOSES

Many different types of instability exist, and as each should be approached in its own way, an exact definition of each patient's problem is essential.

Severity

Dislocation

A dislocation means a complete loss of contact between the two joint surfaces, with the two bones remaining in this dislocated position for a period of time varying from a few seconds to hours or days. In many patients with previous episodes of dislocations, x-ray films of the dislocated joint exist as a proof of the pathology, but very often when the surgeon is assessing an unstable shoulder, no clear proof exists of whether a complete dislocation has ever occurred. However, even though the patient has never needed medical assistance to reduce the joint, the possibility of a complete dislocation at some point still exists; in such a patient, if the surgeon is not convinced by the history and clinical findings alone, further investigations should be employed such as examination under anesthesia (EUA) or arthroscopy (or both) to assess the details of the instability.

Some surgeons still expect patients to "earn" the operation by proving a certain minimum number of dislocations before a stabilization procedure is offered. However, since complete dislocations can often be reduced by patients, they may not be able to provide this proof; the indications for surgical treatment should be reconsidered in such a situation.

Subluxation

Subluxators are rarely able to provide radiographic proof of instability, but they may still be severely impaired for sporting activities. Their complaints should lead to a careful investigation to reveal the nature of the instability. The only complaint might be a clicking, sometimes painful, sensation in critical positions of the arm. They might not even be aware that the shoulder is unstable. They might experience the "dead arm" syndrome (an almost paralyzing pain shooting down the arm, or sudden heaviness and numbness in the arm). In these patients, an EUA and preferably also an arthroscopy should be obligatory before deciding on treatment. Pathologies that can be treated by surgery are often found.[62]

Etiology

Traumatic Onset

Usually a patient with a traumatic onset of instability gives an exact history of a specific incident that caused the first dislocation. As a rule the contralateral shoulder is normal. The direction of the instability is often given by a detailed description of the injury. In these patients a well-defined lesion of the joint is usually present, and repair is therefore usually successful. In some patients with lax joints minor trauma may convert a hyperlax but yet "controllable" joint into an unstable one.

Atraumatic Onset

Some patients with generalized joint laxity (see below) also have shoulder instability that is usually painless. Although often quite severe, this form of instability can remain relatively asymptomatic for a long time. These patients often adapt their activities to their shoulder disorder. The numerous subluxations or dislocations suffered rarely inflict damage to the joint and are usually pain-free due to the very lax capsule and soft tissues around the joint. However, this instability may turn symptomatic, either because the patient assumes new activities or because a minor injury leads to protection of the shoulder for a period of time, after which the normal movement pattern previously enabling the patient to control the shoulder has been lost.

Such patients can suffer traumatic dislocations that inflict soft tissue damage to the joint and may thus need surgical treatment of the lesion in question. However, in most instances atraumatic instability is preferably treated with rehabilitation alone. In these patients, the laxity almost always affects both shoulders, although only one may be symptomatic; therefore the doctor should always examine the "normal" shoulder first to assess its degree of laxity.

Acquired Injury

Repetitive stretching can lead to microtrauma to the capsule and muscles, mainly the infraspinatus and the subcapularis. It is seen in competitive swimmers.[57] Although not the result of a single episode, it is in effect a traumatic disorder and can be treated successfully with surgery, although rehabilitation should always be tried first.

Patients with acquired laxity often have bilateral symptoms and signs (depending on their activities) but usually have major complaints from one side only.

Acute or Chronic Injury

Acute Dislocation

The term *acute* simply describes a dislocation that has occurred recently, say within the last few hours or days.

Chronic Locked Dislocation

A dislocation may be locked (i.e., the humeral head has remained dislocated for a long period of weeks, months, or years); although movement and function are often severely limited, some patients manage surprisingly well for long periods with an established locked dislocation. These dislocations are very difficult to manage if treatment is delayed beyond 6 weeks, due to the secondary changes in the soft tissues.

Chronic Recurrent Dislocation

The most common type of chronic dislocation is the recurrent one. After one or more previous dislocations have inflicted such soft tissue damage to the joint the humeral head tends to dislocate increasingly more easily, the patient ends up adapting daily living to the limits set by the shoulder, "losing confidence" in the arm. The joint is often so lax that the dislocation is easily reduced by the patient or reduces spontaneously. This condition is severely disabling, but the authors have seen a number of patients who have tolerated the situation by never lifting the arm above shoulder level.

Direction

Anterior Instability

Anterior instability is by far the most common form of instability. The patient does not always know the direction in which the shoulder dislocates. However, patients will nearly always explain that their symptoms appear when they abduct and externally rotate the arm, or else they report that the initial injury took place with the arm in this position. The clinical findings are usually very clear.

Posterior Instability

A history of symptomatology with the arm flexed, internally rotated, and adducted may suggest a diagnosis of posterior instability, a less common condition. It is usually seen as recurrent subluxations rather than recurrent dislocations, and is often associated with a lax shoulder joint, often highlighted by a sulcus sign. Recurrent posterior dislocation is commonly seen as a form of voluntary dislocation (described below).

Sports typically associated with posterior instability are swimming and gymnastics. In both sports, a large ROM is essential for high-level performance, and athletes with lax joints and excessive movement can achieve better results. The training also aims to develop this ROM further, and the athlete therefore tends to go to a level of laxity that is very easily (by either additional capsular stretching or a single episode of trauma) converted into an instability.

Swimmers develop posterior instability mainly because of capsular stretching. The butterfly stroke in particular seems to stretch the posterior capsule. If at the same time the athlete's training program focuses mainly on strengthening the anterior muscles of the shoulder (the subscapularis and the pectoralis major) and if the posterior muscles (the infraspinatus and the teres minor) are neglected, leaving them comparatively weak, the static as well as the dynamic posterior stabilizers of the shoulder can no longer control the position of the humeral head in the glenoid. The authors have seen previously asymptomatic elite swimmers develop posterior instability so severe that high-level performance was impossible after having hit the side of the pool with the arm during a turn. This minor trauma might be sufficient either to add more capsular stretching or to inflict a capsular avulsion, causing disabling instability.

High-level gymnasts, very often in their teens, generally have very lax joints; since the shoulder joint has only poor intrinsic stability, in these athletes the shoulder is on the verge of instability. Trauma inflicted during very forceful exercises or additional stretching from repetitive exercises often leads to symptomatic instability.

Weightlifters can develop posterior capsular stretching, especially during the bench-press maneuver.

Throwers such as javelin throwers or baseball pitchers may also develop posterior shoulder instability if the deceleration phase of the throwing movement is not perfectly coordinated. Unless the posterior muscles are strong, the athlete will tend to "throw the arm away" during this phase and stretch the posterior capsule. Again, the importance of a balanced training program that builds up both the posterior and the anterior muscles cannot be overemphasized.

Racket sports athletes, like those in the throwing sports, often have an unbalanced training program that focuses on the anterior muscles. When striking the ball in what corresponds to the deceleration phase of the throwing movement, a similar stretching injury is inflicted on the posterior capsule unless the dynamic stabilizers are strong.

The acute posterior dislocation is often caused by violent trauma or convulsions and is frequently overlooked (especially if only an anteroposterior [AP] radiograph is obtained), complicating the subsequent treatment.[26] A marked reduction of external rotation with a fixed internal rotation deformity following trauma should always raise the suspicion of a posterior dislocation.

Inferior Instability

Inferior instability with the humeral head dropping downward is rarely seen as a solitary symptom but rather in combination with instability in other directions. It can be associated with neuromuscular conditions such as deltoid palsies and is frequently seen in the first week after a humeral neck fracture.

Superior Instability

The tissues superior to the shoulder joint (the acromion and the coracoacromial ligament) prevent a complete superior dislocation unless the acromion is fractured. If muscular control of the humeral head is lost as a result of a supraspinatus or infraspinatus weakness or a rotator cuff tear, the humeral head will tend to move upward, and impingement will result. Thus, in young individuals with impingement, instability or cuff weakness should be suspected; it should be treated before surgery such as an acromioplasty is considered. Impingement due to rotator cuff degeneration in these young patients is extremely rare, and this diagnosis should only be considered when superior instability has been carefully ruled out. Acromioplasty will only allow the humeral head to ride even higher, and the impingement pain secondary to instability will still be present.

If impingement due to subacromial inflammation has resulted from overhead activity such as throwing or swimming, the treatment of choice should first be guidance by an experienced physiotherapist or the trainer to correct the throwing or swimming movement, followed by specific cuff strengthening exercises and perhaps injection of steroids into the subacromial bursa. The tendon itself should never be injected. Only if this treatment fails should acromioplasty be considered.

Multidirectional Instability

Multidirectional instability should always be borne in mind when diagnosing shoulder instabilities. The humeral head is often hypermobile in an anteroinferior or posteroinferior direction, but if hypermobility is seen in anterior, inferior, and posterior directions true multidirectional instability exists. Patients with acquired or congenital laxities and the voluntary dislocators are most commonly seen in this group. Extremely careful assessment is necessary before deciding which treatment should be carried out, since selecting the wrong procedure may be likely to aggravate the problem rather than relieve it.

These patients are seen relatively frequently among athletes, since laxity of the shoulder joints is the basis of high performance in many disciplines of sports. Throwers, swimmers, and gymnasts are examples; their inherent joint hypermobility can sometimes be highlighted by their ability to take their abducted arm into 110 to 120 degrees of external rotation. Since their muscles are well trained and provide good dynamic stability, the laxity is initially well controlled and does not cause symptoms. However, an injury, even a minor one, or loss of muscular stability due to reduced training may make the shoulder symptomatically unstable.

Such patients often suffer from generalized joint laxity. Typically the asymptomatic shoulder may be as lax as the symptomatic one, but often laxity in other joints is seen. If the patient can hyperextend elbows and knees, if the fifth metacarpophalangeal joint hyperextends to 90 degrees, and if the thumb can be brought to lie along the volar aspect of the forearm, generalized joint laxity is clearly present. Since results from surgery in these patients tend to be less good (in our hands, at least), conservative treatment should be tried first.

Often these patients have developed an abnormal movement pattern that has caused their very lax shoulder to be symptomatically unstable; by restoring a normal movement pattern the shoulder can be restored to an asymptomatic lax state. This can be achieved by an intensive rehabilitation program under the supervision of physiotherapists with a special insight into this condition. Of course, patients with multidirectional instability can suffer acute injuries to their shoulder joint and may even be more susceptible to injuries due to their excessive ROM. If a relevant trauma has occurred, arthroscopy is recommended to detect any intra-articular injuries. If lesions are found, these should be treated as for any injured shoulder, and the patient then taken through an intensive planned rehabilitation program.

If surgery is indicated, usually the capsular shift procedure as described by Neer and Foster,[50] or a modification of it, is the method of choice. It can be carried out from either an anterior or posterior approach, depending on the main direction of the instability. Care should be taken not to create an imbalance with the surgical repair (i.e., if the joint is made too tight anteriorly, it will tend to become even more unstable in a posterior direction). For some patients this condition is so disabling that they are prepared to accept a shoulder with restricted movement rather than an unstable one, but it should be remembered that tight repair of shoulder instabilities seems to increase the risk of late secondary arthritis.

Voluntary or Involuntary Dislocation

Voluntary (Intentional) Dislocation

A patient with a lax shoulder may occasionally learn how to dislocate and reduce the glenohumeral joint and may do this as a kind of trick. If this maneuver causes no pain, the habit may develop into an abnormal movement pattern of the shoulder, resulting in dislocations that occur unwillingly. The condition has now converted into that of involuntary dislocations. As muscular slings do not work in these patients, rehabilitation should be considered before surgery.

In some of these patients a psychological factor contributes to the syndrome, and although it appears that the patient is "voluntarily" dislocating the shoulder, it is actually occurring as a result of a subconscious activity. The primary aim of treatment is therefore to get the patient out of the habit of dislocating the shoulder voluntarily. Surgery will have no effect until the movement pattern is corrected and is then usually no longer indicated.

Involuntary (Unintentional) Dislocations

Unintentional dislocations often occur with the arm in certain positions. If little pain is associated, the condition can sometimes turn into that of voluntary dislocations. Although a major anatomic abnormality might exist in these patients, rehabilitation often proves beneficial, particularly building up the rotator cuff muscles—the dynamic stabilizers.

During very forceful convulsions in epileptic patients shoulder dislocations are sometimes seen, often associated with large bone lesions of the glenoid or the humeral head. They may occur anteriorly or posteriorly, and conventional repairs seem to have a high failure rate. This is partly due to the large bony defects and partly because repeated convulsions tend to tear the surgical repairs apart.

How to Define a Dislocated Shoulder

Using the terms described above, the doctor can now very clearly describe any individual dislocation. For example, *acute, traumatic, recurrent, anterior dislocation* describes a situation in which the shoulder dislocates completely (anteriorly) after a trauma; it has done so on a number of occasions, and a dislocation is present. *Chronic, recurrent, involuntary, multidirectional subluxation* describes an unstable shoulder that does not completely dislocate; the problem is long-standing, disabling, and (due to the multidirectional instability) difficult to treat (described below).

TUBS/AMBRI

The terms *TUBS* and *AMBRI* have been introduced to distinguish between the two main groups of instabilities, their characteristics, and their management. They are defined as follows: *TUBS*: *t*raumatic, *u*nidirectional, *b*ankart procedure and *s*urgery usually necessary; *AMBRI*: *a*traumatic, *m*ultidirectional, *b*ilateral, *r*ehabilitation and *i*nferior capsular shift if surgery is necessary.

EXAMINATION OF THE UNSTABLE SHOULDER

The examiner should establish a standard procedure for shoulder examination and should use this routine in every patient. Making a diagnosis from a shoulder problem is both difficult and complicated, since many pathologies have similar symptoms often located on the same spot. The examiner must be careful not to make the final decision before all the different diagnoses have been considered; although the diagnosis may seem obvious from the history alone, a careful clinical examination often reveals additional findings. Only tests related specifically to problems of instability are discussed below, but it should be remembered that a shoulder examination should always include a full assessment of the patient.

History

A careful history should always be obtained before examining the patient. It is important to remember that shoulder pain may originate from the neck, and questioning the patient on neck pain and changes in sensation or power in the arm is important to elucidate symptoms. In obtaining the history, it is helpful to follow a fixed pattern and to clarify the following points.

1. *Onset of symptoms*: Was there an injury? Did the symptoms start in relation to a certain event, or was the onset gradual?
2. *Subsequent symptoms*: When does the patient experience symptoms? Are they related to specific activities or positions of the arm?
3. *Character of symptoms*: What is the character of the symptoms and their exact location? Are radiating symptoms present?
4. *Consequences of symptoms on daily living*: Has the condition forced the patient to give up sports? Have activities been altered because of the symptoms? If dislocations occur, can the patient reduce the shoulder, and what maneuver is used to do this?

Clinical Examination

In the examination of an unstable shoulder, it is very important to remember that the patients are often apprehensive and have developed firm habits to protect the shoulder from dislocating. As no careful examination can be carried out in a patient who is not relaxed, it is necessary to perform the examination gently and proceed at a speed that leaves the patient confident that a maneuver can be stopped before it reaches a point of severe discomfort. The examiner has to make sure that this trust is established before the examination takes place.

When the problem is unilateral, the asymptomatic shoulder should be examined first. This will allow the examiner to establish "normal" values against which the findings in the symptomatic shoulder can be compared. As in other clinical examinations, the sequence Look-Move-Feel is logical.

Look

When inspecting the patient, both shoulders should be studied at the same time, and the arms should also be exposed, to allow unrestricted movement. In women the bra is retained. The examiner then looks for wasting of the muscles around the shoulder. Atrophy can be a sign of nerve lesions, or it might be caused by wasting following disuse of one or more of the shoulder muscles.

Move

When assessing movement, the active and passive movements must be compared. Usually the standard movements of forward flexion, abduction in the plane of the scapula (30 degrees anterior to the coronal plane), and extension are recorded. Internal and external rotational movements are tested with the elbow by the side. External rotation in 90-degree abduction should also be measured. The standard of recording movement as described by the American Academy of Orthopaedic Surgeons[3] is recommended.

Starting with the active movement, the examiner observes the rhythm of the scapulothoracic and the glenohumeral joints during active forward flexion and during active abduction when the patient simultaneously moves both shoulders; a comparison of the two shoulders can then be made. The patient may try to protect the glenohumeral joint by transferring more movement to the scapulothoracic joint. The movement of the humeral head should be observed from the front to see whether it performs a smooth movement or if it makes any sudden visible subluxations.

When testing the passive ROM, the patient must be completely relaxed. The movement is then tested in the same planes as was the active movement, and the examiner notes the difference between active and passive.

When testing the muscles, abnormal findings may be either reduced power or pain during resisted movement, but combinations are commonly seen. The techniques described by Cyriax[16] are recommended. The three parts of the deltoid are tested separately, all with the arm hanging down: the anterior third is tested by resisted flexion, the middle third by resisted abduction, and the posterior third by resisted extension. The muscles of the rotator cuff are then also tested with resisted movement. With the elbow flexed to 90 degrees and stabilized at the patient's side by one hand of the examiner and with the shoulder in neutral rotation, the subscapularis is tested by active resisted internal rotation, and the infraspinatus by active resisted external rotation. The supraspinatus is tested by active resisted movement of the straight arm in a position of around 20 degrees of abduction and 20 degrees of flexion.

An important differential diagnosis to consider when assessing for shoulder instability is acromioclavicular joint problems, and this joint should always be carefully examined. In patients aged above 40 years, dislocations are often associated with rotator cuff lesions; in these patients the rotator cuff should be assessed, even if the patient reports no symptoms of cuff disease.

Feel

Finally, the examiner carries out various tests to try to reveal details of the instability. In most of them the examiner, by trying to push the humeral head in the direction of instability, will either provoke the patient's usual symptoms or be able to feel the head subluxing. These tests, especially the stress tests, should be performed with care, as a risk of dislocating the shoulder exists.

Drawer Test

With the patient's arm hanging down relaxed, the examiner, standing behind the patient, firmly stabilizes the shoulder girdle by gripping the spine of the scapula and the clavicle with the opposite hand (Fig. 4-2). With the other hand the examiner holds the humeral head and feels if it can be pushed forward or backward on the glenoid—the drawer sign. The translation detected by this maneuver is graded in three stages: grade 1, the humeral head is hypermobile, but cannot be subluxed; grade 2, the humeral head can be subluxed or nearly dislocated, but reduces spontaneously; and grade 3, the humeral head can be dislocated and stays dislocated after the examiner stops pushing.[24]

Inferior Laxity Test (Sulcus Sign)

In pulling the arm downward, if inferior joint laxity is present, a sulcus sign may appear. As the head subluxes downward, the soft tissues are sucked into the subacromial space, leaving a sulcus under the acromion (Fig. 4-3). The presence of a sulcus sign only indicates a lax shoulder joint; it is not diagnostic of instability, and the patient may be free of symptoms and have a stable shoulder.

Anterior Apprehension Test

The patient may be either sitting or supine. The arm is abducted to 90 degrees with the elbow flexed to 90 degrees and is passively brought into external rotation by rotating the forearm (Fig. 4-4). During the test the examiner, who is in front of the patient, carefully

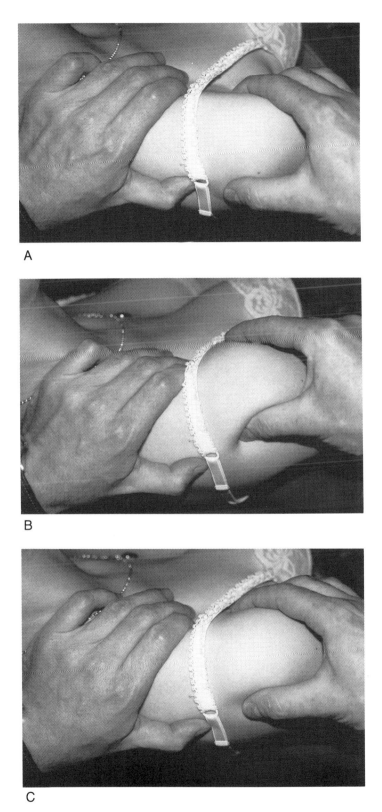

Fig. 4-2. The drawer sign in a patient with multidirectional instability. **(A)** The humeral head is translated posteriorly. **(B)** It is in neutral position. **(C)** It is translated anteriorly.

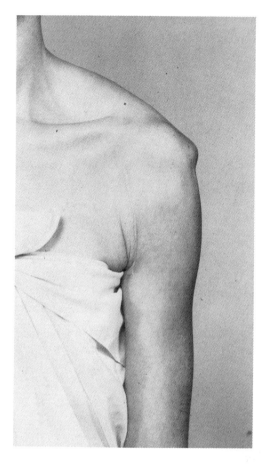

Fig. 4-3. The sulcus sign appears when the humeral head can be pulled inferiorly, creating a space under the acromion.

4-5). If this relieves the patient's typical symptoms, anterior subluxation is assumed to have taken place with the apprehension maneuver. The test can be extended, if the signs of the first part are not clear. The backward pressure on the humeral neck usually allows the humerus to be externally rotated another 10 degrees, and another point of pain is reached. Eventually, when the backward push on the humeral neck is suddenly removed, the humeral head bounces back into the subluxed position, and the patient experiences sudden return of pain or discomfort. (C. Jobe, personal communication).

Anterior Stress Test

Sometimes it is possible to perform the anterior stress test in a nonanesthetized, apprehensive patient, although with difficulty. The patient is asked to lie supine and the examiner fixes the scapula with the contralateral hand and the elbow with the ipsilateral hand. With the shoulder in 90 degrees of abduction and maximal extension, an axial load is applied to the humerus while gently rotating the arm, in an attempt to sublux the head anteriorly. While maintaining this load the arm is taken from the abducted position across the chest to a flexed/adducted position (Fig. 4-6A). If the humeral head was caused to sublux initially, it will relocate during this maneuver with a palpable and often audible click (Fig. 4-6B). The test should be performed in various positions of abduction, guided by the findings of the anterior apprehension test.

watches the patient's face to detect signs of pain or discomfort. This test can also be done from behind but with a mirror in front of the patient to allow observation of the face. The test is positive if apprehension is provoked, or if muscle spasms prevent the same amount of external rotation as is seen on the asymptomatic side. These clinical signs are strongly suggestive of anterior instability.

By moving the shoulder from 60 to 140 degrees of abduction while the maximal external rotation is maintained, the point at which instability is at its maximum can be identified.

Jobe Relocation Test

With the patient supine, and the humerus abducted 90 degrees and externally rotated to the point of pain, the examiner pushes backward on the humeral neck (Fig.

Posterior Stress Test

In a similar way as above, the shoulder can be tested for posterior instability. Usually patients with posterior instability are not experiencing the same discomfort as patients with anterior instability, and this test is easier to perform in the nonanesthetized patient. With the patient supine and the humerus in 90 degrees of flexion, the examiner stabilizes the scapula by placing the contralateral hand behind the scapula and the glenohumeral joint (Fig. 4-7A). By gently pushing the humerus backward, the examiner may sublux the humeral head posteriorly. Sometimes the subluxation can be felt by the hand holding the scapula. While the axial load on the humerus is maintained, the arm is now brought into abduction; if the humeral head has been subluxed or dislocated the head of the humerus will suddenly relocate with a clunk or click (Fig. 4-7B).

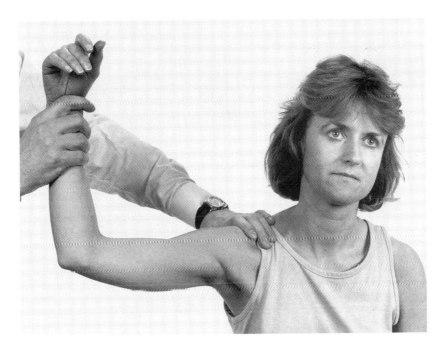

Fig. 4-4. The position of the arm when performing the apprehension test.

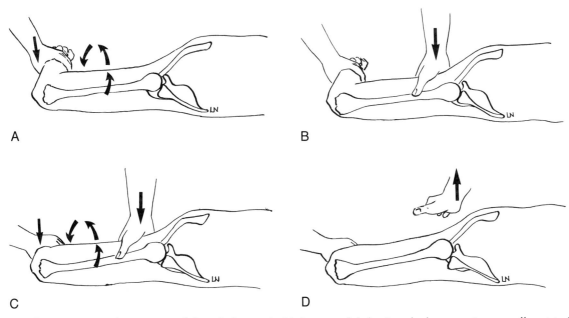

A

B

C

D

Fig. 4-5. The Jobe relocation test. **(A)** With the arm in 90 degrees of abduction, the humerus is externally rotated to the point of pain. **(B)** Firm pressure is applied to the humeral neck, which reduces the joint and relieves the pain. **(C)** While maintaining pressure further external rotation can be achieved, until another point of pain is reached. **(D)** When the pressure on the humeral neck is suddenly removed, the patient experiences a sudden increase of pain and may experience the sensation of instability.

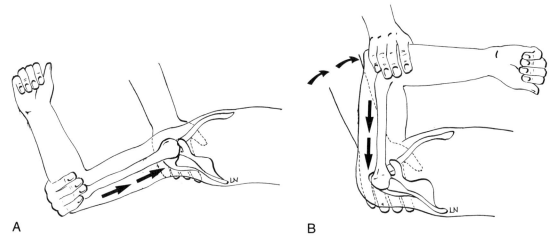

Fig. 4-6. The anterior stress test. **(A)** The humeral head is subluxed anteriorly with the arm in extension, abduction, and external rotation. **(B)** While an axial load is maintained, the arm is brought from abduction into a flexed position. The test is positive if reduction of the joint is felt by the examiner.

Generalized Joint Laxity

If bilateral lax shoulders are diagnosed, or if an excessive inferior laxity exists, generalized joint laxity should be suspected. Different scoring scales for grading generalized joint laxity have been developed and should be used in these patients.[42]

Voluntary Dislocators

If voluntary dislocation is suspected, the patient should be asked to carry out the maneuver, during which the shoulder usually dislocates, and any subluxations or dislocations are noted. The maneuver is then repeated during resisted movement. For instance, if a posterior

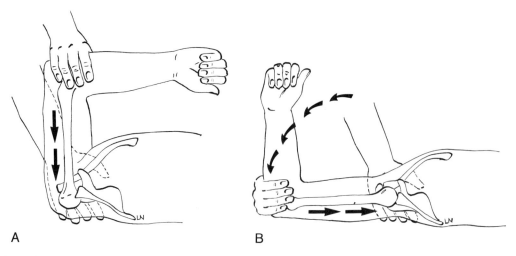

Fig. 4-7. The posterior stress test. **(A)** The humeral head is subluxed posteriorly with the arm in flexion. **(B)** The arm is taken from the flexed into an abducted position while maintaining an axial load. If reduction is felt by the examiner, the test is positive.

dislocation takes place during forward flexion, this movement is carried out in conjunction with resisted external rotation. If the joint now does not dislocate during the movement due to the contracted infraspinatus muscle, the examiner has confirmed that the patient has an abnormal movement pattern and may be a voluntary dislocator.

The stress and apprehension tests should be carried out with great care, since a risk of dislocating a very lax shoulder exists when they are used. The senior author has had the embarrassment of having to reduce a shoulder under general anesthesia following such a test.

Sometimes no definite diagnosis can be made from these tests and it is then necessary to perform the tests again during an EUA. With the patient relaxed, a clear clinical diagnosis should be made. Part of any examination under general anesthesia must include executing the anterior and posterior stress tests.

Additional Examinations

Based on the findings of the clinical examination, further investigations can now be considered. The authors believe that the vast majority of diagnoses of unstable shoulders can be made clinically, and that additional tests are usually used for confirmation only.

Plain Radiography

Conventional radiographs are of course mandatory in the acute situation to clarify the direction of the dislocation and, even more important, to reveal any associated fractures or avulsions. Radiographs are also useful in the elective situation, since secondary changes to bone can often be seen. Usually AP and axillary views are sufficient. If the previous dislocations have damaged the glenoid rim, fragments can often be seen in the avulsed capsule next to the glenoid rim (Fig. 4-8) or as loose bodies (Fig. 4-9). With repeated dislocations, abrasion of the glenoid rim can be detected on the axillary view (Fig. 4-10). This lesion can very often also be picked up on the AP view as a defect in the condensed line indicating the location of the anterior glenoid rim (Fig. 4-11).

The Hill-Sachs[29] lesion is often visible on the axillary view as an impression in the humeral head posteriorly in shoulders with anterior instability (Fig. 4-12) and anteriorly (the reversed Hill-Sachs lesion) in posterior

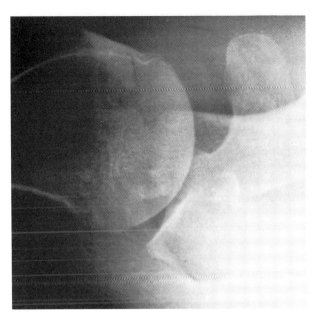

Fig. 4-8. Bony Bankart lesion. In this axillary view a small fragment of the anterior glenoid rim is seen in the avulsed anterior labrum and capsule.

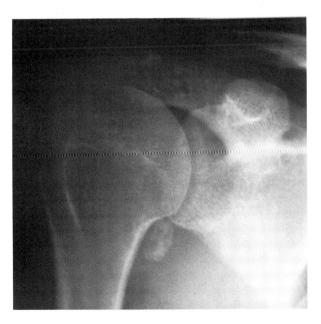

Fig. 4-9. A loose body in the inferior recess of the glenohumeral joint suggests a bony lesion of the joint.

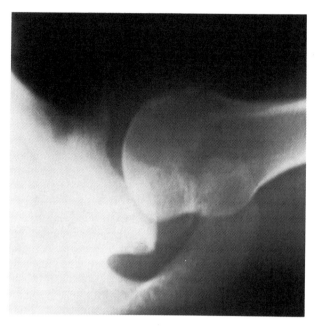

Fig. 4-10. In this axillary view, the anterior glenoid rim appears flattened and concave due to wear from a large number of anterior dislocations.

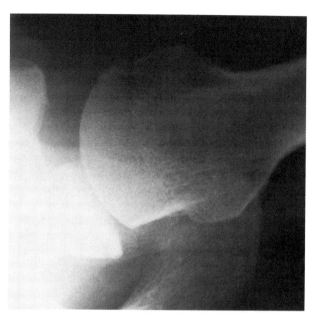

Fig. 4-12. The humeral head in this axillary view has a posterior fracture—a Hill-Sachs lesion—caused by impaction of the head on the anterior glenoid rim during an anterior dislocation. (Compare with Fig. 4-14)

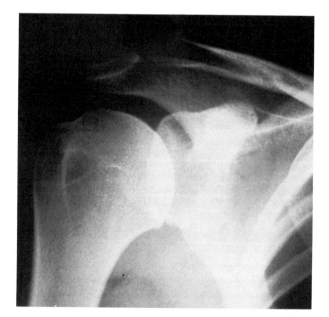

Fig. 4-11. In an AP view of the shoulder in Figure 4-10, the condensed line normally indicating the location of the anterior glenoid rim is missing. (Compare with the shoulder in Fig. 4-15, in which this line is present.)

instability. Special views, such as the West Point view or Stryker view, may sometimes be necessary.

As discussed in the section on anatomy, certain normal values are established for the relative angles and shapes of the glenoid and humeral head. The x-ray film obtained should always be of a quality that will allow assessment of these structures, so the examiner can detect any dysplasia. However, for detailed information on this subject a computed tomography (CT) is necessary.

The pain in a dislocated or recently reduced shoulder or the presence of a sling may prevent the radiologist from obtaining a conventional axillary view. This view is, however, of great importance, as it not only reveals the direction of the dislocation, but very often also shows associated lesions not visible on the AP view. In such patients, the modified axillary view (the Nottingham view) can be useful. Figure 4-13 shows such a view of a shoulder after an anterior bone block operation in a patient still in a sling with blocked abduction and external rotation.[68]

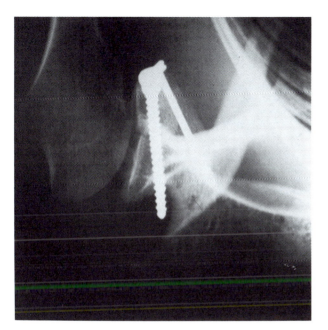

Fig. 4-13. A modified axillary view—Nottingham view—of a shoulder with a large bone defect of the anterior glenoid rim, treated with a tricortical iliac crest graft. The graft was fixed with two 4.5-mm cortical screws, and the small fragment screw was used for reattaching the coracoid process. It is seen that the graft acts as a glenoid extension.

Computed Tomography

CT provides excellent detailed information about the osseous structures in the shoulder and is the examination of choice if dysplastic changes such as retroversion of the glenoid are expected or to assess the extent of fractures of the glenoid or humeral head.

Magnetic Resonance Imaging

The accuracy of MRI in identifying labral tears has been shown to be as high as 92 percent with a 95 percent sensitivity and a 86 percent specificity.[35] This examination may in future be the investigation of choice. Unfortunately, in most clinics this examination is not yet readily available.

Arthrogram—Conventional and With CT Scan

A conventional double-contrast arthrogram can be of use, especially if additional cuff pathology is suspected. However, if detailed information on the soft tissues is required, a CT arthrogram is the investigation capable of giving the most detail, not only of the cuff but also of the labrum (and its relation to the glenoid rim) and of bony lesions of the glenoid and humeral head.[19] CT arthrography has a very high accuracy. Callaghan and co-workers[12] have shown that the sensitivity in detecting anterior labral lesions was 90 percent and the specificity 100 percent.

Arthroscopy

A diagnostic arthroscopy carried out in conjunction with an EUA will clarify the exact nature of any laxity and the associated intra-articular lesions. This has become a routine procedure; it gives the surgeon an excellent preoperative assessment of the lesions in the shoulder prior to treatment and allows for good preoperative planning.

TREATMENT
Acute Dislocations
Anterior Dislocation

An anterior dislocation is most often seen when the patient's arm has been forced into external rotation and abduction. Clinically, the patient presents with a painful shoulder, often with a fixed external rotation. In muscular individuals it is not always possible to see the bulk of the humeral head in front of the shoulder, but an epaulet sign is present, with a square shoulder and a prominent acromion, as well as a palpable hollow defect behind the shoulder.

Before carrying out reduction of the dislocation, a clinical examination should always be performed to determine the condition of the two nerves at most risk of damage from the dislocation (the axillary and the radial nerves), particularly as these nerves may also be damaged during reduction. Due to the risk of associated vascular injury, the peripheral pulse should also be checked. A prereduction radiographic examination should be carried out to see whether any associated fractures are present such as humeral neck fractures or avulsion fractures of the tuberosities. In the elderly patient, acute dislocations may be associated with rotator cuff tears.

Usually reduction can be carried out under relaxation with diazepam or using morphine, but it may require general anesthesia. If a fracture of the humeral neck or the tuberosities is present, reduction should only be carried out under general anesthesia. The maneuver should be gentle; the method with the least risk of inflicting additional damage to the joint is Hippocrates's method, in which a firm longitudinal pull in the axis of the arm along the body is carried out. It may be necessary to maintain this pull for several minutes until reduction occurs. Kocher's method has been very popular for reduction without anesthesia for many years. It is the authors' view that the Kocher's method should be avoided, as it may inflict damage to the cartilage of the humeral head or cause a previously undisplaced tuberosity or humeral neck fracture to displace.

Aftertreatment consists of a broad arm sling or Gilchrist[23] sling, usually for 4 weeks. Controversy exists about whether this immobilization has any preventative effect on recurrences.[32] Indeed, the recurrence rate is very high, especially in younger patients.[41,66]

Traumatic anterior dislocation is nearly always associated with one or both of the following lesions:

1. The Bankart[6] lesion, which in an avulsion of the anterior capsule and glenoid labrum from the front of the scapular neck. Sometimes an additional fracture of the glenoid rim is seen—the bony Bankart lesion (Fig. 4-8) or the rim is worn down by the repeated dislocations, creating a lesion visible on an x-ray film (Fig. 4-10).
2. The impression fracture created in the posterior portion of the humeral head by the anterior glenoid rim—a Hill-Sachs[29] fracture or a Broca[10] lesion—when the front of the glenoid is impacted into the humeral head (Fig. 4-14). This fracture may be an important reason for recurrences, as spontaneous or easy reduction cannot take place when the impression catches the glenoid rim and transforms a subluxation into a dislocation. However, the presence of a Hill-Sachs lesion was noted by Rowe[60] to have no effect on recurrence rate.

Reeves[55] demonstrated the different injuries inflicted on the shoulder suffering an anterior dislocation. The first result of the trauma is a stretching and tearing of the anterior capsule, and then a Bankart lesion is created, avulsing the labrum from the glenoid rim and eventually stripping the capsule and periosteum from the anterior scapular neck. The first lesions seem to

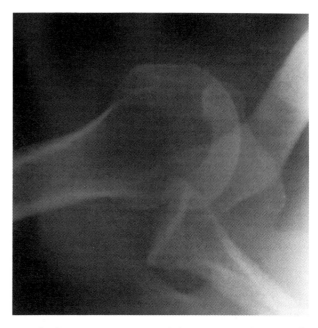

Fig. 4-14. An acute anterior dislocation, in which a Hill-Sachs lesion of the humeral head is caught on the anterior glenoid rim.

heal quickly, whereas the labral detachment leads to recurrences of the instability episodes.

Posterior Dislocation

Posterior direction of dislocation is rare, and is more commonly seen as a sequel to convulsions. Clinically, the patient presents with a fixed internal rotation, but may otherwise show very few signs of dislocation. The same precautions as those mentioned above should be taken (i.e., careful clinical examination and radiographs before reduction). In these cases, the axillary view is of extreme importance, as sometimes very little abnormality may be seen in the AP view.

Reduction requires general anesthesia and is carried out by traction on the arm at 45 degrees of abduction during which firm pressure is applied behind the dislocated humeral head. The arm should be gently rotated internally during this maneuver to allow the humeral head to "unlock" from the back of the glenoid. After reduction the patients are either immobilized in a spica in 45-degree external rotation for 4 to 6 weeks or an operation is carried out to repair the soft tissue lesions. In these dislocations, a *reverse Hill-Sachs lesion* can be seen, that is, an impression fracture in the anterior portion of the humeral head caused by the posterior glenoid rim. Although the posterior glenoid labrum is small compared with the anterior, a posterior Bankart lesion can also be seen. The recurrence rate after posterior dislocations has been reported to be 38 percent[58] but is even higher in patients with fits. A posteriorly unstable shoulder, even when it does not fully dislocate, is a very disabling condition and may prevent the patient from performing a normal forward flexion of the arm.

Inferior Dislocation

In rare cases an anterior dislocation can be anteroinferior; in these cases, the humeral head is caught under the inferior pole of the glenoid, causing luxatio erecta, whereby the patient keeps the arm in nearly full elevation while it is dislocated and cannot bring the arm back down to his side. Reduction takes place under general anesthesia, and traction is applied in the direction of the arm (i.e., in the nearly full elevation). Treatment after reduction is similar to the treatment after reduction of an anterior dislocation.

Chronic Dislocations

Locked Dislocations

A locked dislocation is irreducible using ordinary maneuvers, and open reduction is usually necessary. Possibly the dislocation has been present for such a long time that the soft tissues have adapted to the situation, and they thus maintain the dislocated position. Other reasons why closed reduction might be impossible may be that an avulsed fragment of the greater tuberosity blocks reduction, or the humeral head cannot be kept in position due to the loss of function of the muscles attached to the fragment. In addition, entrapment of soft tissues like the long head of the biceps tendon or a very large impression fracture in the humeral head interlocking firmly with the glenoid might also necessitate open reduction.

At the time of open reduction, the goal is to restore the anatomy as closely as possible to normal. Often in posterior-locked dislocations the treatment must include obliteration of the reversed Hill-Sachs lesion by transpositioning the insertion of the subscapularis into the defect.[44]

Recurrent Dislocations/Subluxations

A chronic condition that may have developed after the initial injury presents either as a tendency for the glenohumeral joint to dislocate completely or as a tendency of the glenohumeral joint to sublux. In anterior subluxations this may only be indicated by the "dead arm" syndrome. The therapist should always beware of the "sprained shoulder," which is often a result of a subluxation or a spontaneously reduced dislocation. In the subluxing shoulder, Rowe and Zarins[62] demonstrated the presence of intra-articular pathologies or a widened rotator interval (which is the separation between the supraspinatus and the subscapularis muscles) in a large number of the patients, so even without complete dislocations, joint damage is present that may need repair. Since the rate of recurrence of dislocation in young patients is very high and since clear pathology can often be identified on radiographs or by arthroscopy and EUA, the authors do not stipulate any minimum number of dislocations before surgery in the athlete.[41,60,66] Instead, they prefer to assess each patient carefully, and if clear clinical findings confirm the presence of joint laxity with subluxation, or if damage to the joint likely to cause instability is suspected, early examination under anesthesia, arthroscopy, and surgical treatment are considered.

The principle of the patient needing to "earn" treatment by having had either at least three recorded dislocations or instability symptoms for more than 12 months cannot be applied to the elite athlete: a long career break might prevent return to the previous performance level. If a Bankart or Hill-Sachs lesion can be demonstrated by arthrograms or arthroscopy, the likelihood of recurrence is so high that the surgical stabilization procedure considered most suitable for the particular case should be carried out early.

Conservative Treatment

When the exact diagnosis and etiology of the instability has been established, patients suitable for conservative treatment can be selected. In the authors' view bracing is useless in an active athletic individual. Most braces available today, if they provide reliable stabilization of an unstable shoulder, also cause such an amount of limitation of movement of the shoulder as to prevent its use in competing sports. As mentioned earlier, the large ROM of the shoulder is essential to most athletes when performing their sports, and any limitation is unacceptable. If the instability is so small that it can be sufficiently braced, it is highly likely that it can also be satisfactorily treated with a rehabilitation program.

Traumatic instabilities are rarely rehabilitated satisfactorily, although improvement may be seen in some patients.[5] In most nontraumatic instabilities, however, when the exact extent of the instability and its directions have been established, and when a tailor-made rehabilitation program for that particular patient has been set up, good results can usually be achieved.

Since surgical treatment of multidirectional unstable shoulders is difficult, rehabilitation should always be tried before surgical stabilization. The program is demanding for the patient as well as the physiotherapist. Even though the patient may be a well-trained athlete, the assessment very often reveals a severe imbalance in the shoulder muscles. A swimmer who concentrates mainly on the butterfly stroke is a typical example: the anterior muscles (the pectoralis major and subscapularis) are extremely well trained, whereas the posterior muscles (mainly the infraspinatus) may have been forgotten in the training program. Likewise, a weightlifter who has concentrated on exercising the pectoralis major muscles often forgets to build up the subscapularis, which is necessary for a balanced shoulder. If the weightlifter then gradually stretches the posterior capsule by doing bench presses, very little posterior stabilization is left, and posterior instability is likely to develop. Focusing on the posterior cuff muscles in the rehabilitation program is very likely to solve this problem. The patient should of course be encouraged to maintain this strength, when it has been regained, or symptoms will recur. *It often requires considerable reinforcement to convince these well-trained athletes that additional strengthening exercises can solve their instability problems.*

Open Surgical Procedures

Scores of surgical procedures for stabilization of the glenohumeral joint have been designed. Only a limited number have gained widespread use, and they generally fall into the groups previously mentioned. Some methods are aimed at repairing the lesion(s) created by the initial injury or the repeated dislocations, while others aim to compensate for the lack of stabilizing effect of the capsule and muscles. It has become clear in recent years that some of these procedures have either short-term morbidity with loss of ROM and overtightness of the shoulder, or longer-term morbidity such as arthritis. In some of the open procedures a risk of inflicting damage to nerves, especially the musculocutaneous nerve, is present. Development of new surgical techniques such as suture anchors has made some of these procedures much easier to perform and reduced the risk of complications, making open procedures still the preferred choice of many surgeons. By using an open procedure, the surgeon can customize the repair for each particular patient depending on the pathology found.

Seventy years ago A.S. Blundell Bankart[6] gave an opinion that should still be borne in mind by any surgeon performing surgical stabilization of the shoulder:

> To anyone who has seen this typical lesion (i.e., the Bankart lesion) exposed at operation, it must be obvious that the only rational treatment is to reattach the fibrous capsule to the glenoid ligament whence it has been torn. It is clear that a plication or similar operation performed at some distant part of the capsule can only have the effect of drawing the detached edge outwards and further away from the glenoid margin. No doubt, if the capsule is sufficiently diminished in size, it may prevent displacement of the head of the humerus notwithstanding the defect at the glenoid margin, but this is in expense of free movement of the joint.

Capsular and Labral Repairs

The Bankart Repair

The Bankart procedure was described most clearly by Blundell Bankart in 1938.[7] Its aim was to repair the injury caused by the trauma of a dislocation, and it is therefore primarily suited for use in traumatic anterior dislocations. However, if a posterior capsular avulsion has been diagnosed, a similar repair can be carried out for posterior traumatic dislocations.

By using sutures through drill holes in the glenoid rim, the avulsed labrum and capsule are taken back to where they were torn off. Clearly it seems logical to treat a disability by eliminating the pathology. However, as the procedure is complicated and difficult to perform, many surgeons have preferred other methods. With the introduction of suture anchors, some of the difficult and time-consuming details of the operation have been eliminated, and it is now regaining popularity. Another advantage of the use of anchors is that they are only placed in the glenoid rim. The glenoid joint surface, which may already have been slightly reduced in size due to wear during dislocations or due to fracture of the rim, is not additionally reduced by sutures taken through it. Figure 4-15 shows a Bankart repair carried out using Mitek anchors. Using suture anchors instead of sutures taken through drill holes, the Bankart procedure is the authors' method of choice for patients with traumatic dislocations, but this operation may be combined with other procedures such as a capsular shift or even a Bristow procedure.

Rowe in his 1978 paper[61] reported only a 3.5 percent recurrence and excellent results in 74 percent of patients treated with a conventional Bankart repair. Hovelius et al.[30] reported a 2 percent recurrence rate. Of great importance is that by using this procedure, reduction of external rotation after the operation is minimal. Rowe[61] saw normal external rotation in 69 percent of the shoulders he re-examined.

The surgical approach is through a vertical 6- to 7-cm incision from just below the tip of the coracoid in the direction of the anterior axillary fold. In women, the procedure can also be carried out through a bra-strap incision for cosmetic reasons. The deltopectoral

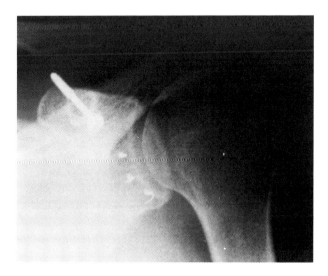

Fig. 4-15. A Bankart repair performed with Mitek anchors. The entry points of the drill holes for the anchors are just on the glenoid rim, the location of which is indicated by a vertical condensed line. The coracoid osteotomy and subsequent reattachment with a screw are optional.

groove is opened, and the coracoid is drilled and tapped with a 4-mm cancellous screw. With an oscillating saw the coracoid is then osteotomized 1 cm from its tip. If a bony defect of the anterior glenoid rim is expected, a bigger fragment may be taken off to allow for an alternative Bristow repair to be used. The conjoined tendons are reflected medially and inferiorly, taking care not to damage the musculocutaneous nerve, which is entering the muscles on the medial side usually 4 to 7 cm below the coracoid. The subscapularis is now exposed, and with the arm in external rotation, it is secured with stay sutures under vision. The brachial plexus is quite near, and the stay sutures act as the protectors of the plexus during the operation until the muscle is later repaired. The subscapularis is then divided vertically at a distance 2 to 3 cm from its insertion on the lesser tuberosity, from distal to proximal all the way to the base of the coracoid process. The capsule is opened at the level of the glenoid rim. It is crucial not to go too laterally with the capsulotomy, as this will cause shortening of the capsule at the time of the repair and subsequent loss of external rotation. The medial capsule with the avulsed labrum is then retracted to expose the glenoid rim. The rim is prepared by removal of any fibrous tissues and by the creation of a rough bony surface, care being taken not to remove glenoid bone. The suture anchors—usually three—are then inserted with the entry point of the drill holes just next to the rim. The sutures should be inserted as far apart as possible to allow all detached capsule to be securely fixed to bone. The lateral capsule can then be sutured down to the glenoid rim. At this stage there should be at least 45 degrees of external rotation. The medial flap can then be brought laterally on top of the repair for reinforcement using the sutures attached to the anchors (Fig. 4-16). The subscapularis is repaired, usually without shortening, and if the rotator interval is widened, it should be closed, too. The coracoid is reattached with a screw, and the wound is closed.

If a large bony defect is found in the anterior glenoid rim, the coracoid can be transferred to the anterior scapular neck and thus (as a Bristow-type repair) aid in the stabilization achieved by the capsular reattachment.

Our aftertreatment consists of 2 weeks in a broad-arm sling with blocked external rotation. Patients start mobilizing at their own pace, taking care not to strain the repair. At 3 months, when scar formation has taken place, the patient is allowed to return to noncontact

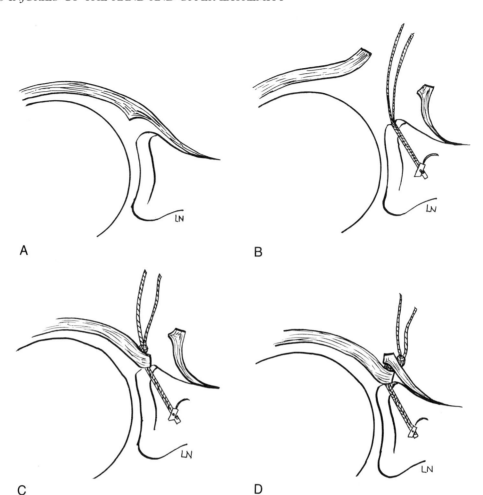

A

B

C

D

Fig. 4-16. Bankart repair with Mitek anchors. **(A)** A Bankart lesion. The anterior labrum is detached from the glenoid rim, and the capsular attachment and periosteum are stripped from the anterior scapular neck. **(B)** The capsule is opened just next to the glenoid rim, and the suture anchors are inserted in drill holes on the rim. **(C)** The lateral capsule is taken down onto the glenoid rim with the sutures attached to the anchors. **(D)** Using the same sutures, the medial flap reinforces the repair.

sports, and at 4 months contact sports such as rugby or football are allowed. It is important to abstain from pushing the rehabilitation at an early stage, as there is a considerable risk of tearing the repair apart before a strong scar formation unites the capsule and anterior glenoid.

In posterior traumatic dislocations, we use an approach through a vertical incision just medial to the location of the joint. The posterior third of the deltoid is usually retracted and detached from the scapular spine, and the infraspinatus is divided like the subscapularis in the anterior procedure. At this stage the supra-scapular nerve is very close as it passes around the lateral margin of the scapular spine. The repair itself is carried out quite like the anterior repair.

Capsular Shift Procedures

In 1980 Neer and Foster[50] described the capsular shift procedure for the treatment of involuntary inferior and multidirectional instability. This procedure has, in most centers, become the method of choice for surgical treatment of these difficult cases. As previously mentioned, before deciding on surgery, it is extremely important to exclude voluntary dislocations, unidirectional instabilities, neural or psychological disorders, and bony abnormalities of the joint. Such patients should all be managed by different methods.

Following the information obtained from the EUA, the surgeon chooses an anterior approach if the instability is mainly anteroinferior, and a posterior approach if the instability is mainly posteroinferior. Often it is advantageous to carry out an arthroscopy before finally deciding on the surgical approach. If no labral tear is present, a capsular shift procedure with a lateral capsular detachment should be carried out. The initial surgical approach is the same as for the Bankart procedure described above, but avoiding a coracoid osteotomy if a lateral capsular shift is planned. The capsule is incised vertically close to its attachment to the humeral head, detaching it as far as can be done under vision. By externally rotating the humerus the incision can be extended onto the posteroinferior attachment also, but the surgeon must always protect the axillary nerve, which is in considerable danger during this procedure. A horizontal incision is then made in the capsule at the level of the equator of the humeral head and a T-shaped opening created. Two triangular flaps—one proximally, one distally—are now created. By taking the distal flap as far proximally as it will go and suturing it to the lateral stump of the capsule, the inferior recess and the inferior glenohumeral ligaments are tightened. The superior flap is then taken down to cover the inferior flap partially, thus double-breasting the repair (Fig. 4-17).

If an additional Bankart lesion is present, it can either be repaired through the lateral T-shaped incision created for the capsular shift, or the T can be reversed, so the vertical part of the incision is made along the glenoid rim as in a conventional Bankart procedure. The capsular shift can then be performed by double-breasting the flaps medially; the sutures attached to the anchors used for the Bankart repair can thus also be used for fixing the flaps (Fig. 4-18). Altchek and co-workers[?] published very good results using this procedure in 42 shoulders with anteroinferior instability. The loss of external rotation was only 5 degrees, although throwing athletes found that they were unable to throw a ball with as much speed as before the operation.

In all these capsular shift procedures, at the time of repair of the subscapular muscle care should be taken to close a widened rotator interval, as this may play an important role in the stabilization of the shoulder.

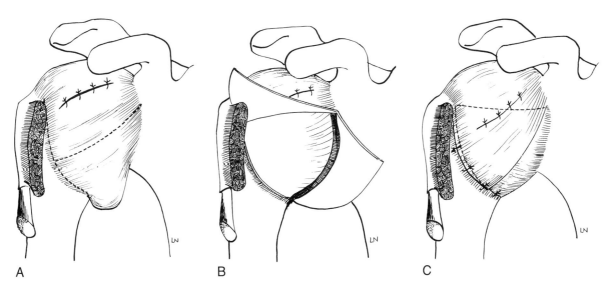

Fig. 4-17. Inferior capsular shift at the humeral insertion of the capsule. **(A)** After closure of any defects in the anterosuperior capsule, the capsule is cut some 3 to 4 mm from its insertion on the humerus and split horizontally. **(B)** This creates a T-shaped incision and a superior and inferior flap. **(C)** The inferior flap is then mobilized proximally and sutured to the lateral capsular remains. The superior flap is then taken distally to double-breast and reinforce the capsular shift.

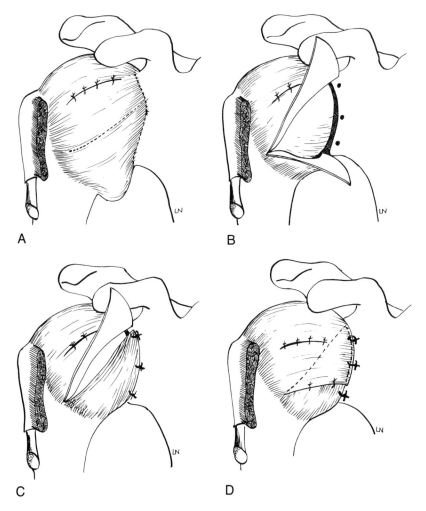

Fig. 4-18. Inferior capsular shift at the glenoid insertion of the capsule. **(A)** A horizontal split of the capsule in addition to the capsular opening of the conventional Bankart repair creates a T-shaped incision. Any defects of the capsule must be repaired before mobilizing the flaps. **(B)** A superior and an inferior flap are created, and the glenoid rim is prepared as in a Bankart repair with drill holes for the suture anchors. **(C)** The inferior flap is taken proximally down onto the anterior rim with the sutures attached to the anchors. **(D)** The superior flap is taken distally to double-breast the repair, once more using the sutures attached to the anchors.

Tendon Transfers

The Bristow Procedure

Originally described by Helfet in 1958[27] and usually performed with the modifications introduced by May in 1970,[43] the Bristow procedure has gained widespread acceptance; Hovelius et al.[31] have shown that it is crucial for the success of this operation that it be carried out with extreme attention to detail.

A high success rate has been reported, with recurrences of only 3 percent according to Lombardo et al.[38] However, it is also associated with some limitation of postoperative external rotation, and therefore should not be the method of choice in athletes doing overhead activities. The loss of ROM in external rotation with the shoulder abducted is usually no more than 10 degrees, but as full ROM in this position is crucial to some athletes, even a minor loss may terminate a career at the top level.[38,56]

The effect of this procedure is to create a "dynamic sling." In the critical position of external rotation in abduction the transferred conjoined tendons act as a sling in front of the humeral head. At the same time, the transposed bone acts as a glenoid extension, preventing contact between a Hill-Sachs lesion and the glenoid. Finally the lower third of the subscapularis is kept inferiorly in relation to the humeral head in external rotation in abduction, thus supporting the dynamic stabilization of the joint.

The authors reserve this method for use in patients for whom a minor loss of external rotation is not crucial and who have a bony Bankart lesion with a deficient anterior rim reducing the surface area of the glenoid. This is usually due to either wear of the rim by repeated dislocations or to a fracture.

The same approach as for the Bankart procedure described earlier is used. However, a larger fragment of the coracoid process (around 1.5 cm) should be taken off. The subsequent fixation of the coracoid is made much easier if the coracoid is drilled and tapped before it is osteotomized. The superior two-thirds of the subscapularis is divided just medial to its musculotendinous separation, and through a capsulotomy just lateral to the glenoid rim the joint is inspected. If any Bankart lesion is present it is repaired as described above, or an additional capsular shift procedure might be carried out. The coracoid is then positioned on the anterior aspect of the glenoid. The capsulotomy allows the positioning of the coracoid in relation to the joint to be carried out under vision, as this positioning is extremely important.[31] The coracoid must be placed below the "equator" of the glenoid, preferably in the lower third, and the bone on which it is placed should be carefully cleared of all soft tissues to allow a solid bony union. The transposed bone should be positioned just next to the joint line, without causing impingement on the humeral head during movement of the arm. The screw used for fixation should be of the lag type, providing solid compression, and it should have a firm grip in the anterior and the posterior cortex of the scapular neck. The correct position of the coracoid and the screw is seen in Figure 4-19.

In small coracoids we usually use a 4-mm, half-threaded cancellous screw for this purpose, as larger sizes of screws cause risk of fracturing the coracoid. In large individuals a 4.5-mm malleolar screw is preferred. The capsule is then repaired; shortening of the subscapularis must be avoided.

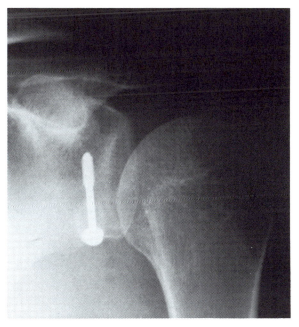

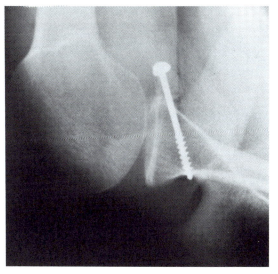

A   B

Fig. 4-19. (A & B) The correct position of the transferred coracoid tip in the Bristow repair. It should be at the lower third of the glenoid, close to the joint line without impinging on the humeral head, and the screw should grip the posterior cortex of the scapular neck.

Postoperatively the patients keep the arm in a broad arm sling with blocked external rotation for 2 weeks and are then allowed to mobilize at their own pace as with the Bankart procedure. As in any procedure involving insertion of metal implants near the shoulder joint, there is a risk of complications, and implant breakage, migration, or wrong positioning causes a certain morbidity.[72] Figure 4-20 shows a screw placed in the joint during a Bristow procedure.

The Boytchev Procedure

The Boytchev procedure[9] is usually performed today with the modifications introduced by Conforty,[15] who reported no recurrences in a series of 18 patients. However, Conforty did not consider limitation of external rotation by up to 20 degrees as a significant loss of mobility. This view cannot be justified when treating athletes.

In this procedure the conjoined tendons, after osteotomy of the coracoid, are tunneled under the subscapularis muscle and the coracoid is then reattached at its original site. Since the conjoined tendons need to be mobilized quite far distally, a risk exists of damaging the musculocutaneous nerve, which will severely disable any athlete.[69] If recurrent dislocations are seen after a Boytchev procedure, reoperation is extremely difficult, since the musculocutaneous nerve may be deeply embedded in scar tissue.

The Magnuson-Stack Procedure

Introduced in 1943, the Magnuson-Stack method, by transferring the insertion of the subscapularis muscle from the lesser tuberosity to the greater tuberosity and slightly distally, prevents further dislocations by reducing the range of external rotation.[39] The recurrence rate in different papers varies from 5 percent[1] to 17 percent.[46] Loss of external rotation, although limited, makes this method unsuitable for athletes involved in overhead sports.[56]

The McLaughlin Procedure

In patients with posterior dislocations and a large anterior humeral head defect, the McLaughlin[44] procedure can be used. The insertion of the subscapularis, with or without a small fragment of bone, is transferred into the defect in the humeral head and attached either by sutures or by a screw. Hawkins and co-workers[26] recommended this procedure in patients with humeral defects involving between 20 and 45 percent of the articular surface. Postoperative ROM and strength were satisfactory. The presence of a large defect will make it difficult to achieve a high success rate using conven-

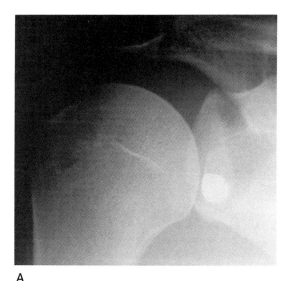
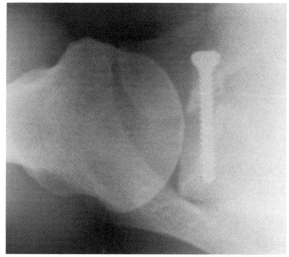

A   B

Fig. 4-20. During a Bristow repair, the screw has been placed so close to the joint that it has later migrated into the joint.

tional repairs, and in these cases the stability obtained justifies the reduced ROM.

Bony Procedures

The Eden-Hybinette Procedure

The Eden-Hybinette procedure, which has been used for many years with numerous modifications, was introduced by Eden in 1918[21] and Hybinette in 1932.[33] By inserting a bone graft into a subperiosteal pouch anterior to the glenoid, the surface of the glenoid is effectively extended anteriorly.

The recurrence rate has been found to be as high as 18 percent by Øster,[53] who also concluded that the main effect of the operation results from scarifying the anterior joint structures, as the graft had disappeared on follow-up in one-half of the cases. Concern has also been raised by Paavolainen's[54] report of late degenerative joint disease in 10 percent of the cases.

Lange's modification,[36] in which an extra-articular graft is placed in an osteotomy parallel to and just medial to the glenoid rim, adds a slightly more posterior orientation of the glenoid surface as well as the anterior extension of the glenoid surface. Zimmermann and Böhler[71] found a recurrence rate of 4 percent in this procedure, but they also reported late arthritis in 50 percent.

Based on the rate of late complications, this procedure and its modifications can no longer be recommended for use in athletes, even though the short-term results are good, with minimal loss of ROM and a low recurrence rate for the Lange's modification.

Bone Block Procedures

For recurrent posterior dislocations, McLaughlin[45] advocated in 1962 the application of a bone block to the posterior glenoid aspect. Mowery and co-workers in 1985[49] reported good results in a small series. To avoid the development of late arthritis, it is important that the block be flush with the glenoid surface and thus act as an extension of the glenoid rather than a bony stop. The method may be a good alternative to a McLaughlin procedure in patients with large humeral impression fractures.

We have used a similar procedure in anterior dislocations in patients with epileptic fits who typically have large Hill-Sachs lesions or extensive glenoid defects. An allograft or a tricortical iliac crest autograft is fixed to the anterior scapular neck with two 4.5-mm cortical screws. This graft must be flush with the joint surface of the glenoid. The capsule is attached to the anterior margin of the graft, making this a true intra-articular joint extension. Figure 4-13 shows a modified axillary (Nottingham) view of an anterior glenoid bone block. Despite using this method in epileptic patients suffering from quite violent dislocations during fits, in the 15 patients operated on to date no recurrences have been seen.

Osteotomies

Glenoid Osteotomies

Glenoid osteotomies have been advocated by several authors to prevent both anterior and posterior dislocations. Hawkins and co-workers[25] reported a recurrence rate of 41 percent after posterior glenoid osteotomy for posterior subluxation. Evidence of a tendency to anterior subluxation and impingement of the rotator cuff on the coracoid following posterior glenoid osteotomy has been shown by Gerber et al.[22] Saha[63] advocated an anterior osteotomy to adjust the tilt of the glenoid in anterior dislocations.

These procedures are technically difficult; complications such as a intra-articular fracture of the glenoid may cause irreparable damage to the joint, and they should not be considered standard procedures. Furthermore, whether "wrong" orientation of the glenoid surface is of importance in most patients is still being debated. It is our belief that most instabilities are caused by soft tissue lesions, or by bony lesions following such soft tissue changes. Glenoid osteotomy should only be carried out in patients after a CT investigation that provides proof of an abnormal glenoid orientation, thus assisting the surgeon in planning the procedure and the amount of correction of glenoid tilt required.

Humeral Osteotomies

Rotational osteotomy of the humeral neck has been popularized by Weber et al.[70] in patients with large Hill-Sachs lesions and anterior instability. By performing a transverse osteotomy of the humeral neck, internally rotating the head 25 degrees and then fixing the fragments with an angled plate, the defective area of the head is brought out of contact with the anterior glenoid rim. This method provided excellent results in Weber's[70] own follow-up of 180 patients, with only 5.7

percent recurrence and limitation of external rotation above 10 degrees only seen in 3.9 percent of the shoulders. However, the procedure is extensive, and frequently an additional surgical operation is required to remove the plate. Recently Broström and Kronberg[11] have improved the technique; in a series of 25 cases they reported a 100 percent success rate.

Soft-Tissue Plication Procedures

The Putti-Platt Procedure

The Putti-Platt procedure was first described by Osmond-Clarke in 1948[52] but was developed independently by Putti in Italy in 1923 and by Platt in England in 1925. The effect of this procedure depends on tightening a slack anterior capsule and the subscapularis tendon. Regan et al.[56] found more than 20-degree restriction of external rotation and Leach et al.[37] found 12- to 19-degree loss of external rotation. Morrey and Janes[48] had a 13.6 percent recurrence rate in 132 shoulders and Hovelius et al.[30] had 19 percent recurrence rate in 68 patients. Angelo and Hawkins[4] reported on eight patients who all had marked arthritis and some also had posterior subluxation following Putti-Platt repairs. For these reasons we have abandoned the use of this procedure completely. The reverse procedure, shortening the infraspinatus and the posterior capsule, remains popular for posterior dislocations.

Arthroscopic Repair

In recent years the arthroscopic management of shoulder instabilities has gained increasing popularity. The methods in use are still being refined, and further developments can be expected in the years to come. Selection of the patients is crucial. Patients with Bankart lesions are well suited for this type of repair, whereas more dispute exists concerning shoulders with no obvious lesions but the appearance of joint laxity only. Of course, huge Hill-Sachs lesions or glenoid defects demanding bony operations, tendon transfers, or rotational osteotomies cannot be managed arthroscopically, although the enthusiastic arthroscopist may try to do so. In long-standing disease with a large number of dislocations, the labrum may have been worn away, or the anterior capsule so much stretched and deformed that repair cannot be performed using the arthroscope.

The early arthroscopic repairs of Bankart lesions were performed by Johnson in 1982, using a metal staple. In his later series of 147 shoulders, recurrence was seen in 31 (21 percent).[34] However, the complication rate from the use of metal staples in the region of the joint is high and their use is no longer recommended.[72] In a smaller series, Maki[40] saw recurrences or painful instability in one-third of the shoulders. Biodegradable staples or tags are being developed, and these are likely to revive the stapling type of repair. Most arthroscopists today use the technique described by Morgan and Bodenstab,[47] in which sutures are passed through the capsule, labrum, and glenoid from the front and then through a hole in the scapular neck to be tied on the posterior side of the scapula. In Caspari's[13] series of 49 arthroscopic repairs, 2 recurrences and 2 cases of persistent subluxations were noted. A patient who requires a capsular shift procedure and a refixation of the capsule to the anterior glenoid rim will currently be treated by an open procedure, but even capsular shift-type procedures are now being performed arthroscopically, as reported in a small series by Duncan and Savoie[20] that showed good results in 10 shoulders with multidirectional instability.

With the continuing development of techniques and equipment and the improved surgical training seen in recent years, arthroscopic repairs in experienced hands are beginning to produce results closer to those achieved in open repairs; no doubt in the future these procedures will be the ones of choice. However, the technique is difficult, the learning curve is long, and the good results seen so far have been achieved by surgeons very experienced in performing arthroscopic procedures. For most surgeons the open procedure remains the best way to achieve good results.

GENERAL MANAGEMENT PRINCIPLES

First Dislocation

For an athlete suffering the first traumatic shoulder dislocation, management is still being debated. However, the authors believe in treating these individuals aggressively, since it has been shown that, once dislocated only a few shoulders in the young age group remain stable after reduction and conservative treatment.[66]

Since the results of stabilization procedures such as Bankart repairs and capsular shifts are excellent, with very few recurrences and a normal or near-normal ROM postoperatively, we believe these athletes should be offered surgery at an early stage. If a top-class athlete goes through a rehabilitation program after a traumatic dislocation and then suffers another dislocation some months after the first, the delay in restoring shoulder stability may cause severe damage to a sporting career.

For these patients we prefer to investigate further immediately either with an arthrotomogram or by arthroscoping the shoulder. Arthroscopy is the method of choice in these cases, in combination with an EUA. In addition, by carrying out the investigations personally, the surgeon gains a much more balanced view of the problem. Findings from EUA and arthroscopy then form the basis of treatment. In the athlete, for whom it is crucial to restore a shoulder as close to normal as possible, we believe that the surgeon should be able to choose between a number of different methods and to select the best for each individual patient and the particular problem.

Recurrent Dislocations

When an athlete experiences dislocation of a shoulder that has been dislocated before (as a result of moderate or severe trauma), surgical repair (as soon as possible) should be considered. Whether the second dislocation took place following trauma or was atraumatic, a definite recurrent instability is present that calls for treatment. We base our selection of surgical procedures on EUA and arthroscopy findings, although often the detailed diagnosis is so obvious from the EUA alone that arthroscopy might be unnecessary.

The same principles apply to athletes who suffer recurrent dislocations after previous surgical repairs. If such a repair has proved deficient, further surgery is necessary to restore stability. These revision procedures are technically difficult and should only be carried out by surgeons with special interest in these problems. Scarring and distorted anatomy demand a surgeon with sufficient experience to restore stability using the sometimes limited possibilities provided by the tissues already compromised by the previous procedure.

REFERENCES

1. Aamoth GM, O'Phelan EH: Recurrent anterior dislocation of the shoulder: a review of 40 athletes treated by subscapularis transfer (modified Magnuson-Stack procedure). Am J Sports Med 5:188–190, 1977
2. Altchek DW, Warren RF, Skyhar MJ et al: T-plasty modification of the Bankart procedure for multidirectional instability of the anterior and inferior types. J Bone Joint Surg [Am] 73A:105–112, 1991
3. American Academy of Orthopaedic Surgeons: Joint motion. A method of Measuring and Recording. American Academy of Orthopaedic Surgeons, 1965
4. Angelo RL, Hawkins RJ: Osteoarthritis following an excessive tight Putti-Platt repair. Orthop Trans 12:728, 1988
5. Aronen JG, Regan K: Decreasing the incidence of recurrence of first anterior shoulder dislocations with rehabilitation. Am J Sports Med 12:283–291, 1984
6. Bankart ASB: Recurrent or habitual dislocation of the shoulder joint. BMJ 2:1132–1133, 1923
7. Bankart ASB: The pathology and treatment of recurrent dislocation of the shoulder joint. Br J Surg 26:23–26, 1938
8. Basmajian JV, Bazant FJ: Factors preventing downward dislocation of the adducted shoulder joint. J Bone Joint Surg [Am] 41A:1182–1186, 1959
9. Boytchev B: The treatment of recurrent shoulder instability. Minerva Orthop 2:377–379, 1951
10. Broca A, Hartman H: Contribution à l'étude des luxations de l'épaule. Bull la Soc Anat Paris 4:312–336, 1890
11. Broström L-Å, Kronberg M: Surgical and methodological aspects of proximal humeral osteotomy for stabilisation of the shoulder joint. J Shoulder Elbow Surg 2:93–98, 1993
12. Callaghan JJ, McNiesh LM, Dehaven JP et al: A prospective comparison study of double contrast computed tomography (CT) arthrography and arthroscopy of the shoulder. Am J Sports Med 16:13–20, 1988
13. Caspari RB, Savoie FH, Meyers JF: Arthroscopic management of the unstable shoulder. Presented at the meeting of the American Academy of Orthopaedic Surgeons, Las Vegas, 1989
14. Clark JM, Harryman DT II: Tendons, ligaments and capsule of the rotator cuff. J Bone Joint S [Am] 74A:713–725, 1992
15. Conforty B: The results of the Boytchev procedure for treatment of recurrent dislocation of the shoulder. Int Orthop 4:127–132, 1980
16. Cyriax J: Textbook of Orthopaedic Medicine. Vol. 1 8th Ed. Ballière Tindall, London, 1982
17. Dempster WT: Mechanisms of shoulder movement. Arch Phys Med Rehabil 46A:49, 1965
18. De Palma AF, Callery G, Bennett GA: Variational anatomy and degenerative lesions of the shoulder joint. AAOS Instructional Course Lecture. 16:255, 1949

19. Deutsch AL, Resnick D, Mink JH et al: Computed and conventional arthrotomography of the glenohumeral joint: normal anatomy and clinical experience. Radiology 153:603–609, 1984

20. Duncan R, Savoie FH III: Arthroscopic inferior capsular shift for multidirectional instability of the shoulder: a preliminary report. Arthroscopy 9:24–27, 1993

21. Eden R: Zur Operation der habituellen Schulterluxation unter Mitteilung eines neuen Verfahrens bei Abriss an inneren Pfannenrande. Deutsche Z Chir 144:269–280, 1918

22. Gerber C, Ganz R, Vinh TS: Glenoplasty for recurrent posterior shoulder instability. Clin Orthop 216:70–79, 1978

23. Gilchrist DK: A Stockinette-Velpeau for immobilisation of the shoulder girdle. J Bone Joint Surg [Am] 49A:750–751, 1967

24. Hawkins RJ, Saddemi SR: Mini-symposium: the shoulder (IV). Shoulder instability. Curr Orthops 4:242–252, 1990

25. Hawkins RJ, Koppert G, Johnston G: Recurrent posterior instability (subluxation) of the shoulder. J Bone Joint Surg [Am] 66A:169–174, 1984

26. Hawkins RJ, Neer CS, Pianta RM et al; Locked posterior dislocation of the shoulder. J Bone Joint Surg [Am] 69A:9–18, 1987

27. Helfet AF: Coracoid transplantation for recurring dislocation of the shoulder. J Bone Joint Surg [Br] 40B:198–202, 1958

28. Helmig P, Suder P, Søjbjerg JO, Østgaard SE: Glenohumeral instability following puncture of the joint capsule: an experimental study. J Bone Joint Surg [Br], suppl. 1.74B:10–11, 1992

29. Hill HA, Sachs, MD: The grooved defect of the humeral head. Radiology 35:690–700, 1940

30. Hovelius L, Thorling J, Fredin H: Recurrent anterior dislocation of the shoulder. Results after the Bankart and Putti-Platt operations. J Bone Joint Surg [Am] 61A:566–569, 1979

31. Hovelius L, Körner L, Lundberg B et al: The coracoid transfer for recurrent dislocation of the shoulder. Technical aspects of the Bristow-Latarjet procedure. J Bone Joint Surg [Am] 65A:926–934, 1983

32. Hovelius L, Eriksson K, Fredin H et al: Recurrences after initial dislocation of the shoulder. J Bone Joint Surg [Am] 65A:343–349, 1983

33. Hybinette S: De la transplantation d'un fragment osseux pour remédier aux luxations récidivantes de l'épaule; constations et résultats opératoires. Acta Chir Scand 71:411–445, 1932

34. Johnson LL: Arthroscopic stapling capsulorrhaphy. Presented at the Fourth International Conference on Surgery of the Shoulder, New York, 1989

35. Lagan JM, Burkhard TK, Goff WB, Balsara ZN: Tears of the glenoid labrum: MR imaging of 88 arthroscopically confirmed cases. Radiology 179:241–246, 1991

36. Lange M: Die operative Behandlung der Gewohnheits-mäsigen Verrenkung der Schulter, Knie und Fuss. Z Orthop 75:162, 1944

37. Leach RE, Corbett M, Schepsis A et al: Results of a modified Putti-Platt operation for recurrent shoulder dislocations and subluxations. Clin Orthop 164:20–25, 1982

38. Lombardo SJ, Kerlan RK, Jobe FW et al: The modified Bristow procedure for recurrent dislocation of the shoulder. J Bone Joint Surg [Am] 58A:256–261, 1976

39. Magnuson PB, Stack JK: Recurrent dislocation of the shoulder. JAMA 123:889–892, 1943

40. Maki NJ: Arthroscopic stabilisation for recurrent shoulder instability. In Post M, Morrey BF, Hawkins RJ (eds): Surgery of the Shoulder. Mosby Year Book, St. Louis

41. Marans HJ, Angel KR, Schemitsch EH et al: The fate of traumatic anterior dislocation of the shoulder in children. J Bone Joint Surg [Am] 74A:1242–1244, 1992

42. Marshall JL: Joint looseness: a function of the person and the joint. Med Sci Sports Exerc 12:189–194, 1980

43. May VR Jr: A modified Bristow operation for anterior recurrent dislocation of the shoulder. J Bone Joint Surg [Am] 52A:1010–1016, 1970

44. McLaughlin HL: Posterior dislocation of the shoulder. J Bone Joint Surg [Am] 34A:584–590, 1952

45. McLaughlin HL: Follow-up notes on my articles previously published in the journal. Posterior dislocations of the shoulder. J Bone Joint Surg [Am] 44A:1477, 1962

46. Miller LS, Donahue JR, Good RP et al: The Magnuson Stack procedure for treatment of recurrent glenohumeral dislocations. Am J Sports Med 12:133–137, 1984

47. Morgan CD, Bodenstab AB: Arthroscopic Bankart suture repair: technique and early results. Arthroscopy 3:111–122, 1987

48. Morrey BF, Janes JM: Recurrent anterior dislocation of the shoulder. J Bone Joint Surg [Am] 58A:252–256, 1976

49. Mowery CA, Garfin SR, Booth RE et al: Recurrent posterior dislocation of the shoulder: treatment using a bone block. J Bone Joint Surg [Am] 67A:777–781, 1985

50. Neer CS, Foster CR: Inferior capsular shift for involuntary inferior and multidirectional instability of the shoulder. J Bone Joint Surg [Am] 62A:897–908, 1980

51. Ovesen J, Nielsen S: Anterior and posterior shoulder instability. Acta Orthop Scand 57:324–327, 1986

52. Osmond-Clarke H: Habitual dislocation of the shoulder. The Putti-Platt operation. J Bone Joint Surg [Br] 30B:19–26, 1948

53. Øster A: Anterior dislocation of the shoulder treated by the Eden-Hybintte operation. Acta Orthop Scand 40:43–52, 1969

54. Paavolainen P, Björkenheim J-M, Ahovuo J et al: Recurrent anterior dislocation of the shoulder. Results of the Eden-

Hybinette and Putti-Platt operations. Acta Orthop Scand 55:556–560, 1984

55. Reeves B: Arthrography of the shoulder J Bone Joint Surg [Br] 48B:424–435, 1966

56. Regan WD Jr, Webster-Bogaert S, Hawkins RJ et al: Comparative functional analysis of the Bristow, Magnuson-Stack and Putti-Platt procedures for recurrent dislocation of the shoulder. Am J Sports Med 17:42–48, 1989

57. Richardson AB, Jobe FW, Collins HR: The shoulder in competitive swimming. Am. J Sports Med 8:159–163, 1980

58. Roberts A, Wickstrom J: Prognosis in posterior dislocation of the shoulder. Acta Orthop Scand 42:328–337, 1971

59. Roberts SNJ, Foley APJ, Swallow HM et al: The geometry of the humeral head and humeral prosthesis design. J Bone Joint Surg [Br] 73B:647–650, 1991

60. Rowe CR: Prognosis in dislocation of the shoulder. J Bone Joint Surg [Am] 38A:957–977, 1956

61. Rowe CR: The Bankart procedure. A long-term end-result study. J Bone Joint Surg [Am] 60A:1 16, 1978

62. Rowe CR, Zarins B: Recurrent transient subluxation of the shoulder. J Bone Joint Surg [Am] 63A:863–872, 1981

63. Saha AK: Theory of Shoulder Mechanism. Charles C Thomas, Springfield, IL, 1961

64. Saha AK: Mechanics of elevation of the glenohumeral joint. Acta Orthop Scand 44:668–678, 1973

65. Schwartz E, Warren RF, O'Brien SJ et al: Posterior shoulder instability. Orthop Clin North Am 18:409–419, 1987

66. Simonet WT, Cofield RH: Prognosis in anterior shoulder dislocation. Am J Sports Med 12:19–24, 1984

67. Turkel SJ, Panio MW, Marshall JL et al: Stabilizing mechanisms preventing anterior dislocation of the glenohumeral joint. J Bone Joint Surg; 63A:1208–1217, 1981

68. Wallace WA, Hellier M: Improving radiographs of the injured shoulder. Radiography 49:223–229, 1983

69. Warren-Smith CD, Wallace WA, Ebrahimzadeh AR, Pailthorpe CA: Pitfalls with the Boytchev operation for recurrent anterior dislocation. In Post M, Morrey BF, Hawkins RJ (eds): Surgery of the Shoulder. Mosby Year Book, St. Louis, 1990

70. Weber BG, Simpson LA, Hardegger F: Rotational humeral osteotomy for recurrent anterior dislocation of the shoulder associated with a large Hill Sachs lesion. J Bone Joint Surg [Am] 66A:1443–1450, 1984

71. Zimmermann R, Böhler N: 21 Jahre Lange-Plastik in der Behandlung der chronisch rezidivierende Schulterluxation. Orthop Praxis 180–182, 1984

72. Zuckermann JD, Matsen FA: Complications about the glenohumeral joint related to the use of screws and staples. J Bone Joint Surg [Am] 66A:175–180, 1984

5

The Impingement Syndrome in the Athletic Shoulder

ROBERT E. LEACH
SUSAN ZECHER

INTRODUCTION

In 1972 Dr. Charles Neer[17] published an article on the coracoacromial arch and its role in producing the impingement syndrome of the shoulder. Now we see that this landmark article somewhat simplified the problem. The basic concept was that when the arm was elevated to 80 to 90 degrees of forward flexion in some individuals the rotator cuff would be caught between the unyielding humeral head and the anterior undersurface of the acromion, the distal end of the clavicle, and/or the coracoacromial ligament. This position of impingement would, over time, cause the rotator cuff to become compromised: tendinitis, bursitis, rotator cuff degeneration, and finally rotator cuff tears could occur.

Thanks to the continuing work of Dr. Neer[18] and his associates as well as that of many others, and because many athletes have had major problems with rotator cuff impingement, we now realize that this basic problem has many facets[1,3,10,12,19,23] The original concept remains, however. The rotator cuff is compromised because of the basic anatomy of the shoulder and the vascularity of the cuff, and this leads to changes in the cuff, which may produce pain and dysfunction of the shoulder.

Many sporting activities involve repetitive lifting of the shoulder above 80 degrees of forward flexion; elevation of the arm above this level, usually combined with internal rotation, leads to the sequence of events we term the impingement syndrome (Fig. 5-1). Not all athletes who use their shoulders in sports are prone to develop this syndrome. It is the manner in which the shoulder is used in sport which causes problems, not simply the act of throwing a ball or using the shoulder a great deal. Baseball pitchers in particular have a multitude of shoulder problems, one of which is the impingement syndrome.[1,6,23] However, a pitcher in another sport, softball, infrequently experiences shoulder problems. Softball pitchers throw the ball about as fast as any baseball pitcher, and yet they can pitch for 10 days in a row, and some have had careers lasting more than 30 years. Softball pitchers rarely have shoulder problems because they pitch underhanded (i.e., the arm is not elevated or forward flexed much above 60 degrees until the ball is released after force is dissipated). It appears that this underhanded motion causes far less stress than the overhand throwing motion (Figs. 5-2 and 5-3).

Swimmers are another large group of athletes who have shoulder problems; again, the impingement syndrome is a major cause of pain and disability.[5,14,20] The problem with swimming appears to be not so much the extraordinary force that is exerted by the rotator cuff muscles during each stroke, as occurs with each baseball pitch, but the repetitive stress placed on the shoulder muscles in practice sessions. The competitive swimmer may swim over 13,000 yards in practice multiple times each week. In all the swimming strokes, the shoulder goes above the 80 degrees of forward flexion level, and the arm is then forcefully brought back down toward the body. The freestyle, butterfly, and backstroke cause the most problems. The overhead motion and the forceful internal rotation required combine to

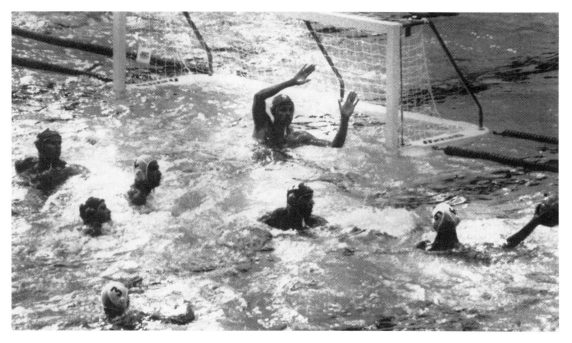

Fig. 5-1. Water polo player with arms overhead; swimmers are subject to the impingement syndrome.

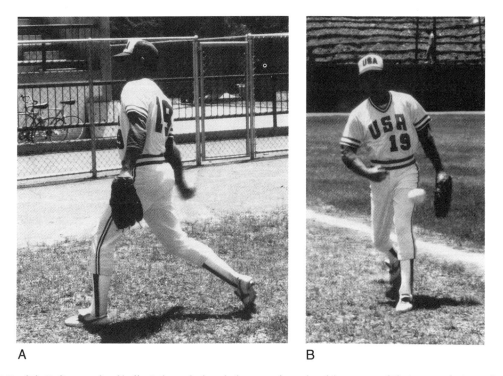

A   B

Fig. 5-2. (A) Delivery of softball pitch underhanded causes less shoulder stress. **(B)** At completion of softball pitch, shoulder stays below 80 degrees.

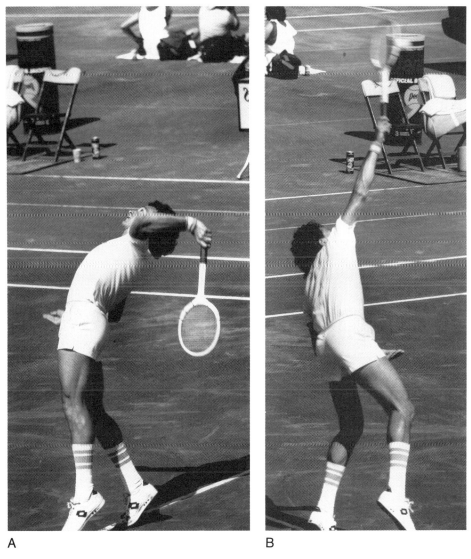

A   B

Fig. 5-3. (A) Tennis server demonstrates shoulder internal rotation, arched back, and laying back of wrist to gain power. **(B)** Arm and shoulder extended as internal rotators bring arm forward and cause external rotators to act eccentrically.

provide the biomechanics for an impingement syndrome.

The tennis serve and overhead shot are other sporting movements that can cause symptoms of the impingement syndrome. Here the motion has some similarities to that of a baseball pitcher, but the magnitude of forces acting on the shoulder capsules and muscles is less in the tennis serve than it is in the baseball pitch. The tennis racquet provides a long lever arm, which allows the tennis player to produce great racquet speed and thus increase the service velocity without the great stress of baseball pitching being produced on the shoulder muscles (Fig. 5-3). While shoulder pain is a common complaint in tennis players, particularly younger players, it is unusual that shoulder injuries end a career or interfere seriously with playing tennis, as commonly happens in baseball pitching.

Most of the general population and indeed, most

athletes, go through life without ever experiencing the symptoms of an impingement syndrome, even though they frequently use the arm in an overhead position. We all have the anatomic possibilities inherent in our shoulders that could subject us to this syndrome, but few individuals out of the total population ever become symptomatic. Even most baseball pitchers, tennis servers, and swimmers practice and compete without ever having significant symptoms. It appears that a combination of the repetitive use of the overhead motion plus the major forces needed to compete in these sports sets the scene for the symptoms of impingement.

ANATOMY

Several anatomic factors could lead to an increased incidence of the impingement syndrome. Bigliani et al.[2] described three anatomic variations of the acromion; it is their belief that the so-called type 3 acromion, with an anterior hook, is a major cause of the impingement syndrome. An anteriorly hooked acromion would make it more likely that the rotator cuff would impinge. Most individuals with a type 3 acromion are over the age of 45, and some authorities wonder whether the hooked acromion starts early in life as an anatomic variant or whether it is a consequence of age and continuous anterior traction by the coracoacromial ligament. The type 3 acromion is a less common cause of the impingement syndrome in the younger athlete. Rockwood and Lyons[22] noted that many of their patients had anterior proliferation of bone on the acromion that created an irregular surface. They wondered if this was the result of osteophytes coming from the acromion's anterior aspect.

Ventrally directed osteophytes on the lateral end of the clavicle at the acromioclavicular joint can impinge on the subacromial space and may cause rotator cuff symptoms. In some instances, this may be combined with degeneration of the acromioclavicular joint, which may cause a problem in determining whether the shoulder condition is an impingement syndrome or degeneration of the acromioclavicular joint. The authors have seen patients in whom, with abduction and some internal rotation, a small defect in the rotator cuff matched up exactly with a ventrally directed osteophyte off the distal clavicle (Fig. 5-4). Again, this finding is more likely to occur in the older athletic group than in younger athletes.

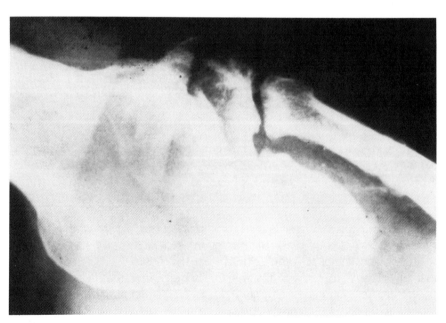

Fig. 5-4. The acromioclavicular joint is narrowed, and a small ventral osteophyte is seen on the distal clavicle.

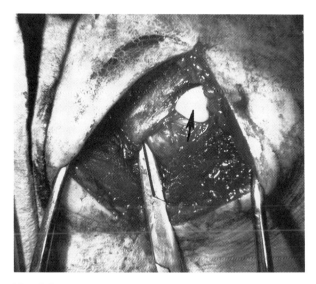

Fig. 5-5. Coracoacromial ligament completes tight anterior aspect of coracoacromial arch. White rice body (*arrow*) came from proliferative bursitis secondary to impingement.

While a thickened coracoacromial ligament has been mentioned as a possible cause of impingement, it seems unlikely that the thickness of this ligament would be the sole direct cause, or even a common cause, of impingement. The coracoacromial ligament does contribute to impingement by helping to tether the anterior aspect of the acromion process, and it is in itself a firm structure that may impinge on the rotator cuff (Fig. 5-5).

PATHOMECHANICS

Overall, the impingement syndrome, particularly in athletes, seems to be caused more by subtle problems that occur within the glenohumeral joint and the rotator cuff than by simple anatomic variants. We take the view that frequently either an acute episode or (more likely) a chronic stress to the rotator cuff has caused some alteration in the integrity of the cuff, which then leads to weakness of the rotator cuff muscles, particularly of the supraspinatus. It is accepted that one of the prime functions of the rotator cuff is to depress the humeral head in the glenoid as the deltoid contracts prior to bringing the arm into abduction or forward flexion. With any cuff problem, due to either pain or structural alteration, weakness may and usually does ensue, and with abduction or forward flexion, the humeral head may not be depressed the requisite amount in the glenohumeral joint. If this were to happen on a chronic basis, the very thin subdeltoid bursal membrane, which acts as a lubricant rather than as a cushion between the distal rotator cuff tendons and the undersurface of the acromion, would become inflamed. When bursal inflammation is present, we would expect some increased thickness of bursal tissue, and this would increase the possibilities of impingement. With increasing use and further cuff weakness, the cycle is repeated, and the possibilities of an impingement syndrome become greater. This gradual onset of the syndrome seems to be the most likely way that most swimmers, tennis players, and indeed, most athletes develop it.

Other causative factors are distinctly possible, however. Many tennis players have a tight posterior shoulder capsule as a consequence of intermittent stress applied to the capsule by forceful internal rotation of the arm and shoulder during the serve and other strokes. With a tight posterior capsule as the arm is elevated, it may not be possible for the humeral head to drop down into the glenoid. The posterior capsule would push the head somewhat forward and superiorly, leading to encroachment on the subacromial space. With this tight posterior capsule, the possibility also exists of some excess anterior movement of the humeral head, which would then lead to an element of instability in the same athlete who is showing signs and symptoms of the impingement syndrome.

Sports medicine physicians are well aware that many overhead throwing athletes have a subtle, underlying anterior instability problem that may coexist with and contribute to a rotator cuff impingement problem (C. J. Dillman, personal communication).[9] Only a little anterior movement of the head can produce pain in the athlete, and this pain is frequently in the same region during many of the same activities as the pain that occurs during the impingement problem. If the athlete has a feeling of instability or a clicking in the shoulder or any type of "dead arm" syndrome, then one is more likely dealing with instability than with an impingement syndrome. However, the two problems may coexist.

Anything that leads to irritation of the shoulder and to adhesive capsulitis will increase the possibility of

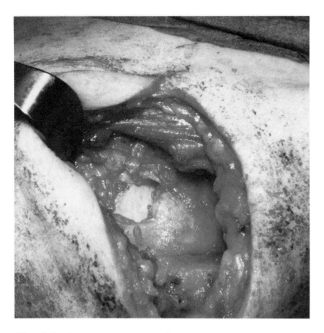

Fig. 5-6. Degenerative tear of supraspinatus tendon in 61-year-old swimmer.

the impingement syndrome. The basic concept is that if the capsule is made tight, the head of the shoulder is unable to drop down into the usual voluminous inferior capsule and the humeral head will be forced upward, causing pressure against the anterior arch of the acromion. Even small losses of motion may lead to the gradual onset of symptoms.

Hawkins and Janda[9] discussed microtrauma and macrotrauma as mechanisms for producing the impingement syndrome. In the baseball pitcher, the possibilities of macrotrauma are greater. The pitcher puts severe stress on the rotator cuff with each pitch, and the stress may be severe enough that part of the musculotendinous cuff may give way microscopically. This acute macrotrauma, which can come about by throwing just one pitch, could lead to cuff weakness and subsequently to a rapid development of impingement syndrome.

The pathology of the rotator cuff in the impingement syndrome has been well described by Neer[18] and others.[10] Younger athletes are usually in stage 1, reversible edema and hemorrhage in the rotator cuff. Progressive thickening and fibrosis comprise stage 2. Later in life, particularly after the age of 40, we see more degenera-

tion of the cuff and small bone spurs. This leads to degeneration and later tendon ruptures and is termed stage 3 (Fig. 5-6).

SYMPTOMS

Most athletes with an impingement syndrome do not have acute pain nor do most go to a doctor at the first sign of pain. The athlete gradually becomes more symptomatic and usually complains of some stiffness, occasionally weakness, and usually pain when the arm is brought into the forward flexed and internally rotated position. Sometimes pure abduction with rotation may produce the same symptoms, but it is definitely the overhead motion of which most athletes complain. Acute onset is less common; in this case, a detailed history is called for to see if the underlying pathology can be corrected immediately. The overuse pattern is far more common. The athletes usually say that throwing or swimming will cause pain, and that following practice or competition this pain is intensified. Sleep at night may be uncomfortable after practice or competition. Many will continue to practice and compete, accepting some discomfort. Gradually, however, the discomfort becomes pain or begins to interfere with performance; at that point, they usually seek medical attention. In taking the history, it is important to get as much detail as possible because an accurate diagnosis may be made based on the exact moment that pain occurs or is intensified. For example, if the pain occurs anteriorly in the shoulder during the cocking phase of the throwing maneuver, then it is more likely due to some anterior instability than to the impingement syndrome.

A few patients complain of local tenderness, which is more likely to occur over the bicipital groove or perhaps over the acromioclavicular joint. The latter may be due to degenerative changes in that joint and radiographs should show appropriate changes. We find that a number of athletes have some tenderness over the bicipital groove, but it is rare in our experience for the biceps tendon to be the major cause of shoulder dysfunction. In some older patients with degenerative changes of the cuff or even a cuff tear, the biceps becomes more subject to use and may suffer the same type of attritional changes as the cuff.

Many athletes have lost some shoulder motion; because of their sports, a number of athletes will have excessive motion in other planes. Swimmers and throwers generally have more external rotation than nonathletes, and this must be taken into account when examining the shoulder. We find that some athletes have a decrease in forward flexion or abduction, or both, and some loss of internal rotation is seen in many. The involved shoulder must be compared with the other shoulder, with careful measurement and recording, to mark progression. As the shoulder is brought into forward flexion from 80 to 100 degrees, and then some internal rotation is added, the patient usually feels pain in the anterior aspect. This has been characterized as the impingement sign. Viewing the patient from the rear as the arm is brought up in forward flexion or in abduction, we often see asynchrony of the scapular muscles; the patient attempts to make the humeral head duck under the acromion when going from 80 to 100 degrees. Asking the patient to reach across the body to the opposite shoulder, which adducts and internally rotates the arm, often produces local pain. Neer[18] and others[10] have suggested an impingement test with the subacromial space injected with a local anesthetic. Relief of pain upon the usual impingement maneuvers is considered an excellent diagnostic sign. We have been somewhat less impressed with this test than other authors, but we will use it at times.

It is very important to determine if anterior instability is a concomitant problem or if it is the major problem. We have tried to translate the humeral head in the glenoid by literally moving it in the anterior, posterior, or inferior directions. Abduction of the arm to 90 degrees and then external rotation may produce pain due to anterior subluxation. Hawkins and Kennedy[10] describe a relocation test after the patient's shoulder is placed in abduction and external rotation. They then use one hand to try to force the humeral head back into its normal anatomic relationship in the glenohumeral joint. If this maneuver decreases the patient's symptoms, it is positive and provides good evidence that anterior instability is a major problem.

Muscle atrophy is not usually seen in the early stages of the impingement syndrome. It is difficult to detect muscle atrophy of the rotator cuff muscles because they are well covered by subcutaneous tissue. In the older patient with a tear of a degenerative cuff, muscle atrophy is much more easily seen and is a negative prognostic factor.

RADIOGRAPHIC EVALUATION

Routine radiographs have seldom been of significant help to the authors, although subacromial sclerosis may be seen. The supraspinatus outlet view may be helpful in viewing the anterior aspect of the acromion, although Rockwood and Lyons[22] have found this to be less satisfactory than another view (Fig. 5-7). They suggest an anteroposterior view of the shoulder, with the patient standing. The 30-degree caudal tilt of the x-ray beam gives a good view of the anterior aspect of the acromion. We have found this more helpful in most patients than the outlet view.

An arthrogram can be diagnostic, particularly in older patients in whom a suspicion exists of a complete tear of the rotator cuff. It is less helpful in diagnosing partial-thickness cuff tears, which are frequent. It can be combined with computed tomography (CT) and is

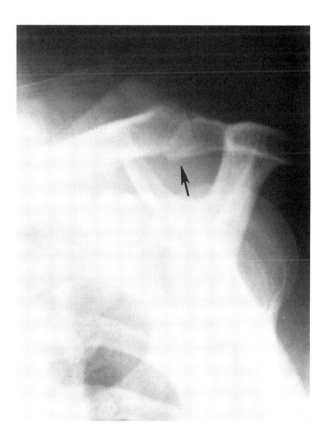

Fig. 5-7. Supraspinatus outlet view showing type I acromion (*arrow*).

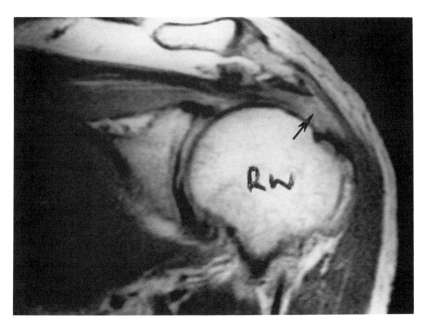

Fig. 5-8. MRI shows rotator cuff tear (*arrow*) in 46-year-old tennis player with long-term impingement.

useful for diagnosing a variety of disorders occurring within the joint.

Ultrasonography is popular in Europe and can be helpful in demonstrating tears and alterations in the structure of the rotator cuff. It has a high specificity, but results depend on the examiner. The results vary greatly from hospital to hospital and even from country to country.

To some extent, the same can be said for magnetic resonance imaging (MRI). It is also operator dependent, but it may show inflammation of the cuff and give a good idea of the location and size of any lesions (Fig. 5-8). As time goes on, it is likely that MRI will become the imaging procedure of choice, since it seems to give detailed information. However, MRI is very expensive. All these tests should be adjuncts only to the history and physical examination, since diagnosis of the impingement syndrome and its associated damage still depends on those modalities.

OTHER SPORTS

Although we have primarily discussed baseball pitching, tennis, and swimming as the principal sports in which the impingement syndrome is seen, it is obvious that the condition could occur in a variety of other sports. We have had patients who are weightlifters, javelin throwers, mountain climbers, football quarterbacks, gymnasts, and wrestlers (Fig. 5-9). In all these athletes, both chronic and acute stress occurs in the muscular and capsular tissues of the shoulder. In some of these sports, one acute episode may lead to changes in the integrity of the cuff, which later lead to an impingement syndrome. In many sports, the chronicity of athletic use causes the symptoms. In each instance, a good history and physical examination should make the diagnosis possible.

TREATMENT

Prevention

Since it is obvious that a number of athletic activities lead to shoulder trouble, and specifically to the impingement syndrome, prevention should be a concern of all those who care for athletes. We can be helpful in three basic areas. First, we can try to ensure that the athlete maintains a full range of motion so that a tight posterior capsule or adhesive capsulitis, which may force the humeral head up and anterior into the glenoid, do not develop. Since we know that certain sports lead to tightness of the capsule, we can recommend that all those athletes participating in these sports work

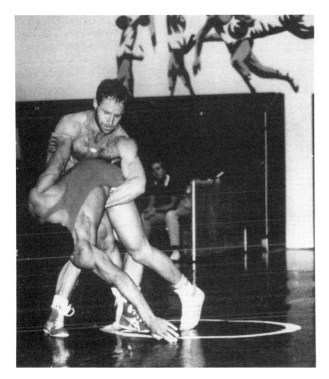

Fig. 5-9. Wrestling can place both acute and chronic stresses on the rotator cuff, which could lead to a later impingement syndrome.

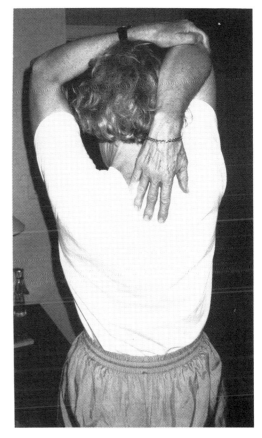

Fig. 5-10. Stretching the shoulder capsule.

on their stretching exercises assiduously. A few minutes each day may go a long way toward preventing future problems (Fig. 5-10).

Second, we can advise the athlete to maintain strength in all the muscle groups around the shoulder. Generally speaking, the internal rotators are stronger than the external rotators, and it is important to keep the external rotator muscles strong so that they are not overpowered. In certain throwing activities, these muscles act as the decelerators; if they become damaged, the sequence of events occurs that can lead to impingement syndrome. We recommend that the athletes work on maintaining their endurance strength and increasing their power. This can be done by the use of rubber tubing, free weights, or machines (Fig. 5-11). Time spent in preventing strength and endurance loss is worthwhile; the external rotators need most of the work. This does not mean that work is not also needed on the internal rotators and the shoulder elevators.

Finally, it is important that all athletes who have problems with the shoulder examine the technique of their sport. In many instances it will be found that the tennis serve, baseball pitch, javelin throw, and so forth are producing major stresses that vary from athlete to athlete. Analyzing and advising on the stresses requires a great deal of knowledge of the sport and ability to relate to and cooperate with the athlete and coach. Nothing is worse than doctors who think they know the sport advising athletes on performance without a sufficient coaching or athletic background. On the other hand, doctors who understand the sport and can discuss it intelligently with athlete, parents, and coaches may be of great help in alleviating specific stresses.

Nonoperative Treatment

Most athletes do not take to the most obvious treatment for impingement syndrome—rest. Rest is needed for the cuff and surrounding tissues to lose the inflammatory component and to allow time to repair micro-

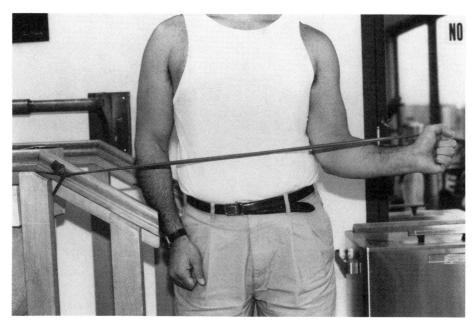

Fig. 5-11. External rotators being strengthened with rubber tubing.

scopic damage. This means that most athletes with an impingement syndrome need a period of time away from the sport that has caused the symptoms. Decrease or modification of activity may sometimes be possible, but in many instances only rest will suffice.

Directed physiotherapy is the cornerstone of any treatment. This therapy has two major goals: regaining range of motion and strengthening rotator cuff muscles. First the range of motion in all directions is accurately measured and then complete range of motion is sought for the injured shoulder. Forward flexion is usually gained relatively quickly, as is abduction, but it is important to regain the full arc of motion. Regaining internal rotation may be more difficult. The loss of motion may be relatively small, but this small loss may be part of the condition that continues to produce symptoms. Restoring full range of motion will allow the humeral head to descend in the glenoid as the arm is elevated, and symptoms should abate. Once full range of motion has been regained, it is important that all athletes be taught a program of stretching to be performed daily whenever they are active in their sport.

Strengthening the muscles of the rotator cuff is no less important. We direct our attention primarily to the internal and external rotators; the latter muscle group is usually weaker and needs more work. We have found

that rubber tubing and bungee cords are very helpful. We begin with low-resistance exercises and gradually increase the number of repetitions before increasing the resistance. We ask that the patient initially keep the arm below 45 degrees of forward flexion. Once the repetitions have reached a reasonable level, we then work on increasing strength and again increase the number of repetitions. Provided that all goes well, the arm can gradually be elevated above 45 degrees; it is hoped that eventually the exercises will be performed at 90 degrees, which is a more appropriate position for most sports. Resistance is gradually increased and then free weights or machines are added. In a well-established impingement syndrome, it may take 10 to 16 weeks of physiotherapy for the rotator cuff muscles to recover completely, since they have often been gradually weakened over time. Once the patient is doing well, maintenance therapy must be continued. We also recommend that the scapular stabilizers be strengthened during this period, since they are often weakened, which can lead to some painful syndromes.

Most athletes prefer to be active, so they can stay in physical condition during rehabilitation. The physician cannot allow a baseball pitcher to continue throwing the ball during the acute rehabilitative phase, nor can swimmers continue as usual, although sometimes training benefit may be gained by changing the stroke. We do not mean changing the mechanics of a particular stroke (unless the coaches perceive this to be appropriate); we mean changing to a different swimming discipline. Of course it is possible for the pitcher or the swimmer or any other athlete to change to some other type of physical conditioning such as biking, jogging, and so forth, which will permit them to stay in physical shape while allowing the injured shoulder to heal gradually.

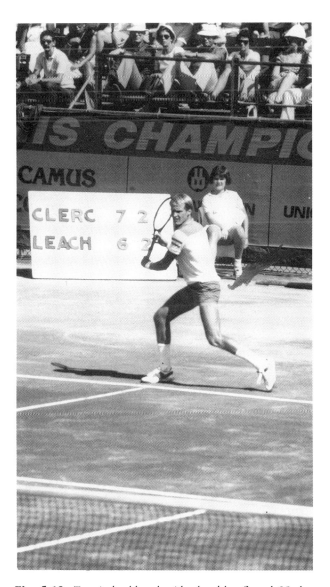

Fig. 5-12. Tennis backhand with shoulder flexed 35 degrees; supraspinatus is still active.

The authors had always assumed that the serve and overhead alone were the major causes of impingement in the tennis player and that hitting groundstrokes would cause no problems during the rehabilitative phase. Some recent work by Dr. Charles Dillman (personal communication) has caused us to wonder whether a tennis player should continue to hit many groundstrokes during the early rehabilitative phase. Dr. Dillman's data show that the supraspinatus muscle, which is critical in the impingement process, is active throughout the groundstroke phase and thus this muscle would be under stress, even when hitting only forehands and backhands (Fig. 5-12). This could be deleterious for the muscle tendon unit during the early rehabilitation phase.

During the past decade, physicians have gradually moved away from the use of corticoid steroids in shoulder conditions such as the impingement syndrome and chronic tendinitis. This popular method of treating many problems of the shoulder and rotator cuff was based on the concept that injection of corticoid steroids into the subdeltoid bursa would decrease inflammation of the bursa and the underlying cuff tissue. Although the corticoid steroid use does cause a decrease in local inflammation and while it may be helpful, particularly in allowing patients to pursue physiotherapy, it must not be looked upon as the only or major treatment of an impingement syndrome. If steroid injections are used to decrease inflammation, the authors believe that the tissues should be allowed a 14-day rest period to let the collagen tissue return to normal. Then exercises, including strengthening ones, may be restarted. Range of motion exercises are acceptable during this period of rest. If one injection has not been helpful, it is unlikely that a second would do any better. Note that tendons may rupture when multiple corticoid steroid injections are used in one area.

The vast majority of young athletes who have the impingement syndrome will improve with nonoperative methods. Nonsteroidal anti-inflammatory drugs (NSAIDs) may help to decrease pain (particularly a great deal of early pain) during the rehabilitation phase. We see these medications as facilitators during rehabilitation. We do worry about the use of medications that mask the underlying disease process and by so doing allow the athlete to continue unlimited practice and competition. In the less painful cases, continued competition while using NSAIDs is perhaps reasonable. However, we must be sure that these patients are following their rehabilitation regimen and that they are gradually improving. The medication must not be seen as an end in itself.

SURGERY

Most young athletes will eventually do well with nonoperative methods. A number of older athletes, particularly those with degenerative cuffs, and a few of the younger ones may fail conservative treatment; then operative intervention should be considered. More than 40 years ago, Hammond[7] performed complete acromionectomies for patients with chronic rotator cuff tendinitis. These patients were mostly nonathletes, but the relief of pain and the return of function was surprisingly good. Precise strength measurements were not made, and most of them probably lost a certain amount of strength. Nevertheless, for everyday functions, these patients did well. In the 1970s, the senior author (R.E.L.) did partial acromionectomies, taking off the anterior third of the acromion and meticulously repairing the deltoid; he found that these patients did very well.[15] A number of athletes, including professional tennis players, were able to return to competition. In the 1970s Neer advocated an anterior acromioplasty in which only a small portion of the undersurface of the anterior acromion was removed. He was thus able to decrease the pressure of the rotator cuff against the anterior aspect of the acromion and the coracoacromial ligament. Neer's concept of anterior acromioplasty has been popularized by a number of other surgeons and continues to be used by many.[8,16] The literature supports this approach.

Rockwood and Lyons[22] recently reported on a series of 71 patients with shoulder impingement syndrome. They performed what they called a modified acromioplasty, which in essence was a removal of the anterior part of the acromion back to the acromioclavicular joint. They then rounded off this distal end of the acromion by removing part of the inferior portion. They found that this two-step acromioplasty gave them even better results, and they were able to solve the problem of deltoid repair by carefully preserving the delto-trapezius fascia and the periosteal fibrous tissue of deltoid origin. This had been emphasized by both Hammond and Leach in their previous articles and by Rockwood's precise anatomic drawings. Follow-up has shown that a very good repair can be made, even with

partial resection of the acromion. Jackson[11] advocated a simple resection of the coracoacromial ligament, although the long-term results of this operation have not proved as effective in the hands of most surgeons.[13] This method may perhaps be considered for younger, nonthrowing patients.

Each of the operations mentioned above has had success, but for the athlete, the anterior acromioplasty or a small partial resection of the anterior acromion seem to be the most efficacious. In any case, the surgery must be followed by a vigorous and directed rehabilitation program. The athlete should not return to action until complete range of motion and virtually full strength of all of the muscle groups around the shoulder have been restored.

During the last decade the concept of arthroscopic decompression of the acromion has gained in popularity.[4] The surgeon first inspects the glenohumeral joint and debrides any internal damage of the rotator cuff. The subacromial space is then visualized, most of the undersurface of the anterior aspect of the acromion removed, and any osteophytes on the distal end of the clavicle also cleared. The coracoacromial ligament is resected. Arthroscopic decompression seems to be easier on the patient, particularly with regard to starting a rehabilitation program, which still remains absolutely essential. Arthroscopic decompression is not without its problems, and certain complications have ensued. At this point, the results of anterior acromioplasty or partial resection are available over a longer term, and most patients are doing well. It is possible that arthroscopic decompression may prove to be as useful over the next few years.

In older patients with impingement syndrome and a degenerated cuff, we would advise both a decompression and a repair of the rotator cuff. We feel that most rotator cuffs can be repaired, particularly in athletic individuals, and that the addition of a partial anterior resection, as advocated by Rockwood,[21,22] would allow the best possibilities of a return to full function. It may be that in the near future an arthroscopic repair of the cuff will become easier, but at the present time the open repair seems better. One key aspect of the open repair is to follow closely the precepts of previously mentioned authors in terms of splitting the deltoid and going down to repair the cuff tissues. Repair of the cuff tissues is essential, but so is repair of the deltoid back to its original position. As more and more individuals continue to participate in athletics for longer periods, it is likely that we will see more and more people with an impingement syndrome. Sports such as swimming and tennis, which can be done throughout a lifetime, are likely to produce a number of patients with shoulder symptoms that will be due to the impingement syndrome. Preventive medicine may prove efficacious, but in those patients who do not do well, operative therapy is indicated and is likely to be successful.

REFERENCES

1. Barnes DA, Tullos HS: An analysis of 100 symptomatic baseball players. Am J Sports Med 6:62–67, 1978
2. Bigliani LU, Morrison D, April EW: The morphology of the acromion and its relationship to rotator cuff tears. Orthop Trans 10:228, 1986
3. Cofield RH, Simonet WT: Symposium on sports medicine. Part 2: The shoulder in sports. Mayo Clin Proc 59:157–164, 1984
4. Ellman H: Arthroscopic subacromial decompression: analysis of one-to-three year results. J Arthroscopic Rel Surg 3:173–181, 1987
5. Fowler P: Swimmer problems. Am J Sports Med 7:141–142, 1979
6. Gainor BJ, Piotrowski G, Puhl J et al: The throw: biomechanics and acute injury. Am J Sports Med 8:114–118, 1980
7. Hammond G: Complete acromionectomy in the treatment of chronic tendinitis of the shoulder. A follow-up of ninety operations of eighty-seven patients. J Bone Joint Surg [Am] 53A:173–180, 1971
8. Hawkins RJ, Brock RM: Anterior acromioplasty: early results for impingement with intact rotator cuff. Orthop Trans 3:274, 1979
9. Hawkins RJ, Janda DH: The athlete's shoulder. Perspect Orthop Surg 1:1–27, 1990
10. Hawkins RJ, Kennedy JC: Impingement syndrome in athletes. Am J Sports Med 8:151–158, 1980
11. Jackson DW: Chronic rotator cuff impingement in the throwing athlete. Am J Sports Med 4:231–1240, 1976
12. Jobe FW, Tibone JE, Perry J, Moynes DR: An EMG analysis of the shoulder in throwing and pitching: a preliminary report. Am J Sports Med 11:3–5, 1983
13. Johnson JE, Barrington TW: Coracoacromial ligament division. Am J Sports Med 12:138–141, 1984
14. Kennedy JC, Hawkins R, Krissoff WB: Orthopaedic manifestations of swimming. Am J Sports Med 6:309–322, 1978
15. Leach RE, O'Connor P, Jone RP: Acromionectomy for tendinitis of the shoulder in athletes. Phys Sports Med 7:96–107, 1979
16. Matsen FA, Arnty CT: Subacromial impingement. p. 623. In Rockwood CA, Matsen FA (eds): The Shoulder. WB Saunders, Philadelphia, 1990
17. Neer CS II: Anterior acromioplasty for the chronic impingement syndrome in the shoulder. A preliminary report. J Bone Joint Surg [Am] 54A:41–50, 1972
18. Neer CS II: Impingement lesions. Clin Orthop 173:70–77, 1983
19. Penny JN, Welsh RP: Shoulder impingement syndromes in athletes and their surgical management. Am J Sports Med 9:11–15, 1981
20. Richardson AB, Jobe FW, Collins HR: The shoulder in competitive swimming. Am J Sports Med 8:159–163, 1980
21. Rockwood CA: The role of anterior impingement to lesions of the rotator cuff. J Bone Joint Surg [Br] 62B:274–275, 1980
22. Rockwood CA, Lyons FR: Shoulder impingement syndrome: diagnosis, radiographic evaluation and treatment with a modified Neer acromioplasty. J Bone Joint Surg [Am] 75A:409–424, 1993
23. Tibone JE, Jobe FW, Kerlan RK et al: Shoulder impingement syndrome in athletes treated by an anterior acromioplasty. Clin Orthop 198:134–140, 1985

6

Arthroscopy of the Shoulder

WILLIAM BEACH
RICHARD CASPARI

INTRODUCTION

A significant percentage of sports injuries involve the shoulder, a fact that arises from the diversity of sports available to the population and the advancing age of the participants. The role of the arthroscopist in diagnosis and treatment of shoulder injuries is increasing.

Two common shoulder problems resulting from sports injuries are traumatic anterior instability and rotator cuff disease. This chapter addresses the setup of shoulder arthroscopy, the examination under anesthesia, and the arthroscopic management of anterior instability and rotator cuff disease.

ARTHROSCOPIC SETUP

Standardization of the setup is mandatory for smooth execution of diagnostic and operative arthroscopy. The operative procedure is as follows: the patient is placed in the supine position on a standard operating room bed covered with a bean bag. Induction of general anesthesia is followed by rolling the patient into the lateral decubitus position. The bean bag is deflated. Care is taken to ensure that the patient is rolled slightly (10 to 20 degrees) posterior. This places the glenoid surface parallel to the table and allows access anteriorly for operative intervention via the anterior portals. Support straps or 3-inch adhesive tape provide additional stabilization of the pelvis to the bed.

An examination under anesthesia is simple, quick, and an extremely valuable part of the operative procedure. With neuromuscular blockade, the musculotendinous units provide little support to the ligamentous structures and an accurate assessment of ligamentous

stability can be obtained. This is done by gently abducting the arm to 90 degrees. The humerus is perpendicular to the floor. The elbow is held loosely and the glenohumeral joint is loaded by the weight of the arm. The examiner's opposite hand then gently grasps the proximal humeral shaft. Attempts at subluxing the humeral head anteriorly, inferiorly, and posteriorly are made. Occasionally an assistant may stabilize the clavicle and scapula to improve recognition of humeral head subluxation. This quick maneuver significantly enhances the diagnostic impression.

The arm is prepped and four towels quarter the operative field. A sterile U drape covers the towels. The hand and arm are fit into a sterile sleeve with a distal loop for 10 to 15 lb of traction. An extremity drape is placed over the arm and creates the sterile field.

The monitor is placed in front of the patient and surgeon. A clear, unobstructed view of the monitor is mandatory (Fig. 6-1) A Mayo stand is brought in over the patient's waist or head. All sharp instruments (scalpel and needle) are kept in an emesis basin on the Mayo stand for protection of the surgeon and assistant. A posterior lateral portal is created 2 to 3 cm inferior to the acromion. The arthroscope sheath and sharp trocar are inserted without insufflation. The posterior glenoid neck is palpated with this sharp trocar. The sharp trocar pierces the capsule. The blunt trocar is inserted and the sheath and trocar enter the joint.

GLENOHUMERAL INSTABILITY

Several classification systems have been proposed for shoulder instability. In this review, only traumatic instability is considered. Instability of the glenohumeral

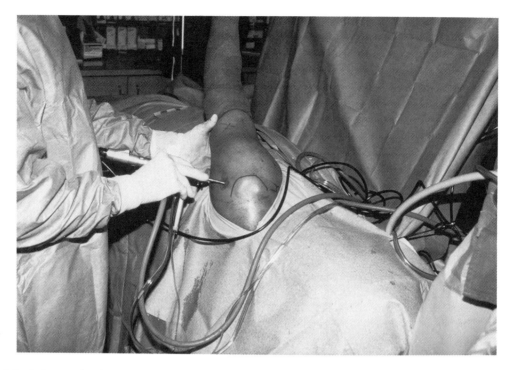

Fig. 6-1. Patient and arthroscopy equipment position are standardized. This allows easy access to the shoulder and an unobstructed view of the monitor.

joint is a common shoulder injury affecting 2 to 8 percent of the population and accounts for approximately one-third of all shoulder-related emergency room visits.[7,12,13,21,26] The risk of recurrent instability may be as high as 88 percent in athletic patients under 20 years of age.[28] Rowe[25] reported a redislocation rate of 74 percent in patients 21 to 30 years of age. Recurrent instability is thus inversely proportional to the patient's age at the initial dislocation.[25]

The pathologic entity responsible for anterior shoulder instability is laxity or incompetence of the anterior inferior glenohumeral ligament.[30] McGlynn and Caspari[16] described several results of chronic instability including Hill-Sachs lesions, labral and subscapularis attenuations, and anterior glenoid flattening.

The primary indication for arthroscopic anterior capsulorrhaphy is recurrent traumatic instability. Additional indications include traumatic or atraumatic subluxations for which conservative treatment or reconstructive procedures have failed. Contraindications to anterior capsulorrhaphy include voluntary shoulder dislocation or generalized ligamentous hyperlaxity.[4] Standard anterior capsulorrhaphy may be

inadequate for multidirectional instability. Additional arthroscopic stabilization procedures are required for the multidirectional, unstable shoulder.

Procedures

Arthroscopic Anterior Capsulorrhaphy

With the arthroscope placed (through a posterior portal) into the glenohumeral joint, an anterior portal is created through an inside-out technique. The portal is located in the triangle created by the glenoid, the biceps tendon, and the subscapularis tendon (i.e., the rotator cuff interval). A sharp trochar placed in the arthroscope sheath is pushed anteriorly, creating the capsular perforation. The sharp trochar is palpated anteriorly under the skin and a small incision exposes the trochar. A membrane-containing cannula is then placed over the sharp trochar. The sharp trochar and cannula are retracted back into the glenohumeral joint. Anterior access is now established. A thorough systematic examination of all interarticular structures is performed, with particular attention to the anterior inferior glenohumeral ligament. If a true Bankart lesion, an anterior labral periosteal sleeve avulsion lesion, or significant ligamentous laxity are present, then instability is confirmed. The presence of a Hill-Sachs lesion or attenuation of the anterior glenoid labrum is also confirmatory.

The capsulorrhaphy begins by releasing the anterior inferior glenohumeral ligament from the anterior glenoid neck. If a true Bankart lesion is seen (Fig. 6-2), then the glenoid labrum is also released off the glenoid. If ligamentous laxity is seen, then a cleavage plane is created between the ligament and the glenoid labrum along the anterior glenoid and glenoid neck (Fig. 6-3). This is done with a high-speed end-cutting shaver through the anterior portal.

The release is carried out, on the right shoulder, from the 2 o'clock to the 6 o'clock position. Special care is given to ensure that the entire ligament is released and that muscle tissue can be seen medial to the release. Once the release has been accomplished, then the end-cutting shaver is removed and a burr is inserted. The anterior glenoid neck is burred to bleeding bone, to provide a healing surface for the soon to be approximated anterior inferior glenohumeral ligament. Once the burring is complete, the burr and the cannula are removed and the anterior portal is then enlarged in line with the delta-pectoral groove.

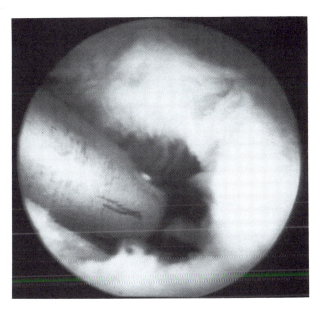

Fig. 6-3. A cleavage plane is created in the anterior inferior glenohumeral ligament (AIGHL) with an end-cutting motorized shaver.

The incision is enlarged to approximately 1 inch. An oval slotted cannula is then placed into the glenohumeral joint with a sharp trochar. The trochar is removed and the suture punch is then placed through the cannula. Six to eight sutures are sequentially placed into the anterior inferior glenohumeral ligament (Fig. 6-4). Inserting the sutures from a superior to inferior position assists in placement and keeps the sutures from obstructing subsequent ones.

Once the sutures are placed, the cannula is removed and a second oval, unslotted cannula is inserted through the same capsular perforation. Through this solid cannula, the double-barrelled pin guide is placed into the glenohumeral joint. Correct pin placement is critical for avoiding complications and optimizing results. The crotch of the double-barrelled drill guide is placed on the glenoid edge (Fig. 6-5). The drill guide is aimed medially and slightly inferiorly to exit the scapula in the infraspinatus fossa. The pin should not be placed transversely across the glenoid because of the risk of superior or lateral exit. The suprascapular nerve is most easily injured as it exits the supraspinatus fossa into the infraspinatus fossa at the base of the scapular spine. With the double-barrelled guide in a proper orientation, a Beath pin is placed through the

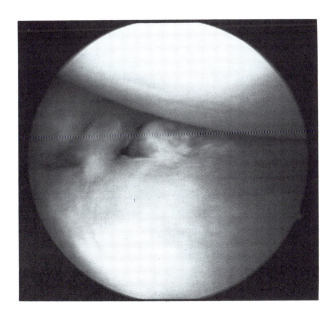

Fig. 6-2. Bankart lesion.

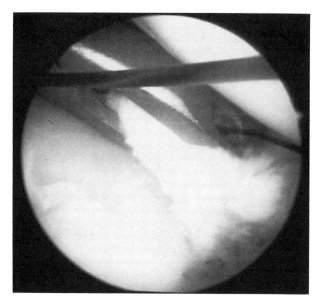

Fig. 6-4. Sutures are placed in the AIGHL using an arthroscopic suture passer.

medial hole; it then exits the scapula inferiomedially. The drill is removed from the Beath pin. The double-barrelled guide is subsequently removed and a loop of suture is placed through the tip of the Beath pin.

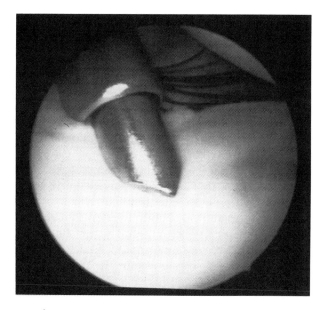

Fig. 6-5. The double-barrelled drill guide is used to place the Beath pin just medial to the glenoid surface.

The pin is pushed through to the subcutaneous tissue, where it is palpated posteriorly.

A transverse incision is then made over the Beath pin posteriorly approximately 2 inches in length. The subcutaneous tissue is elevated off the muscular fascia. The sutures that had previously been placed into the anterior inferior glenohumeral ligament are then passed through the suture loop. The Beath pin is pulled out posteriorly and the sutures are dragged through the drill hole in the glenoid neck. The anterior inferior glenohumeral ligament is shifted, proximally thus retensioning the ligament. The arm is then removed from the traction device. With a free needle, half the sutures are sewn through the infraspinatus fascia. The other half are looped through a separate suture and placed through the infraspinatus fascia. The two sutures bundles are then tied over the infraspinatus fascia. All incisions are closed with absorbable and nonabsorbable sutures. A sterile dressing is applied and the patient is placed in a shoulder immobilizer prior to completion of the anesthetic. The patient is then awakened and extubated, transferred to a stretcher, and taken to the postoperative recovery room.

Postoperative Treatment

Phase I

1. Sling: encourage use of uninvolved joints and ice tid for 0 to 3 weeks
2. Gentle Codman exercises in a sling: start at 1 to 2 weeks
3. Gentle pain-free isometric exercises: start at 1 to 2 weeks
4. Mobilization out of sling, passive range of motion (ROM), mobilization, and supine wand exercises (avoid aggressive anterior and inferior humeral glides and avoid external rotation initially): start at 3 weeks
5. Active assistive ROM against gravity (wand, wall climb, pulley, and so forth; start into flexion and gradually progress to abduction): start at 3 to 4 weeks
6. Active ROM against gravity, same considerations as in step 5; start at 4 weeks
7. Limited arc-resistive exercises, avoiding external rotation beyond 0 degrees, emphasis on anterior shoulder musculature; low-resistance, high-repetition program initially: start at 4 to 5 weeks

Phase II

1. Progressive ROM—begin working into external rotation with arm at side, as appreciation for end-feel is essential; full flexion should be obtained by 10 to 12 weeks: start at 5 to 6 weeks
2. Increasingly rigorous strengthening exercises, avoiding combined position of external rotation and abduction; address both muscle isolation and synergy; a great deal of manual resistance initially, progressing to isokinetic and finally isotonic exercises emphasizing eccentric mode for throwers: start at 6 weeks
3. Mobilize into external rotation with arm abducted: start at 8 weeks

Phase III

1. Vigorous strengthening program—high load, low repetition as indicated and tolerated: start at 10 to 12 weeks
2. Full ROM if indicated for function; may require rather vigorous mobilization and stretching: obtain by 14 to 16 weeks
3. Functional progression: start at 16 weeks

Posterior Instability Technique

After an examination under anesthesia and determination of posterior shoulder instability, routine arthroscopic examination of the glenohumeral joint is carried out. An anterior portal is created with an inside-out technique, as previously noted. The arthroscope, however, is then transferred to the anterior portal for more complete evaluation of the posterior inferior glenohumeral ligament and the posterior labrum. If sufficient laxity or labral-ligamentous instability is noted, then an end-cutting shaver is introduced through the posterior portal and the posterior inferior glenohumeral ligament is released. On a right shoulder, the ligament is released at approximately a 9 o'clock to 6 o'clock position on the glenoid face. A bone burr is then inserted and this area is abraded to bleeding bone to provide a healing surface for the reapproximated ligament. The skin incision is then enlarged and an oval slotted cannula is placed into the glenohumeral joint. Approximately six sutures are then placed into the posterior inferior glenohumeral ligament using the suture punch. The sutures are then withdrawn from the posterior portal. A supraclavicular portal is created and en-

ters the glenohumeral joint just medial to the glenoid face. A loop of suture is then placed down through this supraclavicular portal and out of the posterior portal. The sutures in the posterior inferior glenohumeral ligament are placed through the suture loop and the ligament sutures are then pulled out through the supraclavicular incision. With the sutures in this position, they can be tensioned to ensure that the ligament laxity is abolished and the ligament is approximated to the posterior surface of the glenoid. This supraclavicular incision is then enlarged to expose the distal portion of the clavicle. Once the distal portion of the clavicle is exposed, a drill hole is made through the clavicle and half the sutures are passed up through the clavicle from inferior to superior. The two suture bundles are then tied over the top of the clavicle. In this way, the retensioned ligament is held in intimate opposition to the glenoid and healing then takes place. The skin incisions are subsequently closed after the arm is removed from the traction device.

The arm is then placed in approximately 30 to 45 degrees of abduction and in neutral rotation. No internal rotation is permitted for 4 to 6 weeks.

ROTATOR CUFF DISEASE

Rotator cuff disease is controversial in terms of both etiology and treatment. Two theories exist on the etiology. In 1934, Codman[6] proposed an intrinsic cause; his theory suggests that rotator cuff tears occur as a degenerative process. Uhthoff et al.[31] showed in cadaveric specimens that most rotator cuff tears begin on the articular side and not on the bursal side, as had previously been suggested. Ozaki et al.[22] share the view that most tears are degenerative in nature. Degenerative changes lead to a weakened cuff, which when exposed to trauma may progress to rotator cuff tear.[22] This theory is in contrast to the extrinsic hypothesis, which was proposed by Meyer in 1931[17] and further espoused by Neer in 1972.[19] They postulate that rotator cuff tears are produced by compression, "impingement" of the rotator cuff tendon between the humeral head and acromion or the coracoacromial ligament (the coracoacromial arch). Neer[19] states that 95% of rotator cuff tears are associated with impingement and further describes three stages of impingement: stage I, edema and hemorrhage; stage II, fibrosis and tendinitis; and stage III, significant tendon degeneration or rotator cuff tear.

The authors have favored the term *rotator cuff disease* because of the unclear etiology of rotator cuff tears. The term *impingement* should be reserved to describe rotator cuff compression between the humeral head and the coracoacromial arch rather than a spectrum of disease.

Hawkins and Kennedy[11] have reviewed the diagnostic criteria for the three stages of rotator cuff disease. They accurately describe the stages as an arbitrary determination of a continuum of the disease. Stage I represents minimal pain with activity, no weakness, and no loss of motion. Stage II denotes marked tendinitis with pain and decreased motion. Stage III involves pain, weakness, and rotator cuff tearing.[11] Neer and Welsh[20] describe a clinical test for impingement by which the humerus is placed in 90 degrees of forward flexion and adduction with internal rotation, causing impingement of the greater tuberosity on the coracoacromial ligament. This test will significantly increase the pain of rotator cuff disease and has been designated the *impingement sign.* Further confirmation of rotator cuff disease can be made by injecting 10 ml of lidocaine into the subacromial space and re-interviewing the patient for pain. If this injection relieves the pain, the test is considered positive. Arthroscopic treatment has its place for all stages of rotator cuff disease. Johanson and Barrington[15a] reported a 95 percent satisfactory result with coracoacromial ligament division in patients who have persistent pain and disability with stage I rotator cuff disease. Penny and Welsh[23] also obtained good results with coracoacromial ligament resection with or without acromioplasty. Patients under 40 years of age underwent ligament resection, and only patients over 40 years of age had an accompanying acromioplasty. Hawkins and Kennedy[11] suggested coracoacromial ligament division for patients with unsatisfactory results after 1 year of conservative treatment.

Several authors have reported on their treatment of patients with stages II and III rotator cuff disease. Speer et al.[29] described 25 shoulders in 24 patients with advanced rotator cuff disease (stages II and III without rotator cuff tear). The patients underwent arthroscopic evaluation of the glenohumeral and subacromial space. A thorough bursectomy and acromioplasty were performed 6 to 8 mm deep to include the anterior 2 cm of the acromion. They noted a 92 percent satisfaction rate. One hundred percent of their patients with night pain had complete relief of symptoms at an average of 6 weeks. Esch et al.[9] reported on 11 patients with stage II rotator cuff disease. These patients underwent subacromial decompression of the anterior acromion by 7 to 10 mm. Nine of the 11 were satisfied with their procedure. Ellman[8] performed subacromial decompression in 40 patients with stage II disease. Eighty-eight percent achieved a good or excellent result.

The authors suggest that patients with stages II and III disease (without tears) who have not improved under conservative treatment undergo a thorough arthroscopic examination of the glenohumeral joint to rule out concomitant pathology. An acromioplasty, as described by Caspari and Thal,[5] should be performed (see below).

Treatment of 36 patients with partial-thickness rotator cuff tears in the supraspinatus portion was described by Andrews et al.[2] These patients underwent arthroscopic examination and debridement of the partial thickness tears without acromioplasty. Sixty-four percent were pitchers and were noted to have a high incidence of concomitant glenohumeral pathology including labral tearing, partial biceps tendon tears, or tendinitis. After this limited treatment, 76 percent had excellent results and 9 percent had good results, with only 15 percent poor results. Esch et al.[9] reported on 34 patients with partial-thickness rotator cuff tears. After debridement, 28 were satisfied but only 16 were objectively rated excellent; 10 were rated good, and 8 were rated fair or poor. Gartsman[10] presented 40 patients with partial-thickness rotator cuff tears. Thirty-two tears involved the articular side of the supraspinatus, and four tears were noted on the bursal side. Four were infraspinatus tears, of which 3 were articular sided. These patients underwent arthroscopic debridement and at 28.9 months, 33 of 40 patients had major improvement in pain, activity, work, and sporting activities.

Arthroscopic treatment of full-thickness rotator cuff tears has been controversial. Gartsman[10] reported on 22 patients with 25 rotator cuff tears. He divided the tears into those smaller than 1 cm, those between 1 and 3 cm, those from 3 to 5 cm, and massive tears larger than 5 cm. All patients were treated with acromioplasty, resection of the coracoacromial ligament and subacromial bursa, removal of osteophytes, and minimal debridement of the rotator cuff. At 30 months, he reported 14 satisfactory and 11 unsatisfactory results. Gartsman[10] concluded that arthroscopic treatment of complete tears was inferior to traditional open treatment, but felt that arthoscopic subacromial decompression had a role in selected patients with full-thickness rotator cuff tears. Rockwood and Burkhead[24] reported on patients with massive (larger than 5 cm) tears of the rotator cuff. An aggressive debridement of the rotator cuff was performed, and a 100 percent satisfaction rate was obtained. The criteria for a satisfactory result included pain relief and the ability to return to activities of daily living. Esch et al.[9] divided their patients with complete tears into tears smaller than 1 cm, larger than 1 cm, and massive. All patients underwent subacromial decompression including acromioplasty and coracoacromial ligament resection as well as debridement of acromioclavicular spurs. Esch et al.[9] concluded that all patients with small full-thickness tears achieved an excellent result. Patients with large tears obtained an excellent objective result in only 4 of 13 cases. Ellman[8] also reported on 10 cases of full-thickness rotator cuff tears. He noted eight good and two poor ratings after coracoacromial arch decompression and debridement. Ellman[8] concluded that decompression and debridement should be reserved for selected cases of irreparable rotator cuff tears for which the goal is pain relief and not increase in strength.

Savoie[27] reported on 87 patients with 89 full-thickness rotator cuff tears. Fifty patients were treated with open rotator cuff repair and arthroscopic acromioplasty. Thirty-seven patients were managed by arthroscopic debridement, subacromial decompression, and abrasion of the greater tuberosity. At 1 year no statistical differences were seen between the groups. However, at 2 years the open repair group was statistically much better than the arthroscopic debridement group, prompting Savoie to discontinue debridement only in the treatment of rotator cuff tears.

The authors' treatment regimen is as follows. Patients refractory to conservative treatment undergo an arthroscopic examination of the glenohumeral joint to rule out concomitant pathology, including a close inspection of the glenoid labrum for evidence of instability. The biceps tendon is closely inspected and debridement is undertaken for lesions of less than 50 percent of the thickness of the biceps tendon. Injuries of greater than 50 percent of the biceps tendon are subsequently treated with tendon resection and tenodesis at the level of the pectoralis major insertion into the humerus.

Partial-thickness rotator cuff tears involving the articular side are subsequently treated with debridement. After the arthroscopic debridement, a marking suture can be placed into the area of the tear so that this area is more closely inspected on the bursal side. Once adequate debridement of the articular side has been carried out, the bursal side is inspected. After an adequate arthroscopic bursectomy, the bursal side of the rotator cuff is inspected. An isolated bursal sided rotator cuff tear is also debrided. Inspection of the undersurface of the acromion and the coracoacromial ligament is performed for evidence of abrasion of the undersurface of the coracoacromial arch. If such evidence is found, then an acromioplasty and resection of the coracoacromial ligament are undertaken. Inferior osteophytes of the distal clavicle may also require resection at this point.

Full-thickness tears are debrided from the articular and bursal side and an acromioplasty is performed in all cases. An attempt is made to repair all tears of the rotator cuff tendon. Tears from 0 to 5 cm are normally repairable through a mini-open deltoid splitting approach. Tears larger than 5 cm or tears that cannot be adequately mobilized are aggressively debrided. Prior to treatment of rotator cuff tears, it is extremely important that the patient's expectations be appreciated and often temporized. If a massive tear is suspected, the patient must understand that the possibility of rotator cuff repair may be small and that pain relief is the goal of the treatment, not necessarily improvement of strength or ROM.

Arthroscopic Treatment

With the arthroscope placed in the glenohumeral joint through a posterior portal, and after the anterior portal has been created, a probe is placed anteriorly. The interarticular structures of the glenohumeral joint are palpated. Biceps tendon fraying is noted, as is any tearing of the articular side of the rotator cuff. If fraying or tearing are noted, then a motorized shaver is placed anteriorly and the pathology is debrided. Close inspection is often needed to ensure that the rotator cuff tear is partial and not full thickness. For partial- or full-thickness tears, debridement should extend back to healthy-appearing tissue. If the biceps tendon has an attrition of over 50 percent, then the tendon is released from its attachment on the glenoid/glenoid labrum using a motorized shaver. The labrum is left with a smooth beveled surface. The biceps tendon is debrided as far distally as possible, and then through a separate open incision, a tenodesis can be performed at the level of the pectoralis major insertion.

The arthroscope is removed from the glenohumeral joint and, through the same posterior portal, it is placed into the subacromial space. This is done by placing the blunt trochar into the arthroscope sheath and palpating the posterior edge of the acromion. The trochar is placed just under the acromial edge and advanced toward the anterior lateral tip of the acromion. A small, sweeping motion is sometimes helpful to break up adhesions in the subacromial bursa, but care should be taken not to traumatize the undersurface of the acromion so that an inspection of this surface can be made for evidence of abrasion. Once into the subacromial space, the coracoacromial ligament and undersurface of the acromion are identified. Using a spinal needle, a lateral portal is established in line with the anterior surface of the acromion. Lateral portal placement is important to allow subsequent resection of the coracoacromial ligament and anterior surface of the acromion. Through this lateral portal a bursectomy is performed to allow visualization of the acromion, the rotator cuff, the coracoacromial ligament, and the distal clavicle. A probe is inserted through the lateral portal to palpate the structures noted above. If a full-thickness tear or a bursal sided rotator cuff tear are found, then further debridement, using a motorized shaver, is undertaken. The debridement must be carried back to healthy, bleeding rotator cuff tissue (Fig. 6-6).

For full-thickness tears, the size of the tear is appreciated as well as the mobility of the cuff. A suture punch may be placed laterally and grasping the cuff. This gives the arthroscopist information on the mobility of the cuff and the likelihood of mobilizing the cuff to the greater tuberosity. Once the size of the cuff tear is determined, then the attention is placed on the surrounding structures. An acromioplasty is then performed by inserting the burr through the lateral portal. The anterior lateral corner of the acromion is identified and the burr is placed on the anterior lateral corner. A small portion of the anterior acromion is resected with the coracoacromial ligament to ensure an adequate resection and also to decrease the bleeding, compared with resection of the coracoacromial ligament only. Once this bony resection has been carried medially past the medialmost portion of the coracoacromial ligament, this portion of the acromioplasty is completed.

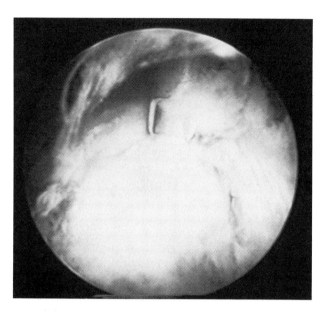

Fig. 6-6. A full-thickness tear is debrided back to healthy tissue.

The arthroscope is then switched to the lateral portal and the burr is placed posteriorly. The posterior portion of the acromion is a flat surface, and by placing a finger under the burr and applying upward pressure on this surface, the burr shaft can be nicely approximated to the undersurface of the acromion. The goal is thus to convert the undersurface of the acromion to a flat surface by keeping the burr shaft against the undersurface of the acromion. The burr is advanced anteriorly with a sweeping type of motion from medial to lateral, converting this surface to a smooth, flat plane (Fig. 6-7). This plane can be extended to the undersurface of the clavicle by removing any inferior osteophytes. Once the coracoacromial ligament, the acromion, and the distal clavicle surfaces have been addressed, attention is returned to the rotator cuff.

The numbers of shapes and types of full-thickness tears are infinite. For tears that are in line with the tendinous fibers of the rotator cuff, the torn portion of the cuff can be debrided and the repair made in a side-to-side fashion. With existing instrumentation, most notably a suture punch, sutures can be placed across the tear and sewn, using a knot pusher. In the vast majority of tears, however, the rotator cuff tendon has been avulsed from the greater tuberosity. For these tears, the tuberosity must be prepared. This is done

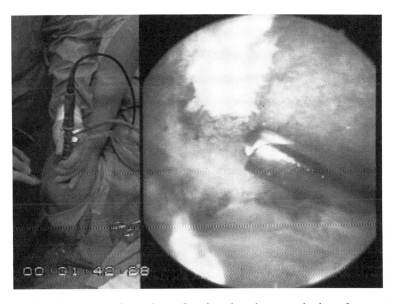

Fig. 6-7. The acromial surface is transformed to a flat plane by advancing the burr from posterior to anterior.

by removing all soft tissues from the original rotator cuff attachment site and creating a trough (Fig. 6-8) for reapproximation of the cuff. With the arthroscope in the posterior portal and the burr in the lateral portal, a trough is created to approximately 5 to 7 mm in depth from the posterior to the anterior portion of the tuberosity. Once the bed has been prepared, arthroscopic suture placement is undertaken. Using a suture punch, sutures are placed in a simple or vertical mattress-type pattern into the rotator cuff (Fig. 6-9). The

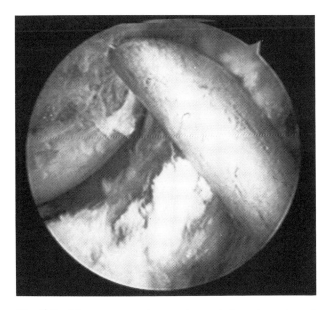

Fig. 6-8. A burr creates a humeral trough for reinsertion of the rotator cuff.

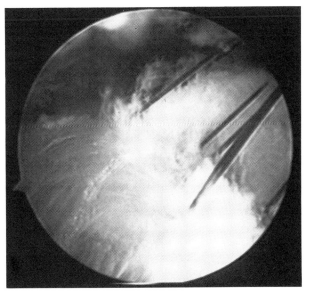

Fig. 6-9. A suture passer is utilized to place multiple sutures in the debrided edge of the rotator cuff tear.

sutures are evenly placed throughout the rotator cuff using sutures from 2-0 to 2, depending on the arthroscopist's preference.

Once the sutures have been placed, a mini-open deltoid splitting approach is used for repair. This is accomplished by removing the arthroscopic instrumentation but leaving the arm in the arthroscopic shoulder holder. An incision is made from the lateral point of the acromion, extending up to 5 cm distally. The deltoid splitting approach is carried down to the proximal humerus. Using rotator cuff repair instruments, a minimum of two bone tunnels are made from inside the trough to the lateral cortex of the humerus for suture transfer. Once the sutures are placed through the bony tunnels, they are tied over bone. Through this small incision, examination of the cuff and the adequacy of the acromioplasty can be assessed. Absorbable and nonabsorbable sutures are used to repair the deltoid fascia, subcutaneous tissue, and skin. The arm is released from the holder, a dressing is applied, and the arm is placed in a sling.

Significant efforts are underway at this time to eliminate the need for the open portion of this repair. Using bone anchors and suture modifications, hopefully the need for mini-open rotator cuff repair will be eliminated.

CONCLUSIONS

Two common pathologic entities, instability and rotator cuff disease, often affect the athlete. Arthroscopic treatment has significantly lessened the morbidity of surgical intervention. The future is likely to include an increasing role for the arthroscopic management of these common shoulder injuries.

REFERENCES

1. Adoffsson, Lysholm J: Arthroscopy and stability testing for anterior shoulder instability. Arthroscopy 5:315–320, 1989
2. Andrews et al: Arthroscopy of the shoulder in the management of partial tears of the rotator cuff: a preliminary report. Arthroscopy 1:117–122, 1985
3. Buss DD, Warren RF, Galinat BJ: Indications for shoulder arthroscopy. p. 465. In McGinty JB, Caspari RB, Jackson RW, Poehling GG (eds): Operative Arthroscopy. New York, 1991
4. Caspari RB, Savoie FH: Arthroscopic reconstruction of the shoulder: the Bankart repair. p. 507. In McGinty JB, Caspari RB, Jackson RW, Poehling GG (eds): Operative Arthroscopy. New York, 1991
5. Caspari RB, Thal R: A technique for arthroscopic subacromial decompression. Arthroscopy 8:23–30
6. Codman EA: Rupture of the supraspinatus tendon and lesions in or about the subacromial bursa. p. 65. In: The Shoulder. Privately printed, Boston, 1934
7. Cofield RH, Kavanagh BF, Frassica FJ: Anterior Shoulder Instability. p. 210. AAOS Instructional Course Lecture, Vol. X. CV Mosby, St. Louis, 1985
8. Ellman H: Arthroscopic subacromial decompression: analysis of 1–3 year results. Arthroscopy 3:173–181, 1987
9. Esch et al: Athroscopic subacromial decompression: results according to degree of rotator cuff. Arthroscopy 4:241–249, 1988
10. Gartsman GM: Arthroscopic acromioplasty for lesions of the rotator cuff. J Bone Joint Surg [Am] 72A:169–180, 1990
11. Hawkins RJ, Kennedy JC: Impingement syndrome in athletes. Am J Sports Med 8:151–158, 1980
12. Hoveluis L, Eriksson GK, Fredin FH, Hagberg MG: Recurrence after initial dislocation of the shoulder. J Bone Joint Surg [Am] 65A:343, 1983
13. Hoveluis L: Anterior dislocation of the shoulder in teenagers and young adults. J Bone Joint Surg [Am] 69A:393, 1987
14. Hurley, JA, Anderson TE: Shoulder arthroscopy: its role in evaluating shoulder disorders in the athlete. Am J Sports Med 18:480–483, 1990
15. Iannotti JP, Zlatkin MB, Esterkai JL et al: Magnetic resonance imagining of the shoulder. J Bone Joint Surg [Am] 73A:17–29, 1991
15a. Johansen JE, Barrington TW: Coracoacromial ligament division. Am J Sports Med 9:11–15, 1981
16. McGlynn FJ, Caspari RB: Arthroscopic findings in the subluxating shoulder. Clin Orthop 183:173, 1984
17. Meyer AW: The minute anatomy of attrition lesions. J Bone Joint Surg 13:341–360, 1931
18. Mok DW, Fogg AJ, Hokan R et al: The diagnostic value of arthroscopy in glenohumeral instability J Bone Joint Sug [Br] 72B:698–700, 1990
19. Neer CS: Anterior acromioplasty for chronic impingement syndrome in the shoulder. A preliminary report. J Bone Joint Surg [Am] 54A:41–50, 1972
20. Neer CS, Welsh RP: The shoulder in sports. Orthop Clin North Am 8:583–591, 1977
21. Neer CS, Foster CR: Inferior capsular shift for involuntary inferior and multidirectional instability of the shoulder: preliminary report. J Bone Joint Surg [Am] 62A:897, 1980
22. Ozaki J, Fujimoto F, Nakagawa Y et al: Tears of the rotator cuff of the shoulder associated with pathologic changes in the acromion. J Bone Joint Surg [Am] 70A:1224–1230, 1988

23. Penny JN, Welsh RP: Shoulder and impingement syndrome in athletes. Am J Sports Med 9:11–15, 1981
24. Rockwood CA, Burkhead WZ: Management of patients with massive rotator cuff defects by acromioplasty and rotator cuff debridement. Orthop Trans 12:190–191, 1988
25. Rowe CR: Dislocations of the shoulder. In Rowe CR (ed): The Shoulder. p. 165. Churchill Livingstone, New York, 1988
26. Rowe CR, Sakellarides HT: Factors related to recurrence of anterior dislocation of the shoulder. Clin Orthop 20:40, 1961
27. Savoie FH: A comparison of open repair vs. arthroscopic debridement for full thickness tears of the rotator. Presented at the 59th Annual AAOS, American Shoulder and Elbow Society, Washington, DC, February, 1992
28. Simonet WT, Melton LT, Cofield RH, Iltrup DM: Incidence of anterior shoulder dislocations in Olmstead County, Minn. Clin Orthop 186:186, 1984
29. Speer et al: Arthroscopic subacromial decompression: results in advanced impingement syndrome. Arthroscopy 7:291–296, 1991
30. Tarkel SJ, Panio MW, Marshall JL et al: Stabilizing mechanisms preventing anterior dislocation of the glenohumeral joint. J Bone Joint Surg [Am] 63A:1208, 1981
31. Uhthoff HK, Loehr J, Saarkar K: The pathogenesis of rotator cuff tears. p. 211. In Takagishi N (ed): The Shoulder. Professional Postgraduate Services, Toyko, 1987
32. Wasilewski SA, Frankl U: Rotator cuff pathology: arthroscopic assessment and treatment. Clin Orthop 267:65–70, 1991

7

Rehabilitation of the Shoulder After Injury

TERRY R. MALONE

INTRODUCTION

The shoulder is the most mobile major joint in the human body and as such requires multiple structures to provide stability. The glenohumeral joint in the body is more dependent on musculature for enhancement and control than any other joint in the body. The inherent dichotomy of mobility and stability requires the rehabilitative specialist to approach these patients cautiously. Few rehabilitative challenges equal the multiple involved shoulder patient. This chapter attempts to provide general principles of rehabilitation based on anatomy in relation to pathology, but placed within the context of the functional demands of the shoulder. Specific pathologies and injuries are addressed elsewhere in this text and thus this chapter is selective in its information. The shoulder complex has many components, which provide the rich functional abilities appreciated by the athletic patient. Rehabilitative specialists must note the many compensatory patterns and positions that evolve in these athletes. The role of the scapula is particularly impressive in overhead throwing athletes, which has been noted and well described by previous authors.[5]

The inter-relatedness of the multiple bony structures (clavicle, scapula, and humerus) allows a single synchronous action, yet multiple sequenced and controlled actions within the trunk and upper extremity are required. The distinct contributions of these individual structures require the clinician to be critical in evaluating the musculofascial structures, which are subject to functional alteration. The tremendous neuromuscular demand on the shoulder complex begins with proximal control (stability of the scapula) and culminates in normal distal activity.[9]

The inherent stability of the complex is the result of active and passive elements; the individual contributions vary with neural action and joint position. A good example of the important interactions of multiple structures with function is given by Terry et al.[10]: "static restraints of the scapulo-humeral joint provide stability for the humeral head in the glenoid cavity, limit extremes of motion of the glenohumeral joint, and guide positioning of the humerus during normal shoulder movement." This definition directly relates to the glenoid labrum, and many of the problems we see with our throwing athletes are due to the inherent demands on the musculature to support the passive structures and to position the humeral head properly during such movements.

Tremendous muscular demands are present during throwing, with the greatest activity seen during deceleration.[2,3] The act of stabilization of the shoulder involves many complex inter-relationships. Many authors have discussed them; Hollinshead[1] nicely delineated the actions as follows: the short muscles act to retain the humerus in its proper orientation, while the longer muscles are responsible for the freedom of movement in the humerus upon the glenoid.[4,7]

Complex force couples are required for normal patterns of movement, and minimal changes result in major adaptive activity. The complex synergistic relationships are often difficult to evaluate, and I believe that the supraspinatus is extremely important to the fine motor control required for athletic performance. The synergistic action of the supraspinatus and the external rotators is vital to the overall complex actions. It should also be remembered that musculature is frequently inhibited by neural mechanisms, appropriate feedback that may be lost following injury to capsular structures, and that rehabilitation may really be more related to neural activity; thus attention to pain-free function in the rehabilitation process must not be overlooked.[6,8]

Techniques for assessment of the shoulder have been presented earlier in this text. The throwing shoulder typically presents multiple soft tissue adaptations involving skeletal positioning (scapular slide) and alterations in functional range of motion (apparent increased external rotation and limitation of internal rotation—tight external rotators or posterior capsule). Thus subtle postural and mechanical alterations are the rule rather than the exception, and these changes may be normalcy to the throwing athlete. The rehabilitation clinician must utilize a functional evaluation of the shoulder, since it is imperative to determine when a specific action creates altered function or pain. This is extremely difficult but is vital to allow appropriate clinical intervention. The clinician should determine if the reaction is due to soft tissue involvement during passive or active sequences and whether the active problem is due to isometric, concentric, or eccentric muscle activation. This information allows the proper structuring of the rehabilitation sequence. A generalized evaluation sequence must be developed by clinicians for the shoulder patient on the initial visit; such a sequence should also reveal the effectiveness of treatment at a later time. A standardized clinical sequence is presented in Table 7-1.

This pattern of assessment allows the clinician to structure the rehabilitation pattern in an appropriate fashion. One of the difficulties in this scheme is the

Table 7-1. Standardized Evaluation for Clinical Decision Making in the Rehabilitation Process of the Shoulder Patient

Observation

Active motion

Palpation

Passive motion

Resisted motion

Joint play

Specific orthopedic tests

Strength (isometric and dynamic assessments)

Functional performance

assessment of strength. Our assessment of muscular output is performed noninvasively and thus does not measure the tension generation capacity of the individual muscle groups. It is not uncommon for clinicians to really be measuring the level of inhibition that may be present with the shoulder-involved patient. It is my opinion that isometric assessment followed by dynamic assessment of both concentric and eccentric muscle activation is required to provide an adequate picture of functional capacity.

An operational definition of strength permits us to communicate with other clinicians as well as with our patients. A frequently used specific methodology includes the type of muscle activation: isometric (muscle

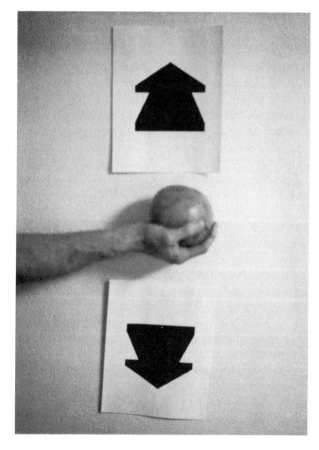

Fig. 7-1. This athlete is attempting to stabilize a ball that has been dropped into his hand. If he is able to hold it and maintain it at that position it is isometric, whereas if his elbow flexes he is exhibiting concentric motion. If he does not hold in place or extends or straightens his elbow, we are then seeing a dynamically controlled eccentric lengthening muscle activation.

is activated but no joint movement other than compression is generated); isotonic (muscle is activated and a distal movement or proximal movement occurs, thus allowing weight to be moved through a specific range of motion [ROM]) concentrically (i.e., moving against gravity in an upward direction) or eccentrically (i.e., lengthening activation whereby the weight is controllably lowered through the ROM). We thus have dynamic assessment involving movement either positively or negatively or isometric assessment stabilizing against the load provided (Fig. 7-1).

In general terms, it is important for the clinician to determine if the difficulties are experienced with concentric, eccentric, or stabilizing actions, since shoulder complex activities require controlled sequencing of all muscle activations. Each muscle activation pattern has inherent problems for the clinician. Isometric techniques of measurement provide feedback on maximal static actions but minimal information on dynamic control. Some of the additional difficulties with manual techniques such as intertester reliability, generation speed in synchronized actions, and lack of objectivity in relationship to function, render isometric

assessment less than optimal. Conversely, isotonic weight lifting involves the movement of weight through a range of motion, but problems include the limitations by neural drive and peripheral interactions, and inherent difficulties with endurance and repeatability. Again, isotonic measurements may not reflect function since most isotonic assessment involves 60 degree/sec actions. It is also quite difficult to assess eccentric levels of performance using isotonic techniques.

To provide further dynamic assessment, the use of isokinetic dynamometry has become popular. This allows evaluation of speed-controlled movements in a variety of shoulder patterns. Relatively new dynamometers allow both concentric and eccentric activation to be utilized. Isokinetic assessment allows us to assess production capabilities of individual muscle groups through stabilized and constrained patterns (Fig. 7-2).

Although isokinetic assessment is quite dynamic, it is not a true functional assessment. As noted in our recommended standardized sequence, functional performance is a critical portion of the overall pattern. This evaluation should be directed toward the specific pursuits of the individual patient and must be related

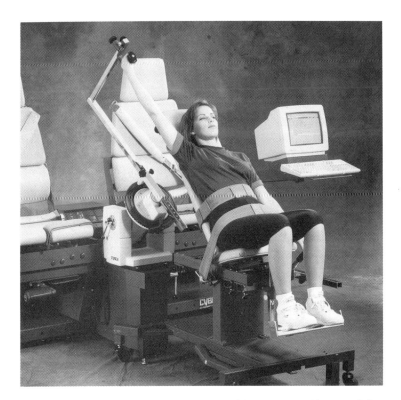

Fig. 7-2. Cybex 6000. Demonstration of a shoulder pattern: adduction-abduction.

to the reason the patient has come for evaluation. Pain that is concentric in activation frequently involves musculotendinous junction injury or impingement of some type of tissue (soft tissue, labral, or bony structure). Eccentric pain is more frequently related to tendinous lesions, frequently seen with decelerative efforts (high eccentric demand). This information is presented in more detail in *The Athletic Shoulder.*[11]

PRINCIPLES OF SHOULDER REHABILITATION

The following seven principles or rules are provided to structure the rehabilitation process (Table 7-2).

Rule 1: Control painful/inflammatory responses

Pain must be recognized as the controlling factor in our rehabilitation program. ROM-specific pain or specific muscular action require the clinician to alter rehabilitation exercises; unless normal pain-free sequences of muscular activity are available, appropriate rehabilitation is impossible. Although pain is frequently a sign of inflammation, the two are not synonymous. Functional pain classification follows a sequence from pain after specific activity, pain during and after activity, on through a sequence culminating in pain at rest (Table 7-3).

Using this type of sequence gives the clinician and patient a common language. I recommend the use of pain- and inflammatory-modulating modalities directed at a specific tissue for a desired response. An example is application of heat in the axilla when attempting to reach the inferior capsular fold of a patient who has restricted abduction. Pain modulation tech-

Table 7-2. Rules of Shoulder Rehabilitation

1. Control painful/inflammatory responses
2. Determine the cause of dysfunction
3. Treat the cause and normalize pain-free exercise sequences (remember range of motion) as treatment permits; muscular activities and retraining permit a normalization sequence to commence
4. Develop/redevelop proximal muscular control
5. Work individual muscles in pain-free portions of the range of motion
6. Work muscle in patterns—integrate actions
7. Functional progression is the rule to the final or culmination of rehabilitation

Table 7-3. Functional Pain Sequence

Level	Definition
1	Pain after specific activity
2	Pain during and after specific activity but not affecting performance
3	Pain during specific activity that affects performance
4	Pain during activities of daily living
5	Pain at rest

niques include manual therapy techniques (oscillations), electrical stimulation patterns, and heat/cryotherapy patterns. Pain modulation and control then permit appropriate rehabilitation activities. Pain modulation or control alone, however, will not provide long-term success.

Unfortunately, clinicians do not recognize the importance of acknowledging that many shoulder conditions are not inflammatory in nature. The clinical appearance may be that of overall inflammation, but the actual condition may be more degenerative and may involve a tendinopathy. Addressing the symptoms frequently does require use of an inflammatory control sequence. Pain is the "inhibitor," whether caused by inflammation or some other reaction.

Rule 2: Determine the cause of dysfunction

As control of pain or inflammatory conditions is achieved, further evaluation and clinical assessment should enable the clinician to delineate the cause of dysfunction. (*Dysfunction* is a good descriptor of the altered neural muscular patterns.) Correction may frequently involve neural retraining as well as muscular strengthening. The smooth coordinated interaction of the shoulder complex requires a great deal of high-level neural and muscular function.

Rule 3: Treat the cause and normalize pain-free exercise sequences (remember range of motion) as treatment permits; muscular activities and retraining permit a normalization sequence to commence

Remember that ROM limitations may need to be addressed, and multiple techniques may be required for normalization of functional pattern.

Rules 4 through 7 guide us through the rehabilitation sequence. It cannot be emphasized enough that pain-free exercise must be the rule.

Rule 4: Develop/redevelop proximal muscular control

Clinicians must learn to address proximal control of the scapula and wait until coordinated actions are present before attempting integrated distal movements.

Rule 5: Work individual muscles in pain-free portions of the range of motion

Individual muscle action allows the clinician to address specific weaknesses and also specific muscle actions required during coordinate movements. The importance of addressing specific muscle groups before attempting to integrate these demands with large or gross muscle actions cannot be emphasized enough. We frequently find eccentric muscle activation to be important in the proximal muscles, as are isometric patterns. It is relatively easy to add an eccentric emphasis by adding the "push" of the other extremity during exercise sessions (Fig. 7-3). It is also quite useful to work lower in the ROM to minimize early demands and to ensure proximal control as individual muscle strengthening sequences are begun.

Rule 6: Work muscle in patterns—integrate actions

Since most shoulder activity involves multiple actions of the shoulder complex, integrative muscular actions lead to the functional component. This allows strengthening activities to be utilized but only in pain-free portions of the ROM. A variety of muscular and neural training patterns may be useful. Also, trunk and lower extremity actions must be coordinated with shoulder function.

Rule 7: Functional progression is the rule to the culmination of rehabilitation

Functional progressions are hierarchically devised sequences of activities from least demanding to most demanding. The specific activities of the athlete must be addressed, including velocity, type of muscle activation, level of resistance, and endurance required for a performance as well as level of participation and individual response. An example of upper extremity progression would be a tennis player working on pain management, then addressing ROM/flexibility needs, progressing to individual and group muscle actions, and ground strokes (volley), culminating in overheads

and serving action. Chapter 19 addresses sport-specific rehabilitation techniques, but the following case studies are provided to illustrate the difficulties in both evaluation and rehabilitation that confront the clinician.

CASE STUDY 1 Swimmer's Shoulder

A 14-year-old female swimmer presented to the clinic with a 4-month history of bilateral shoulder pain. She indicated that the left shoulder was more symptomatic than the right and that she had been doing the exercises provided 3 months earlier through a previous intervention program. Her strengthening sequence primarily involved internal rotation strengthening and chest press and latissimus maneuvers. She had been given anti-inflammatories and told not to swim if she had pain. Her continued swimming difficulties had led to bilateral injections with a corticosteroid with minimal response. The injections were given 3 weeks before she came to our clinic. Her previous radiographs were negative, and she had been told that her problem was common for swimmers in her age group and she would probably continue to have such problems (if she continued swimming!)

We observed a healthy 14-year-old swimmer who was left hand dominant and whose left scapula was somewhat lower than her corresponding right scapula; she had a somewhat forward head posture in a standing position. She had extremely strong internal rotators when assessment was conducted low in the ROM, but her external rotators were weak in maximal output at a 90-degree glenohumeral position. We termed this an internal rotation bias, probably more reflective of internal rotation strengthening than of an absolute weakness of the external rotators. Her present swimming routine consisted of 3,000 to 4,000 m in the morning followed by an additional 3,000 to 4,000 m in the afternoon. Interestingly, her primary stroke was the breast stroke, but she was swimming the vast majority of these multiple hours of exercise in freestyle. She had also added hand paddles to her routine beginning approximately 6 months previously. The onset of her symptoms somewhat corresponded to the addition of hand paddles to her sequence.

ROM evaluation, both active and passive, revealed an internal rotation limitation of ap-

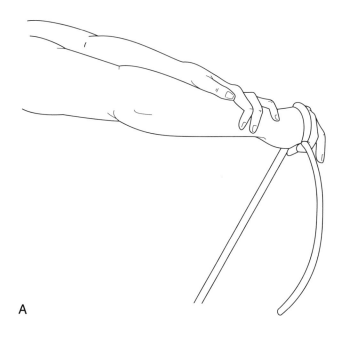

A

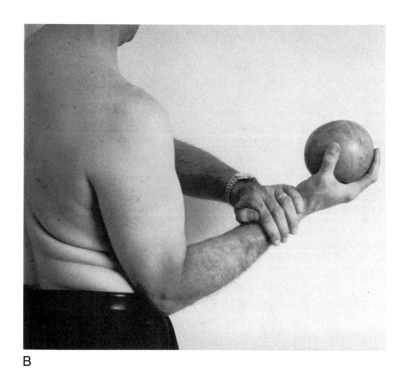

B

Fig. 7-3. **(A)** After lifting/stretching the surgical tubing, the patient makes a greater effort of loading in fighting (resisting) the additional load during the eccentric lowering phase. **(B)** Additional force of the contralateral extremity allows a more maximal eccentric effort.

proximately 10 degrees bilaterally, but she accomplished full rotation through additional compensation of the scapula. Her instability assessment revealed a positive posterior apprehension test on the left as well as a similar apprehension sequence on the right. Impingement testing was positive in both the left and right shoulders, and she had minimal posterior labral tenderness bilaterally. We performed strength assessment both manually and through isokinetics and found her prone external rotation-to-internal rotation ratio to be below 50 percent (40 percent). Functional assessment demonstrated a strengthening routine that had continued to emphasize internal rotation rather than attempting to strengthen her external rotators and in both an absolute maximal as well as endurance pattern. We like to use the prone position for testing, which duplicates her functional position (Fig. 7-4). This patient had been treated as if she had an impingement problem, but the impingement was probably secondary in nature. Her impingement was related to a lack of humeral head control associated with the incredible demands of her swimming routine. This activity-related problem was probably accentuated by her underlying level of passive restraint

but the initiation of hand paddle swimming strokes may also have been a contributing factor.

As her external rotation strength was enhanced and hand paddles were eliminated, her symptoms began to resolve rapidly. When her external/internal rotation ratio achieved a 50 percent level, she became asymptomatic. She remained asymptomatic as long as she was able to balance her dynamic control with her functional demands.

This case highlights the need for integrated intervention for a young swimmer with shoulder pain. The pathology was initially thought to be impingement, but our evaluation pointed to secondary impingement. The actual entity is often not as important as appropriate management is in addressing symptoms clinically and giving attention to causative factors. In this case, the use of hand paddles was somewhat related to the development of symptoms, and we have often seen young individuals who add excessive internal rotation strengthening. Another common mistake is the use of a kick board, which places the arms forward into an impingement pattern during early rehabilitation. The previous intervention had been unsuccessful, since the caus-

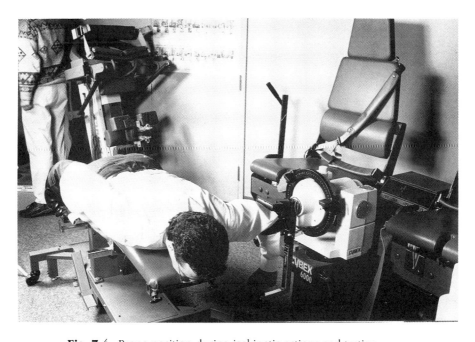

Fig. 7-4. Prone position during isokinetic actions and testing.

ative factors had not been addressed (external rotation weakness, supraspinatus inhibition, and inability to control the humeral head dynamically).

CASE STUDY 2 Thrower's Shoulder

A 21-year-old right hand dominant, intercollegiate NCAA Division One, throwing athlete reported to the clinic with a chief complaint of right shoulder pain during pitching activities. This individual had been a starting baseball pitcher for the past 13 years and had not experienced pain of this nature before. His condition had developed gradually over the previous few weeks. Symptoms worsened during the game (duration related) and were also present during and after certain weight-lifting routines.

Examination revealed that the right scapula was laterally and upwardly biased (as is frequently seen in throwing athletes). He demonstrated a forward head posture and lacked 30 degrees of normal internal rotation, but had a 30- to 40-degree increase in the expected external rotation (Fig. 7-5). Otherwise, his range of motion was within normal limits. Manual muscle testing revealed normal to above normal strength for

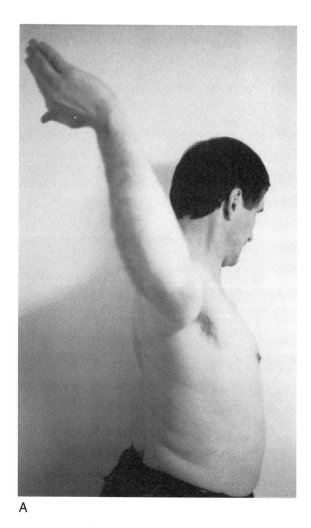

A

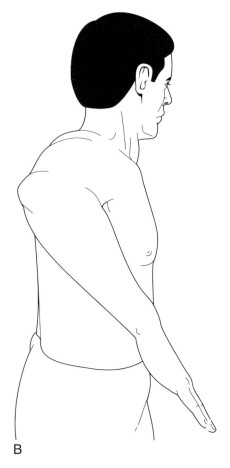

B

Fig. 7-5. (A) Increased external rotation in the throwing athlete. **(B)** Lack of internal rotation in the throwing athlete.

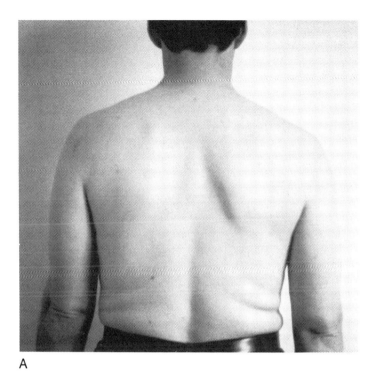

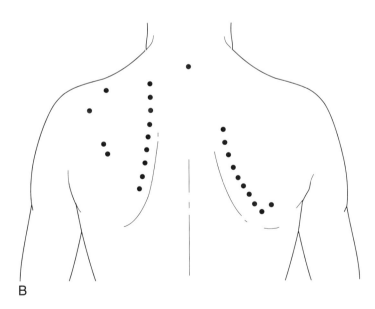

Fig. 7-6. (A) Lower dominant right shoulder. **(B)** Altered scapular position to provide greater throwing efficiency for the throwing athlete.

all muscle groups tested when examination was performed in pain-free areas of the range. At a 90-degree flexion position, certain movements were inhibited by pain, particularly when internal rotation accompanied the action. He demonstrated extremely strong internal rotation on his dominant extremity with an external rotation sequence similar to the opposite side This bias decreased when compared with the enhanced internal rotation of the dominant extremity. He demonstrated a negative apprehension as well as labral test. He had posterior shoulder pain after ball release during the throwing motion as well as a vague feeling of discomfort during throwing or other overhead actions. He demonstrated pain with forced internal rotation when the shoulder was flexed 90 degrees and with overpressure at terminal flexion. His exercise routines emphasized internal rotations and adductor strengthening (bench and military press maneuvers), with a distinct minimum of specific external rotation or rotator cuff (supraspinatus) patterns.

Our general impression was that this patient had a primary impingement pathology. Forward head posture and internal rotation strength bias are very common in such patients, as well as in the "thrower" position scapula. The gradual onset of symptoms also points toward a primary impingement rather than a secondary pattern, which often relates to an underlying level of glenohumeral instability. His ROM limits were related to adaptations for greater throwing/pitching efficiency. The increased external rotation provides a greater distance for acceleration and also potentiates the internal rotation, thus increasing pitched ball velocity. To accomplish these actions, the musculoskeletal system of many athletes' dominant shoulders maintain the scapula in an altered pattern, thus enhancing glenoid position in relation to the humeral head during throwing activities (Fig. 7-6).

Since this athlete was in the middle of his competitive season, an aggressive yet functional medical and rehabilitation sequence was required. His program was as follows: an oral anti-inflammatory (Feldene 20 mg), ice massage after exercise (10 minutes' duration), posterior capsule stretching, external rotation muscular strengthening with an eccentric emphasis, decrease in activities that caused pain (bench/military press), decreased emphasis or attention to the internal rotator muscle strengthening patterns, attention to proximal scapular positioners and stabilizers, specific rotator cuff actions (supraspinatus and external rotators) performed pain-free to allow normal recruitment sequences, and a functional throwing progression. It is interesting to note that these athletes can typically throw from the outfield much more comfortably than they can from the pitcher's mound, which may relate to the position of ball release; the time frame available for humeral deceleration may be minimized. This particular athlete was able to continue with his pitching activities but missed two starts in the pitching rotation. He became less symptomatic, resumed full pitching activities during the second week of treatment, and fortunately responded extremely well to his overall treatment sequence. Not all athletes with impingement will respond this quickly; this case represents a positive result in an athlete who was caught early in the abusive cycle.

CONCLUSIONS

This chapter presents the clinician with seven rules for addressing the athletic shoulder patient. The principles are provided to enable a structured rehabilitation sequence culminating in a return to the functional environment. It is hoped that this framework will allow success with a variety of pathologic shoulder conditions. Readers are urged to be specific as well as eclectic in their approach to rehabilitation of the shoulder patient.

REFERENCES

1. Hollinshead WH: Functional Anatomy of the Limbs and Back. 3rd Ed. WB Saunders, Philadelphia, 1969
2. Jobe FW et al: An EMG analysis of the throwing shoulder in throwing and pitching. Am J Sports Med 11:3–5, 1983
3. Jobe FW et al: An EMG analysis of the throwing shoulder in throwing and pitching. A second report. Am J Sports Med 12:218–220, 1984

4. Kent BE: Functional anatomy of the shoulder complex. Phys Ther 51:867–887, 1971

5. Kibler WB: Role of the scapula in the overhead throwing motion. Contemp Orthop 22:525–532, 1991

6. Kegerris S, Jenkins WL: Throwing Injuries. In Malone TR (ed): Sports Injury Management. Williams and Wilkins, Baltimore, 1989

7. Perry J: Shoulder anatomy and biomechanics. Clin Sports Med, 247–270, 1983

8. Smith RL, Brunolli J: Shoulder kinesthesia after anterior glenohumeral joint dislocation. Phys Ther 69:106–112, 1989

9. Soderberg GL: Kinesiology: Application to Pathological Motion. Williams & Wilkins, Baltimore, 1986

10. Terry GC et al: The stabilizing function of the passive shoulder restraints. Am J Sports Med 19:26–34, 1991

11. Wilk KE: Elements of standardized shoulder examination. In Malone TR (ed): The Athletic Shoulder. Churchill-Livingstone, New York, 1993

8

Acromioclavicular Joint Injuries

JOHN E. SAMANI
PER A. F. H. RENSTRÖM
CLAUDE E. NICHOLS III

INTRODUCTION

Acromioclavicular joint injury in the athlete is a common, complex problem. Although the anatomy, mechanism of injury, and biomechanics have been well described in recent years, the controversy as to how these injuries are best managed in the athletic population rages on. Various methods of nonoperative treatment and more than 30 different operative procedures have been described.[39,44] Furthermore, the natural history of these injuries is not well known. The literature therefore includes many treatment alternatives often employed on anecdotal experience only. A thorough knowledge of the pertinent anatomy and biomechanics, natural history, diagnostic principles, and types of injury is necessary for the implementation of the best treatment option for a given athlete.

A final consideration in the management of these injuries in the athlete is recovery of shoulder strength and function and ultimately return to sport following treatment. Again, no consensus exists as to which method of treatment best preserves strength and range of motion (ROM), but several prospective studies have shed some light on this area in recent years.[41,46]

HISTORY

From a historical perspective, operative management of a complete dislocation remained the treatment of choice for more than 100 years after Cooper first described operative repair for this injury.[13] Indeed, Powers and Bach[35] found that only 9.5% of all orthopaedic residency training programs in the United States in 1979 were recommending nonsurgical treatment. Since that time numerous studies have reported successful management of complete dislocations by nonsurgical techniques; as a result, a distinct trend exists toward managing these injuries nonsurgically.

INCIDENCE

Although the exact incidence of injury to the acromioclavicular joint is not known, it is a common joint injury in sport, especially those sports in which a risk of falling onto the shoulder exists. Most authors have found that incomplete injuries are nearly twice as common as complete dislocations and that the incidence in males is five times that of females.

MECHANISM OF INJURY

The vast majority of acromioclavicular injuries are due to a direct force produced by the athlete falling onto the point of the shoulder with the arm in the adducted position (Fig. 8-1). The force applied drives the acromion downward, causing disruption of the acromioclavicular ligaments, the coracoclavicular ligaments, or both sets in the sequence described by Horn.[21]

Alternatively, fracture of the clavicle might occur as the sole injury or (rarely) in combination with the acromioclavicular joint injury. Although they are uncommon, concomitant ipsilateral fractures such as cor-

121

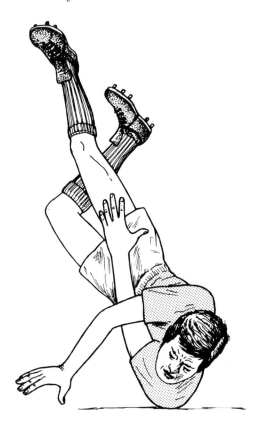

Fig. 8-1. The most common mechanism of injury is a direct force that occurs from a fall on the point of the shoulder.

acoid process fractures should be ruled out during evaluation.

Acromioclavicular joint injury less commonly occurs as a result of an indirect force, for instance when the athlete falls on an outstretched hand. Force is transferred up the arm, through the humeral head, and into the acromion process. The strain is felt by the acromioclavicular ligaments only, and not by the coracoclavicular ligaments, since the coracoclavicular space is actually decreased. In this setting an athlete might also sustain glenohumeral subluxation or even dislocation.

ANATOMY/BIOMECHANICS

The acromioclavicular joint is a diarthrodial joint whose articular surfaces are covered with fibrocartilage. The joint contains an intra-articular cartilaginous disc of variable size and shape that starts degenerating by the third decade; beyond the fourth decade it is essentially no longer functional. Variability in orientation of the joint also exists, and it has been suggested that obliquity of the joint surface may predispose to traumatic disruption. Urist[43] reported that the joint surface was obliquely disposed in 49 percent of normal radiographs and was vertical in 36 percent. Similarly, DePalma[17] has shown marked variability in the plane of the joint from almost vertical to a point where the clavicle may over-ride by as much as an angle of 50 degrees. By contrast, Moseley[30] stated that an under-riding type of inclination may exist, with the clavicular facet under the acromion. He found that athletes with this orientation were the most prone to prolonged disability following acromioclavicular joint injury.

As with other joints, the acromioclavicular joint is enclosed by an articular capsule. The capsule is a primary stabilizer of the joint and is stoutest above, where it is reinforced by the fibers of the trapezius muscle (which span the joint posterosuperiorly) and anteriorly, where it is reinforced by the clavicular head of the deltoid. Because of their proximity to the joint, concomitant tears of the clavicular attachments of the trapezius and deltoid are seen with higher energy trauma. These muscular tears are not only implicated in joint stability, but also in pain and strength recovery following injury.

The acromioclavicular joint is stabilized by two sets of ligaments, the acromioclavicular and the coracoclavicular ligaments (Fig. 8-2). The acromioclavicular ligaments consist of superior, inferior, anterior, and posterior parts; the superior part blends with fibers of the deltoid and trapezius muscles. Most investigators have concluded that the acromioclavicular ligaments function primarily as horizontal stabilizers and play only a small role in preventing vertical displacement of the distal clavicle in acromioclavicular joint injuries.

The coracoclavicular ligament consists of two parts, often separated by a bursa. The conoid ligament is cone-shaped and is the most medial of the two parts. Its apex inserts onto the posteromedial side of the base of the coracoid process, and its broadened base inserts onto the conoid tubercle on the posterior undersurface of the clavicle. The trapezoid ligament, which is strong, flat, and quadrilateral in shape, arises anterior and lateral to the conoid ligament and runs downward from the oblique trapezoid line on the undersurface of the

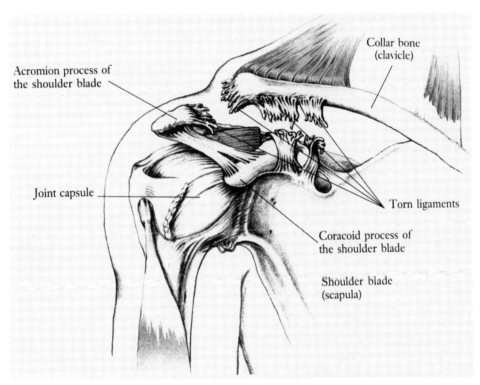

Fig. 8-2. Separation of the acromioclavicular joint with torn ligaments. (From Peterson and Renström[33], with permission).

lateral clavicle to a 2-cm rough ridge on the upper surface of the coracoid process. Most authors agree that these ligaments provide principally for the stability of the acromioclavicular articulation. Several studies have shown that both the conoid and trapezoid ligaments must be divided to produce a complete acromioclavicular joint dislocation in the vertical plane, indicating that the coracoclavicular ligaments are the prime vertical stabilizers of the joint.[10,34,43]

Fukuda et al.[18] further studied the individual contributions of the acromioclavicular and coracoclavicular ligaments in a 1986 load-displacement study with sequential ligament sectioning. The conoid ligament appeared to be more important than previously described. It played a primary role in constraining anterior and superior rotation as well as anterior and superior displacement of the clavicle. Additionally, they found that the acromioclavicular ligaments were the primary restraints to both posterior (89 percent) and superior (68 percent) translation of the clavicle at small displacements. At large displacements the conoid ligaments provided the primary restraint (62 percent) to superior translation, while the acromioclavicular liga-

ments remained the primary restraint (90 percent) to posterior translation. The trapezoid ligament was found to be the primary restraint to acromioclavicular joint compression at small and large displacements.

With glenohumeral motion, acromioclavicular motion is also present. In a classic study, Inman et al.[23] showed that the total range of motion at the joint was about 20 degrees, occurring both in the first 30 degrees of abduction and after 135 degrees of arm elevation. Little motion occurred between these two points. They also found the clavicle to rotate upward 40 to 50 degrees with full elevation of the arm. When a pin was placed to prevent this rotation, arm elevation was restricted to 110 degrees. The authors concluded that the clavicular rotation was fundamental to shoulder motion and that a coracoclavicular screw would limit clavicular rotation, thereby limiting abduction of the arm. Subsequent work showed that a screw placed across the coracoclavicular space in effect gives an arthrodesis but still allows full arm abduction by "synchronous scapuloclavicular rotation."[11,25,26] This explains, at least in part, why patients with coracoclavicular lag screws and even acromioclavicular arthrodesis or heterotopic ossification maintain a surprisingly good ROM.

CLASSIFICATION

In the past, orthopaedists tended to classify or group all complete dislocations together without recognizing the more extensive injuries that can occur to the surrounding soft tissues. Much of the controversy regarding methods of management is found in this group of patients. Thus, a useful classification system must address all pathology present, since it has implications for morbidity, treatment, and prognosis. Ideally, the clinician should be well versed in the natural history of each type of athletic injury as well as in the demands of a particular sport on the shoulder, thus gaining the ability to distinguish patients who would benefit from nonoperative therapy from those better managed by early reconstruction.

Horn[21] described the pathology of acute acromioclavicular joint dislocation as a giving way of several structures in sequence: (1) the superior attachment of the articular disc gives way and the superior acromioclavicular ligament is detached from its proximal attachment, (2) the lateral end of the clavicle is shelled out of the inferior periosteum; (3) the coracoclavicular ligaments and the clavipectoral fascia tear; and (4) the entire clavicular attachment of the deltoid is stripped, with an associated longitudinal tear in the trapezius between the clavicular and acromial attachments in very severe cases. Therefore we feel that injuries to the acromioclavicular joint are best classified not only by the extent of injury to the acromioclavicular and coracoclavicular ligaments, but also by the amount of damage done to adjacent supporting muscles as well.

As proposed by Tossy et al. in 1963[42] and by Allman in 1967,[2] these injuries have classically been termed type I, II, or III depending on the extent of ligamentous disruption to the acromioclavicular and coracoclavicular ligaments. We have found that Rockwood's[32] classification, published in 1984, clarifies the more severe injuries better (Table 8-1; Fig. 8-3).

In addition to the injuries originally referred to as Allman's types I, II, and III, Rockwood[37] recognizes three other types of complete acromioclavicular dislocation. In a type IV injury, the clavicle is grossly displaced posteriorly through the trapezius. In a type V injury, the clavicle is considerably more displaced vertically than in the type III injury, and the deltoid and the trapezius muscle attachments are disrupted. In a type VI injury, the clavicle is dislocated inferiorly under the coracoid process. By far the most common injury types seen in athletes are types I to III; the type III injury has been the topic of great discussion and debate in sports medicine circles in recent years.

DIAGNOSIS

In diagnosing acromioclavicular joint injuries in athletes, it is important to take a complete history first. The patient will usually describe a direct blow to the point of the shoulder, by contact either with another player or with the ground. Pain is usually well localized to the anterior and superior aspects of the shoulder, it usually does not radiate, and the severity is often proportional to the degree of injury.

Physical examination may show swelling, an abrasion, ecchymosis, and/or deformity over the joint. The involved arm is usually held at the side, and all shoulder motion is restricted because of pain. Localized distinct tenderness over the joint will verify the diagnosis. Because of swelling and muscular splinting, dislocation may not be readily apparent on initial physical examination, especially in the supine position. Therefore, when acromioclavicular joint injury is suspected, we feel that the athlete should be examined in the standing or sitting position. The weight of the upper extremity will make the deformity more apparent.

The signs and symptoms seen on initial examination provide valuable information for typing. They also provide insight into expected morbidity, optimal treatment, time to return to sport, and long-term sequelae. Clinical findings by injury type are described below.

Type I Injury

With type I injury the athlete most often has pain in the region of the acromioclavicular joint and minimal pain with shoulder movements. Pain is not present in the coracoclavicular interspace. Tenderness over the joint is mild to moderate in nature and the joint is not displaced. The athlete may or may not leave competition at the time of injury, depending on the nature of the sport and the demands on the upper extremity.

Table 8-1. Rockwood's Classification of Injuries to the Acromioclavicular-Coracoclavicular Complex

Type	Features
I	Sprain of acromioclavicular ligaments
	Acromioclavicular joint intact
	Coracoclavicular ligaments intact
	Deltoid and trapezius intact
II	Acromioclavicular joint disrupted
	Acromioclavicular joint wider; may be slightly separated vertically when compared with the normal shoulder
	Sprain of the coracoclavicular ligaments
	Coracoclavicular interspace might be slightly increased
	Deltoid and trapezius intact
III	Acromioclavicular ligaments disrupted
	Acromioclavicular joint dislocated and shoulder complex displaced inferiorly
	Coracoclavicular ligaments disrupted
	Coracoclavicular interspace greater than the normal shoulder (i.e., 25–100% greater than the normal shoulder)
	Deltoid and trapezius usually detached from the distal clavicle
	In children, a pseudodislocation of the acromioclavicular joint occurs with the coracoclavicular ligaments remaining intact to the intact periosteal tube, and the clavicle displaced from tube
IV	Acromioclavicular ligaments disrupted
	Acromioclavicular joint dislocated and clavicle anatomically displaced posteriorly into or through trapezius
	Coracoclavicular ligaments completely disrupted
	Coracoclavicular space may be displaced, but may appear to be the same as the normal shoulder
	Deltoid and trapezius detached from distal clavicle
V	Acromioclavicular ligaments disrupted
	Coracoclavicular ligaments disrupted
	Acromioclavicular joint dislocated and gross disparity between the clavicle and the scapula (i.e., 100–300% greater than the normal shoulder)
	Deltoid and trapezius detached from distal clavicle
VI	Acromioclavicular ligaments disrupted
	Coracoclavicular ligaments disrupted
	Acromioclavicular joint dislocated and clavicle displaced inferior to the acromion or the coracoid
	Coracoclavicular interspace decreased with the clavicle inferior to the acromion or the coracoid
	Deltoid and trapezius detached from distal clavicle

(From Neer and Rockwood,[32] with permission.)

Type II Injury

The athlete with type II injury presents with moderate-to-severe pain near the acromioclavicular joint and coracoclavicular interspace, and shoulder motion is restricted due to the discomfort. Considerable tenderness is found over both the acromioclavicular joint and the coracoclavicular interspace. The clavicle may be palpably displaced and it may be possible to palpate increased back-and-forth motion when the clavicle is manipulated from its central third. The athlete will usually withdraw from competition at the time of injury.

Type III Injury

In a type III injury the upper extremity is visibly depressed and the distal clavicle may appear to be free-floating, possibly tenting the skin. (Fig. 8-4) As with

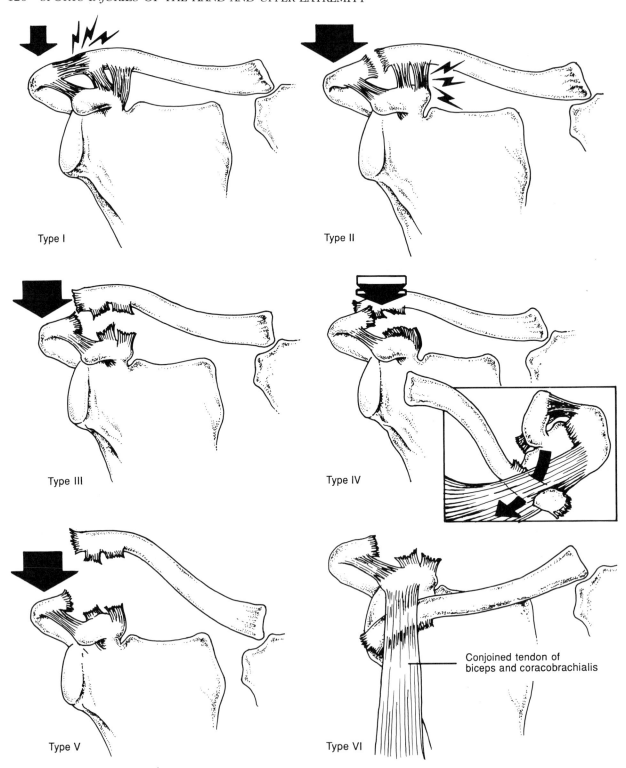

Type I

Type II

Type III

Type IV

Type V

Type VI

Conjoined tendon of
biceps and coracobrachialis

Fig. 8-3. Rockwood's classification of injuries to the acromioclavicular-coracoclavicular complex. (From Neer and Rockwood,[32] with permission.)

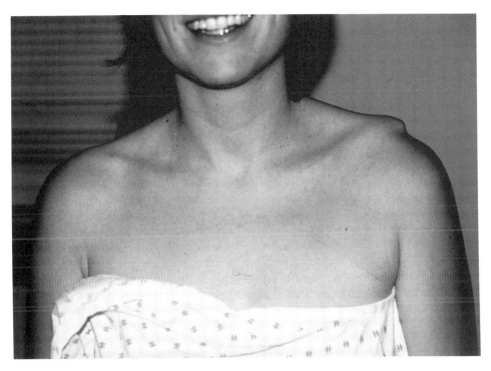

Fig. 8-4. Acromioclavicular joint separation, grade III.

type II injuries, moderate-to-severe pain is present and is increased with any shoulder motion. Tenderness is appreciated over the acromioclavicular joint, the coracoclavicular interspace, and the superolateral one-fourth of the clavicle secondary to trapezius and deltoid disruption. It may be possible to move the end of the clavicle from a dislocated to a reduced position and vice versa. The athlete will be unable to continue sports participation due to painful shoulder motion, especially if the patient is a throwing athlete.

Type IV Injury

Clinical findings in a type IV injury are similar to those found in a type III injury except that more pain is usually present and the clavicle is dislocated posteriorly. The displaced clavicle penetrates into or even through the fibers of the trapezius. The lateral clavicle may be highly movable or locked in its dislocated position. The energy requirements that cause this type of trauma are much higher than those generated in most athletic injuries.

Type V Injury

Again, in a type V injury, the clinical findings are similar to those found in type III. The patient will, however, usually present with more pain and displacement between the distal clavicle and the acromion. Due to extensive soft tissue disruption over the lateral clavicle, severe tenderness will be found in this region. An injury of this severity is rarely seen in the athletic population.

Type VI Injury

The shoulder has a flat appearance superiorly due to inferior displacement of the lateral clavicle. Because of the high amount of trauma necessary to produce a subcoracoid dislocation of the distal clavicle, the type VI injury, too, rarely occurs in athletics. A high incidence of concomitant clavicle and rib fracture, nerve injury, and vascular compromise is present.

RADIOGRAPHIC EVALUATION

Radiographic evaluation of the acromioclavicular joint should consist of an anteroposterior (AP) radiograph of both acromioclavicular joints, taken with one-third to one-half the intensity needed for a quality radiograph of the glenohumeral joint. Zanca[47] recommended that the x-ray tube be tilted 10 to 15 degrees in a cephalic direction to avoid superimposition of the joint on the spine of the scapula. An axillary lateral view should also be obtained to demonstrate any posterior displacement of the distal clavicle and to rule out small fractures not apparent on the AP view as well as associated coracoid fractures. In the setting of significant trauma to the shoulder without obvious clavicular displacement, the scapulolateral radiograph taken with both shoulders thrust forward, causing anterior and inferior displacement of the acromion under the distal end of the clavicle, may confirm dislocation.[1]

Some controversy surrounds the use of stress radiographs to differentiate the type II injury from the type III dislocation, which can be difficult, if not impossible, to do clinically. Rockwood and Young[38] support their use when the physician believes that a type III or greater injury needs surgery, or if the physician wants to make a correct diagnosis of the degree of ligament injury. They emphasize that the radiographic feature of greatest importance in the stress view is not the coracoclavicular interspace distance, but rather the comparison of the interspace between the injured shoulder and the normal one. According to Beardon et al.,[5] a 40 to 50 percent increase in coracoclavicular distance of the injured shoulder over the normal shoulder should be considered a complete coracoclavicular ligament disruption. By contrast, Bossart and colleagues[9] found the use of stress radiographs unjustifiable because of their low percentage yield and, in fact, found that they actually decreased the coracoclavicular distance at times, further clouding the degree of injury.

Because it is our feeling that type III injuries can be managed successfully by nonoperative means in a manner similar to type II injuries, and because of the question of efficacy of stress radiographs, we do not recommend their use in the athletic population. Instead, we have found AP radiographs of the injured and normal shoulders and an axillary view to evaluate AP displacement of the injured shoulder to be sufficient for the evaluation of the athlete's traumatized shoulder in an acute setting.

TREATMENT

Treatment of acromioclavicular joint injuries has been a subject of much debate for many years, especially with regard to type III dislocations. Treatment of these injuries in the athlete has been the object of even more contention, as the demands for performance, quick return to sport, and longevity have never been greater. Residual weakness has been offered as a sequela of untreated acromioclavicular dislocation and a reason for repairing the joint in the athletic population, especially in the overhead throwing athlete.

The literature reflecting these controversies is extensive, and adherents of both nonoperative and operative management have presented justification for their treatment views. In so doing, three schools of thought have evolved: (1) nonoperative treatment of almost all types I to III injuries, (2) surgical repair for all type III or greater injuries, and (3) surgical repair for selected patients. Certainly, the athlete is a special patient for whom many have maintained that operative intervention is better despite recent evidence to the contrary.

Since Cooper[13] first operated for acromioclavicular joint dislocation in 1861, operative management has been the treatment of choice for many authors and remains so even today. Operative fixation has been said to give superior results in manual workers,[21] athletes,[26] and members of the armed services,[24] but comparative results have been described after nonoperative management in similar groups of patients.[20,22,43] Most of these studies have, however, proved inconclusive because most are retrospective in design, lack proper controls, present difficulties in comparing numerous surgical procedures and their associated complications, and lack objective data. Finally, very few studies have specifically addressed these injuries in the athletic population. We will outline our treatment principles below.

Type I Injury

The type I injury is the most common acromioclavicular joint injury in athletes. The acromioclavicular and coracoclavicular ligaments remain intact, but the acromioclavicular ligaments are strained. Frequently, the injury goes unnoticed until later in the day of injury or the day after injury. The athlete may even be asymptomatic until post-traumatic arthritis causes discomfort in the anterior-superior part of the shoulder in the months following injury. Again, the joint is stable, and the athlete maintains full ROM about the shoulder with discomfort usually only at the extremes of motion, especially abduction and flexion.

It is currently, universally agreed that treatment for the type I injury should consist of rest, ice, and anti-inflammatory medication. Some form of immobilization, such as a sling or shoulder immobilizer, may be used for comfort. Early ROM is instituted within the first few days following injury and is increased as tolerated by the athlete, with symptoms usually resolving in 7 to 10 days. Most authors report essentially 100 percent recovery following this injury, and most athletes are able to return to competition within 1 to 2 weeks. High-level throwers may take slightly longer (up to several weeks) to return to their preinjury level of performance. Upon return to competition, athletes should have pain-free ROM and the acromioclavicular joint should be nontender. Padding may be placed directly over the joint for protection if the patient is a contact sport participant.

Type II Injury

The type II injury is also frequently encountered in the athletic population. The damage consists of second-degree sprain of both the acromioclavicular and coracoclavicular ligaments with resultant partial displacement of the acromioclavicular joint less than the width of the clavicle. Because of the degree of pain and functional disability, the athlete is usually immediately aware of this injury and will often withdraw from competition at the time of injury or shortly thereafter. Physical examination will reveal considerable discomfort with and limitation of abduction and adduction of the shoulder. The stepoff between the clavicle and acromion is often readily apparent.

Treatment of this injury is again symptomatic, but many authors feel that the joint must be more aggressively supported due to the degree of ligamentous damage. Considerable differences of opinion exist as to the type and length of immobilization in the athlete. Various types of slings, bandages, adhesive tape strappings, braces, and harnesses have been advocated. Whatever method is used, the goal is to provide continuous compression of the coracoclavicular space to allow for ligamentous healing. This compression, however, is usually difficult to maintain.

In our experience, the shoulder immobilizer pro-

vides the necessary support and comfort to be effective in treatment. The length of immobilization depends on the symptoms and the type of athlete, but as a rule, 1 to 2 weeks of immobilization is sufficient for symptoms to abate in most. Some authors recommend up to 6 weeks of immobilization and avoidance of contact sports for 8 weeks to allow for complete ligamentous healing, thereby preventing conversion of a type II injury to a type III injury. This length of immobilization has, however, not been necessary in our experience. We allow the athlete to return to sport as soon as pain is gone and when the shoulder has full ROM, whenever that may be. The athlete should be informed that the deformity due to subluxation noted on presentation will likely be permanent, but will not interfere with strength or function unless post-traumatic arthritis sets in.

Chronically Symptomatic Type I and Type II Injuries

Although little attention has been paid to the sequelae of type I and type II injuries in past texts, these injuries can cause significant problems for the athlete in the months and years after injury. In considering the fate of acromioclavicular joint injuries in athletes, Cox in 1977[14] and Bergfeld et al. in 1978,[7] performed follow-up studies of midshipmen at the United States Naval Academy; they found a surprisingly large number of persistent positive physical findings as well as radiographic changes and significant symptoms (Table 8-2). The physical findings consisted of thickening and prominence of the acromioclavicular joint. The abnormal radiographic findings included post-traumatic degenerative changes about the joint and, commonly, osteolysis of the lateral clavicle in type I injuries. The late symptoms encountered in these studies consisted

Table 8-2. Long-Term Findings in Grades I and II Acromioclavicular Injuries

	Grade I (%)	Grade II (%)
Positive physical examination	43	71
Abnormal radiograph	29	48
Support system	3.5[a]	13[a]
	9[b]	23[b]

[a] Data from Cox.[14]
[b] Data from Bergfeld et al.[7]

of pain with throwing motions, serving in tennis, bench pressing, and dips between parallel bars. The cause of these symptoms appeared to be incongruity of the acromioclavicular joint as a result of tearing of the meniscus, or else post-traumatic arthritis.

Chronically symptomatic type I and type II injuries should not be taken lightly, because the associated disability might very well prevent return to sport. One should first ensure return of full strength and motion about the shoulder. Anti-inflammatory medication and rest during exacerbations may serve as temporizing measures. Consideration can be given to corticosteroid injection to relieve inflammation, with one or two repeat injections as necessary if the first is effective. In athletes who present with more complex shoulder symptoms, the injections may prove to be diagnostic as well as therapeutic. Ultimately it may be necessary to debride the joint, excise the meniscus, and, if the degenerative arthritis is marked, excise the distal clavicle.

Although many authors have expressed concern regarding loss of strength or function, or both, after the Mumford[31] procedure in the athlete, no report existed on 1 objective muscle testing following the operation prior to 1988, when Cook and Tibone[12] specifically addressed this issue in 23 athletes, including 6 at the professional level. At an average of 3.7 years after the Mumford procedure, all but 1 were satisfied with the procedure, and 16 returned to their same level of sports activity, including 5 of the 6 professional athletes. The most common complaint of those not achieving their previous level of sports was the inability to achieve their previous maximum bench press strength. All athletes demonstrated full motion, and at the faster Cybex testing speeds, little or no weakness or fatigue was demonstrated in the involved shoulder. Therefore the Mumford procedure not only provides for symptomatic relief but appears to allow for return to sport in most athletes, even at the professional level.

Type III Injury

Type III injuries are of higher energy, and the injured athlete usually experiences more significant anterior shoulder pain, limitation of motion, and downward displacement of the acromion and upper extremity. The athlete often leaves the field/court of competition supporting the injured limb with the opposite arm. The clavicle is freely movable and integrity of the acromioclavicular joint and coracoclavicular ligament is completely lost. Partial tears of the deltoid and trapezius from the distal clavicle are frequently associated.

Treatment of the type III injury remains controversial, but a definite trend toward nonoperative management has emerged in the last 20 years. In the 1950s, 1960s, and 1970s, clinicians appeared to be near consensus that the complete dislocation be managed by operative means. In 1974, Powers and Bach[35] surveyed chairman of United States residency programs and found that 95% would treat the injury operatively. Surgical treatment varied, but 60 percent used temporary acromioclavicular fixation, and 35 percent used coracoclavicular fixation. In sharp contrast, an informal 1980s poll of orthopaedic surgeons who treat athletes exclusively revealed that approximately 90 percent advocated nonoperative treatment.[6]

Nonoperative Treatment

Many forms of nonoperative treatment, including adhesive strapping, sling or bandage, sling/brace and harness, figure-of-eight bandage, and casts for acromioclavicular dislocation, have been employed, but the most commonly used method appears to be Kenny-Howard sling and harness immobilization, the sling supporting the forearm and arm, and the harness depressing the clavicle downward to provide reduction. Alternatively, many orthopaedists advocate *skillful neglect* treatment consisting of nothing more than a standard sling. Indeed, this form of management is recommended by many physicians who manage athletic injuries. In 1977, Glick and colleagues[20] reported on 35 unreduced type III injuries treated by skillful neglect and found that none of their athletes were disabled on follow-up. They recommended nonoperative treatment for these injuries, especially for athletes, since it allowed them to return to their event more quickly and "just as safely." The authors stressed the need for a vigorous shoulder-strengthening program. Cox[15] evaluated 13 type III dislocations in an athletic population, focusing attention on the often damaged deltoid and trapezius over the distal clavicle. He also strongly recommended rehabilitation of the injured musculature as an important aspect of nonoperative treatment.

Several recent studies have addressed the nonoperative treatment of type III injuries. In 1980, Darrow et al.[16] obtained good or excellent results in 16 of 19 patients treated by reduction and immobilization in a harness device for 6 weeks. In 1983, Bjerneld and colleagues[8] reported on a 5-year follow-up study with patients treated with a sling and early ROM when pain abated. Thirty of 33 patients obtained good or excellent results. The authors concluded that acromioclavicular joints have considerable potential to alter and adapt to the new position of the clavicle. A more vertical joint space is formed and, in most cases, the new joint is stable.

Although most of the recent orthopaedic literature supports nonoperative treatment of the type III injury even in the athletic population, questions still exist as to the long-term outcome of this treatment modality, especially with regard to persistent symptoms and functional limitations. Wojtys and Nelson[46] reported on 22 patients with type III injuries who were treated nonoperatively with a sling, a sling and swathe, or a Kenny-Howard sling. At 2- to 6-year follow-up many patients reported shoulder pain with activities such as throwing and contact sports, and some even with sleeping. Isokinetic testing showed the injured dominant arm to be significantly stronger than the uninjured nondominant side in adduction at 400 degrees/sec, in external rotation at 400 degrees/sec, and in external rotation at 60 degrees/sec. With isokinetic endurance testing, the uninjured nondominant side performed better on average, but the differences were insignificant. Forty-five percent rated their results as fair or poor. The authors concluded that patients with type III injuries who are involved in activities requiring strength and repetition will continue to function well in these activities but may very well continue to experience symptoms of pain and soreness.

Similarly, Tibone and colleagues[41] reported the results of isokinetic testing of 20 men with nonoperated type III injuries at an average of 4.5 years' follow-up. Testing showed no significant difference in strength for shoulder adduction, abduction, internal rotation, external rotation, flexion, or extension at speeds of 60 degrees/sec and 120 degrees/sec. Subjectively, 31 percent complained of mild pain with throwing but did not feel limited in their sports activities. They recommended conservative (nonoperative) treatment for these injuries.

From these two studies, it appears that active patients who sustain type III acromioclavicular injuries have a significant chance of experiencing pain and soreness with activity and sometimes at rest when treated nonoperatively, but they will not experience significant weakness about the shoulder, nor will they have significant functional limitations even with activities such as throwing.

Operative Treatment

Over the years, many different types of operative procedures have been described for treating type III injuries (Table 8-3). Today, most orthopaedic surgeons use one or a combination of the following four basic procedures: acromioclavicular repair and stabilization; coracoclavicular ligament repair, fixation, or reconstruction; excision of the distal clavicle; and dynamic muscle transfer. Various forms of fixation have been employed including pins or wires inserted through the acromioclavicular joint; loops of wire, resorbable tape, or fascia to connect the clavicle to the coracoid; or a screw introduced through the clavicle and into the coracoid (e.g., Bosworth screw). These operative techniques have met with varying degrees of success in the literature, but overall subjective and functional results appear comparable to those of the previously cited nonoperative techniques. However, complications, especially related to hardware use, arise in all reports of operative treatment modalities for this injury. These include K-wire migration to various locations, deltoid irritation, and accelerated post-traumatic arthritis. Clavicle fracture can occur after surgery with tape or wire around the coracoid.

Table 8-3. Operative Techniques for Type III Injuries

Primary acromioclavicular joint fixation	With pins, screws, suture wires, plates, and so forth, or reconstruction (i.e., with or without coracoclavicular ligament and/or acromioclavicular ligament repair or reconstruction)
Primary coracoclavicular ligament fixation	With screw, wire, fascia, conjoined tendon, or synthetic sutures
	With or without acromioclavicular ligament repair or reconstruction
Excision of the distal clavicle	With or without coracoclavicular ligament repair with fascia, suture, or coracoclavicular ligament repair with fascia, suture, or coracoacromial ligament transfer
Dynamic muscle transfers	With or without excision of the distal clavicle

In an effort to define the best method of operative repair, several authors have compared acromioclavicular and coracoclavicular fixation. The literature is inconclusive. Lancaster and colleagues[27] found a higher complication rate with acromioclavicular fixation but a higher failure rate with coracoclavicular fixation. By contrast, Bargren et al.[4] had superior results using a Dacron coracoclavicular loop when compared with acromioclavicular fixation with pins.[8] Taft et al.[40] found that patients managed with acromioclavicular fixation had a higher incidence of post-traumatic arthritis than those managed with a coracoclavicular screw.

Excision of the distal clavicle, often referred to as the Mumford procedure, has been performed in combination with a variety of procedures as treatment for acromioclavicular dislocations, in both the acute and chronic setting. In 1972, Weaver and Dunn[45] described their technique of excision of the distal 2 cm of the distal clavicle in combination with coracoacromial ligament transfer from its acromial attachment to the intramedullary canal of the clavicle, where it is held in place with suture through cortical holes. Rauschning et al.[36] performed this procedure in 12 patients with acute type III injuries and 5 patients with chronic symptoms following conservative treatment of type III injuries. All 17 cases demonstrated excellent results with painless, stable shoulders and normal shoulder strength on Cybex testing. As cited earlier, Cook and Tibone's[12] testing of athletes following the Mumford procedure met with similar results. Smith and Stewart[39] compared acromioclavicular fixation and coracoclavicular ligament repair with and without distal clavicle excision and found no differences in symptoms, ROM, or strength, but a higher incidence of degenerative changes in patients without distal clavicle excision.

It appears clear that excision of the distal clavicle is a necessary component of any procedure performed in the athlete with chronic symptoms following type III acromioclavicular joint injury. Additionally, it appears from recent studies that good strength and shoulder function can be expected following distal clavicle excision whether in an acute or chronic setting, with the possible exception of weight lifters who perform bench press exercises. What remains unclear is the role of distal clavicle excision in combination with coracoclavicular repair in the acute setting in the high-level athlete.

Operative Versus Nonoperative Treatment

It has long been suspected that failure to reduce and fix a complete acromioclavicular dislocation would result in a loss of shoulder strength and function, and this has been the rationale for many who prefer operative treatment of these injuries. However, none of the surgical methods described have been consistently shown to improve on the outcome following nonoperative management of the type III injury.

In a comparison of operative versus nonoperative treatment of complete acromioclavicular dislocations, Galpin et al.[19] showed that nonoperative treatment provided equal if not superior results, with earlier return to activities when compared with coracoclavicular screw fixation. Using a rating system incorporating subjective, objective, and roentgenographic criteria, Taft et al.[40] compared 52 patients treated with surgical reduction of the acromioclavicular joint with 75 patients treated nonoperatively. They found nearly equal results and a significantly higher rate of complication with operative management at an average of 9.5 years' follow-up. McDonald et al.[29] examined operative and nonoperative groups retrospectively for recovery of strength and function and found that most strength and flexibility tests showed no significant differences between these two groups. Some strength tests did indicate that nonoperative treatment of the complete acromioclavicular dislocation might be superior in restoring normal shoulder function. Similarly, Imatani et al.[22] found that nonoperative treatment gave equal, if not better results than operative treatment.[28]

Authors' Preferred Treatment for the Type III Injury

In light of these studies, it is understandable that many orthopaedic surgeons now favor nonoperative treatment for the complete acromioclavicular dislocation, even in high-level athletes. Comparative results have been attained with nonoperative methods of management. Additionally, contact athletes are at significant risk for reinjury to the shoulder and therefore performing a repair with its inherent risks is not advisable in our opinion. Instead, we advocate nonoperative treatment for the type III injury in the athlete using sling immobilization or a shoulder immobilizer and symptomatic treatment with rest, ice, and anti-inflammatory medication. The sling is discontinued and early ROM is instituted as soon as symptoms allow. The athlete progresses to resistance exercises as soon as they can be tolerated, and when pain-free ROM and strength has been attained, the athlete is allowed to return to competition. Until a specific surgical procedure has been shown to produce consistently better results, we will continue to manage athletes with this injury in this manner.

Long-Term Sequelae of Type III Injuries

Occasionally an athlete may present with chronic pain on overhead arm motion or with bench pressing, or both, following a complete acromioclavicular dislocation. If the pain or disability (or both) interfere with performance, and if the patient fails to evidence symptomatic relief after 2 to 3 months of conservative management, we recommend distal clavicle excision, coracoacromial ligament transfer, and coracoclavicular fixation without use of hardware. This operation eliminates the source of late problems by removal of the distal clavicle, most closely restores normal anatomy by coracoclavicular fixation, avoids complications secondary to use of hardware, and has demonstrated the best results to date of any procedure described in this setting. Bergfeld et al.[7] recommend simple resection of the lateral clavicle for those patients with severe calcification and scarring in the area of the coracoclavicular ligaments, which would otherwise make reduction very difficult.

Types IV, V, and VI Injuries

For the more severe and rare Rockwood types IV, V, and VI injuries, operative reduction and repair is often advocated for the athlete, since the great majority of these patients have chronic pain and deformity when managed nonoperatively.[37] Acromioclavicular fixation with or without distal clavicle excision are often employed following reduction. Special attention should be given to restoration of the deltotrapezius aponeurosis when torn.

Posterior dislocations or type IV injuries deserve special mention in the athletic population. Although they constitute fewer than 5% of acromioclavicular joint dislocations in most series, Bergfeld[6] has reported that they occur more commonly in the skeletally immature athlete, especially wrestlers. He recommends a computed-tomography scan with comparison to the opposite shoulder when posterior subluxation or dislocation cannot be confirmed by physical examination.

Injuries in Children

In general, children younger than 13 years who have sustained acromioclavicular joint injuries would be considered to have distal clavicle fractures and should be treated as such, usually nonoperatively. Children 13 years of age and older are treated as adults in our clinical practice.

CONCLUSIONS

The treatment of acromioclavicular joint injuries has been debated for many years, and the literature reflecting the controversy about the subject is extensive. Contact sport athletes are at considerable risk for sustaining these injuries, and in so doing often place their future participation and even likelihood in jeopardy as the demands for performance and quick return to sport following injury have never been greater.

It is now generally agreed that athletes who sustain type I or II injuries are best managed by some form of nonoperative treatment. The type III injury, however, has been the subject of more contention. The concern is whether an athlete with a completely dislocated acromioclavicular joint has a greater risk of poor function, loss of strength, and chronic symptoms when managed nonoperatively than does the athlete treated by surgical means. Although operative management for this injury continues to have its advocates, recent evidence and our experience suggest that these injuries in athletes are managed as effectively by nonoperative treatment, with equivalent results in terms of shoulder strength, shoulder motion, and return to sport. Occasionally later surgery is needed. The more severe types IV, V, and VI injuries are best managed by operative reduction and repair due to the extensive degree of soft tissue damage.

REFERENCES

1. Alexander OM: Radiography of the acromioclavicular joint. Radiography 15:260, 1949

2. Allman FL Jr: Fractures and ligamentous injuries of the clavicle and its articulation. J Bone Joint Surg [Am] 49A:774–784, 1967

3. Bannister GC, Wallace WA, Stableforth PG, Hutson MA: The management of acute acromioclavicular dislocation. J Bone Joint Surg [Br] 71B:848–850, 1989

4. Bargren JH, Erlanger S, Dick HM: Biomechanics and comparison of two operative methods of treatment of complete acromioclavicular separation. Clin Orthop 130:267–272, 1978

5. Bearden JM, Hughston JC, Whatley GS: Acromioclavicular dislocation: method of treatment. J Sports Med 1:5–17, 1973

6. Bergfeld JA: Acromioclavicular complex. p. 169. In: The Upper Extremity in Sports Medicine. CV Mosby, St. Louis, 1990

7. Bergfeld JA, Clancy WG, Sandrish JT: Evaluation of the acromioclavicular joint following first and second degree sprains. Am J Sports Med 6:153–159, 1978

8. Bjerneld H, Hovelius L, Thorling J: Acromioclavicular separations treated conservatively: a 5-year follow-up study. Acta Orthop Scand 54:743–745, 1983

9. Bossart PJ, Joyce SM, Manaster BJ, Packer SM: Lack of efficacy of 'weighted' radiographs in diagnosing acute acromioclavicular separation. Ann of Emerg Med 17:47–51, 1988

10. Cadenat FM: The treatment of dislocations and fractures of the outer end of the clavicle. Int Clin 1:145–169, 1917

11. Caldwell GD: Treatment of complete permanent acromioclavicular dislocation by surgical arthrodesis. J Bone Joint Surg 25:368–274, 1943

12. Cook FF, Tibone JE: The Mumford procedure in athletes: an objective analysis of function. Am J Sports Med 16:97–100, 1988

13. Cooper ES: New method of treating long standing dislocations of the scapuloclavicular articulation. Am J Med Sci 41:389–392, 1861

14. Cox JS: The fate of the acromioclavicular joint in athletic injuries. Am J Sports Med 9:50–53, 1981

15. Cox JS: The fate of the acromioclavicular joint in athletic injuries. Am J Sports Med 9:50–53, 1981

16. Darrow JC, Smith JA, Lockwood RC: A new conservative method for treatment of type III acromioclavicular separations. Orthop Clin North Am 11:727–733, 1980

17. DePalma AF: Surgery of the Shoulder. 2nd Ed. JB Lippincott, Philadelphia, 1973

18. Fukuda K, Craig EV, An K-N, Cofield RH: Anatomic and biomechanical studies of the ligamentous system of the acromioclavicular joint. J Bone Joint Surg [Am] 68A:434–439, 1986

19. Galpin RD, Hawkins RJ, Grainger RW: A comparative analysis of operative versus nonoperative treatment of grade III acromioclavicular separations. Clin Orthop 193:150–155, 1985

20. Glick JM, Milburn LJ, Haggerty JF, Nishimoto D: Dislocated acromioclavicular joint: follow-up study of 35 unreduced acromioclavicular dislocations. Am J Sports Med 5:264–270, 1977

21. Horn JS: The traumatic anatomy and treatment of acute acromioclavicular dislocation. J Bone Joint Surg [Br] 36B:194–201, 1954

22. Imatani RJ, Hanlon JJ, Cady GW: Acute complete acromioclavicular separation. J Bone Joint Surg [Am] 57A:328–332, 1975

23. Inman VT, Saunders JB, Abbott LC: Observations on the function of the shoulder joint. J Bone Joint Surg 26:1–30, 1944

24. Kato F, Hayashi H, Miyazaki T et al: Treatment of acute complete dislocation of the acromioclavicular joint. p. 67. In Bateman JE, Welsh RP (eds): Surgery of the Shoulder. CV Mosby, St. Louis, 1984

25. Kennedy JC: Complete dislocation of the acromioclavicular joint: 14 years later. J Trauma 8:311–318, 1968

26. Kennedy JC, Cameron H: Complete dislocation of the acromioclavicular joint. J Bone Joint Surg [Br] 36B:202–208, 1954

27. Lancaster S, Horowitz M, Alonso J: Complete acromioclavicular separations: a comparison of operative methods. Clin Orthop 216:80–88, 1987

28. Larsen E, Bjerg-Neilsen A, Christensen P: Conservative or surgical treatment of acromioclavicular dislocation: a prospective, controlled randomized study. J Bone Joint Surg [Am] 68A:552–555, 1986

29. McDonald PB, Alexander MJ, Frejuk J, Johnson GE: Comprehensive functional analysis of shoulders following complete acromioclavicular separation. Am J Sports Med 16:475–480, 1988

30. Moseley HF: Athletic injuries to the shoulder region. Am J Surg 98:401–422, 1959

31. Mumford EB: Acromioclavicular dislocation. J Bone Joint Surg 23:799–802, 1941

32. Neer CS, Rockwood CA: Fractures and dislocations of the shoulder. In Rockwood CA, Green DP (eds): Fractures in Adults. JB Lippincott, Philadelphia, 1984

33. Peterson L, Renström P: Sports Injuries: Their Prevention and Treatment. Martin Dunitz, London, 1985

34. Poirier P, Rieffel H: Mechanisme des luxations sur acromiales de la clavicule. Arch Gen Med 1:396–422, 1891

35. Powers JA, Bach PJ: Acromioclavicular separations—closed or open treatment. Clin Orthop 102:213–223, 1974

36. Rauschning W, Nordesjo LO, Nordgren B et al: Resection arthroplasty for repair of complete acromioclavicular separations. Arch Orthop Trauma Surg 97: 161–164

37. Rockwood CA Jr: Injuries to the acromioclavicular joint. p. 860. Rockwood CA, Green DP (ed): Fractures in Adults. Vol. 1. 2nd Ed. JB Lippincott, Philadelphia, 1984

38. Rockwood CA Jr, Young DC: Disorders of the acromioclavicular joint. p. 413. In: The Shoulder. Vol. 1. WB Saunders, Philadelphia, 1990

39. Smith MJ, Stewart MJ: Acute acromioclavicular separations. Am J Sports Med 7:62–71, 1979

40. Taft TN, Wilson FC, Oglesby JW: Dislocation of the acromioclavicular joint: an end-result study. J Bone Joint Surg [Am] 69A:1045–1051, 1987

41. Tibone J, Sellers R, Tonino P: Strength testing after third-degree acromioclavicular dislocations. Am J Sports Med 20:328–331, 1992

42. Tossy JD, Mead NC, Sigmond HM: Acromioclavicular separations: useful and practical classification for treatment. Clin Orthop 28:111–119, 1963

43. Urist MR: Complete dislocation of the acromioclavicular joint: the nature of the traumatic lesion and effective methods of treatment with an analysis of 41 cases. J Bone Joint Surg 28:813–837, 1946

44. Urist MR: The treatment of dislocation of the acromioclavicular joint. Am J Surg 98:423–431, 1959

45. Weaver JK, Dunn HK: Treatment of acromioclavicular injuries, especially complete acromioclavicular separation. J Bone Joint Surg [Am] 54A:1187–1197, 1972

46. Wojtys EM, Nelson G: General orthopaedics: conservative treatment of grade III acromioclavicular dislocations. Clin Orthop 268:112–119, 1991

47. Zanca P: Shoulder pain: involvement of the acromioclavicular joint: analysis of 1,000 cases. Am J Radiol 112:493–506, 1971

9

Functional Anatomy and Applied Biomechanics of the Elbow

HING-CHUEN TSENG
PING-CHUNG LEUNG
K. M. CHAN

INTRODUCTION

The elbow is a complex joint that serves as a lever for positioning the hand in space, as a fulcrum for power lifting activities, and as a stable linkage to the upper limb for fine and strenuous activities. It is intrinsically stable due to the congruous articulation among the distal humerus, proximal radius, and ulna as well as the soft tissue restraints, consisting of a tough capsule with strong thickened collateral ligaments.

The elbow's chief function (positioning the hand in space) is demonstrated by our ability to subconsciously and effortlessly bend it to raise the hand to the face or extend it to lower the hand to the feet. Its fulcrum and load-bearing function allows actions such as lifting, pushing, and throwing. A mobile and stable elbow joint is necessary for most daily activities and for recreational and professional sports. A stiff, incongruous, or unstable elbow joint that results from fracture malunion or rheumatoid arthritis severely affects function in work and sports.

Besides major traumatic problems in athletics, chronic repetitive stress and overuse account for most elbow syndromes. Overhead activities such as throwing and pitching, racquet sports, swimming, contact sports, and fencing can all produce elbow injuries. These activities share the common demand of valgus strain to the elbow.

In this chapter, we first analyze the anatomic and biomechanical factors that contribute to a stable and mobile elbow. Mechanisms causing elbow injuries are described. Then we look at throwing as an example of sport activities that may contribute to elbow injuries. Special bone and joint problems in young, skeletally immature athletes are briefly discussed. It is a common belief that sports injuries mostly occur in the lower limb. In reality, the elbow is used so often in racquet sports and most other athletic activities that chronic sprain and careless use often lead to long-term problems, ranging from an ailment to disabling trouble. In this chapter, our intention is to bring some of the overlooked sports-related pathologies back to the right perspective.

ANATOMIC AND BIOMECHANICAL BACKGROUND OF ELBOW INJURIES

The basic structures that contribute to the stability of the elbow joint include the following:

1. Osteoarticular surfaces (radiocapitellar, ulnotrochlear, and proximal radioulnar joints)
2. Joint capsule
3. Collateral ligaments (medial and lateral)
4. Tendons and muscles around the joint (medial flexor-pronator, lateral wrist extensors and anconeus, posterior triceps, and anterior elbow flexors)

Osteoarticular Surfaces

The elbow has conventionally been described as a hinge joint. However, the combination of flexion and extension with pronation and supination allows much greater motion flexibility. It is therefore more appropriate to classify this joint as a trochoginglymus joint (*trochus*, a disc; *ginglymus*, a hinge), which carries the meaning of a hinge while at the same time suggests the ability to glide.[7]

The distal humeral trochlear and capitellar condyles articulate with the greater sigmoid notch and the radial head, respectively (Fig. 9-1). The circular margin of the radial head articulates with the lesser sigmoid notch. The tip of the olecranon and the coronoid process fits into the olecranon and coronoid fossae of the humerus during full extension and flexion, respectively. Any irregularity of the radiocapitellar joint, any deformities at the coronoid or olecranon, or narrowed fossae of the olecranon or the coronoid would lead to limitations of flexion and extension. Any abnormality of the radioulnar articulation destroys the congruity of the joint and leads to limitation of pronation and supination. The bony articular configurations of the elbow joint itself contribute to 50 percent of the stability.

The distal humeral condyles lie along a line making a 6-degree valgus angle with the coronal plane (Fig. 9-2A). This line is also rotated about 30 degrees anteriorly in the sagittal plane (Fig. 9-2B). The 30-degree posterior rotation of the articular surface of the ulnar notch matches well the anterior rotation of the distal humerus (Fig. 9-2C). This provides stability in full extension. The articular surface of the greater sigmoid notch is discontinuous in the midsection, which is covered by fatty or fibrous tissue in 90 percent of individuals.[18] As this section is not supported by strong subchondral bone, it is inherently weak and prone to fracture. This knowledge helps us to plan the transolecranon osteotomy to expose the elbow without damaging the hyaline cartilage of the greater sigmoid notch. In arthroscopy, this deficiency of articular cartilage must not be mistaken for a pathologic entity.

Carrying Angle

The carrying angle is formed by the long axis of the humerus and the long axis of the ulna. It is measured in the frontal plane with the elbow extended. The 4-degree proximal ulnar valgus and 6-degree distal humeral valgus angulation combine to produce a 10- to 15-degree valgus carrying angle (average, 10 to 15 degrees in men and 5 degrees more in women). This tends to increase among athletes and must be recognized as a "normal" deviation in this population.[20]

Radial-Capitellar Joint

The capitellum is a 180-degree hemisphere covered anteriorly and inferiorly with cartilage. It buttresses the lateral compression and rotational force during throwing. The articular surface margin of the radial head consists of 280 degrees of articular cartilage and 80 degrees of nonchondral margin. Only the cartilaginous portion articulates with the lesser sigmoid notch of the ulna. The anterolateral nonarticular portion of the radial head lacks the stronger subchondral bone support. Therefore slice or shear fracture of the radial head frequently occurs here. Such extra-articular fractures may not lead to limitation of forearm rotation if displacement is minimal. The 15-degree angulation of the radial neck away from the radial tuberosity, coupled with the bowing of the radius, allows forearm rotation of almost 180 degrees, while the radial head maintains precise axial alignment with the capitellum (Fig. 9-1D). This avoids the impingement of the radial tuberosity on the adjacent ulna during full supination. Another mechanism working to avoid this impingement is the 2-mm lateral displacement of the slightly ovoid radial head during full supination.

Elbow Axis of Rotation

Normal elbow flexion is 0 to 150 degrees. Pronation is 75 degrees and supination is 85 degrees. Most activities of daily living may be accomplished with a functional arc in flexion-extension of 100 degrees (30 to 130 degrees) and in pronation-supination of 100 degrees also (50 degrees of pronation to 50 degrees of supination).[10]

Young throwers may have elbow flexion contractures of up to 12 degrees and valgus deformities of up to 37 degrees. This results from abnormal growth and secondary joint changes due to overuse. These deformities may adversely affect future elbow function and stability and may even result in tardy ulnar nerve palsy.

The axis of elbow flexion and extension passes through the centers of projection of the capitellum and the trochlea, a line connecting the middle of the lateral epicondyle and the anteroinferior aspect of the medial

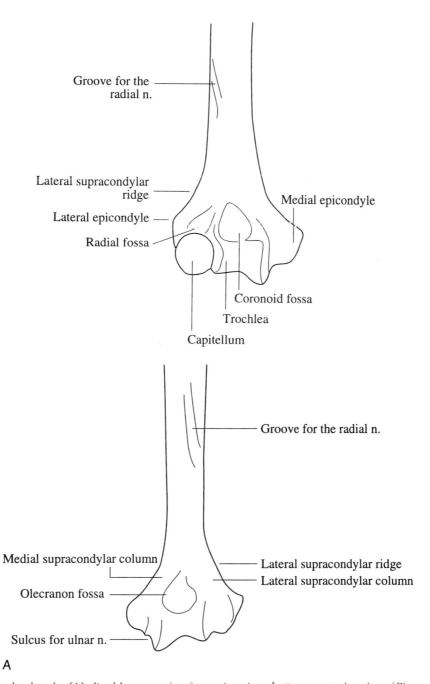

Fig. 9-1. Bony landmarks **(A)** distal humerus (*top*) anterior view; *bottom*, posterior view. (*Figure continues.*)

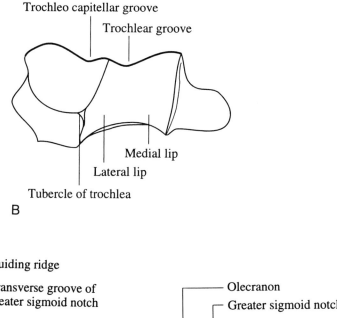

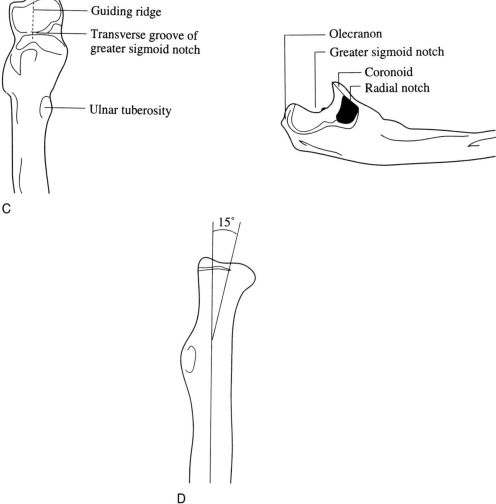

Fig. 9-1 (*Continued*). **(B)** Axial view of distal humerus. **(C)** Proximal ulna. **(D)** Proximal radius.

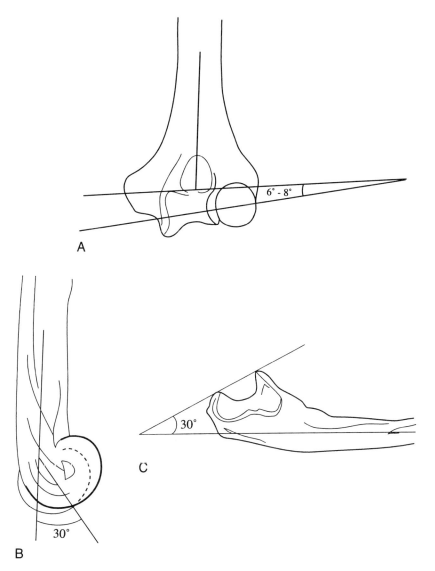

Fig. 9-2. **(A)** Valgus tilt of distal humeral articulation. **(B)** Lateral view of humerus showing 30-degree anterior rotation of humeral articular condyles in the sagittal plane. **(C)** Lateral view of the proximal ulna showing 30-degree posterior rotation of the articular surface of the greater sigmoid notch.

epicondyle, which are the landmarks for the origins of the collateral ligaments.

Axis of Forearm Rotation

The axis of forearm rotation is usually considered to be a line passing through the capitellum and the head of the radius extending to the distal ulna. Ray et al.[15] found slight abduction/adduction of the distal ulna during forearm pronation and supination around an axis through the index finger. Kapandji[5] suggested that the distal ulna is displaced in a small arc consisting of a lateral extension component, whereas the distal radius rotates around a larger arc. The common center of both arcs lies on the axis of pronation-supination (Fig. 9-3).

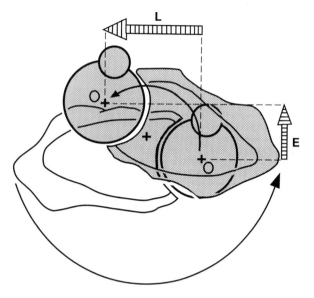

Fig. 9-3. The axis of forearm rotation. (From Kapandji,[5] with permission.)

Collateral Ligaments

The predominant stressor to the elbow in most activities is valgus. Throwing, hammering, and falling on an outstretched hand all subject the elbow to valgus stress. The first line of defense against this valgus stress is the flexor forearm mass. This is rarely injured unless valgus stress is associated with a sudden massive wrist flexion as in throwing.[7]

Medial Collateral Ligament Complex

The medial collateral ligament (MCL) complex is the strongest ligamentous restraint for this valgus force. It consists of anterior and posterior bundles (sometimes named anterior and posterior oblique bands) plus a transverse ligament (Fig. 9-4A).

The transverse ligament spanning the two bundles is a thickening of the caudalmost portion of the joint capsule that serves to expand the greater sigmoid

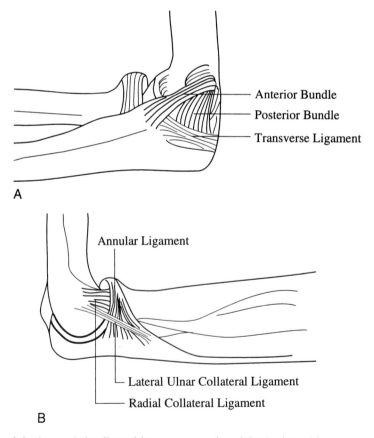

Fig. 9-4. (A) The medial collateral ligament complex. **(B)** The lateral ligament complex.

notch. The anterior bundle inserts into the medial aspect of the corocoid process of the ulna just distal to the articular margin. Its humeral origin is eccentrically located at the inferomedial surface of the medial epicondyle, away from the axis of elbow flexion. It is rectangular, with anterior fibers taut in extension and posterior fibers taut in flexion. This combines to provide stability throughout the full range of motion.[17] Furthermore, the anterior bundle is also the most important factor in resisting valgus stress at the elbow. The posterior bundle of the MCL contributes minimally to elbow stability except in end flexion. In cadaveric specimens, valgus stability is maintained when the posterior bundle is sectioned and the anterior bundle is left intact. This stability is lost if the anterior bundle is sectioned even if the posterior bundle is intact.[17] Hotchkiss and Weiland[2] and multiple investigators concur that the anterior band of the MCL is the most important valgus stabilizer. Excision of the radial head reduces valgus stability by 30 percent which is not improved with silicone rubber replacement.

Lateral Collateral Ligament Complex

The lateral collateral ligament complex (LCLC) consists of a lateral collateral ligament (LCL) and a lateral ulnar collateral ligament (LUCL)[6] (Fig. 4b).

The LCL originates from the lateral epicondyle and fans out to insert into the annular ligament. The origin of the LCL is coincident with the axis of rotation of the elbow. Therefore its tension is constant throughout the range of elbow motion. It does not perform the function of a true collateral ligament, which should have bone-to-bone attachment. Tullos et al.[19] found that the only structure that conforms to a true LCL is the anconeus muscle, which originates in the lateral epicondyle and inserts into the proximal ulna.

Morrey and O'Driscoll[10] noted the importance of the LUCL component of the LCL complex in preventing posterolateral rotatory instability. They proposed a posterolateral rotatory subluxation test to diagnose this disorder. The LUCL is present in 90 percent of the population.[6] It originates at the midpoint of the lateral epicondyle, crosses the radiocapitellar joint, and inserts into the tubercle of the crista musculi supinatorus on the ulna. If the LUCL is released, the remaining intact LCL cannot prevent the elbow from subluxating in an inferior rotatory type of mechanism (pivot shift phenomenon of the elbow joint).[14] Conversely, releasing the LCL while preserving the LUCL does not allow this instability. The LUCL complements the MCL in providing varus stability to the ulnohumeral joint, independent of the LCL or the presence of the radial head. The annular ligament stabilizes and holds the radial head tightly against the ulnar.

Tendons and Muscles

The elbow flexors are the brachialis, biceps, brachioradialis, and the flexor pronator that originates from the medial epicondyle. The main elbow extensors are the triceps and the anconeus. Since the flexor muscles act through a short moment arm, a large muscle force is needed to hold a weight in the hand at greater distance from the center of elbow flexion. A large joint reaction force is created, especially when lifting at full extension. This may predispose the joint to injury and degeneration. Therefore, some consider the elbow to be a weight-bearing joint. However, rapid joint motion, as in throwing, can easily be facilitated.[1]

The actively contracting common extensors that originate from the lateral epicondyle are commonly injured by excessive or repeated stress transmitted from the tendons that insert into the wrist. An electromyographic study by Morrey[6] showed that:

1. The biceps is less active in full forearm pronation because of its secondary role as supinator.
2. The brachialis is the workhorse of flexion, as it is active in most ranges of function.
3. Triceps activity increases with elbow flexion. Different heads of triceps and biceps are active in the same manner through most motions.
4. The anconeus is active in all positions. Therefore it is considered to be a dynamic joint stabilizer.

Elbow Joint Capsule

The capsule is bonded anteriorly to the biceps and brachialis and posteriorly to the triceps muscle and tendon. Although the anterior elbow joint capsule is thin and filamentous, its fibers become taut in extension. It functions to limit elbow extension and provides significant varus-valgus stability when the elbow is in full extension.

The normal maximal elbow joint capacity of 25 ml occurs with the elbow in 80 degrees of flexion. Therefore patients hold their elbows in 80 to 90 degrees of flexion after an injury with hemarthrosis. This is also the commonest position for elbow ankylosis, and the extension night splint has thus been advocated to prevent this problem after elbow injury.[13]

The capsule's resistance to disruption is low, and mechanical fluid pumps should be used cautiously in arthroscopic procedures. Though normally thin, the anterior capsule will respond to injury with aggressive repair, fibrosis, and contracture, especially with injudicious passive mobilization. This may be complicated by the development of a dense, thick, and later calcified capsule.

Joint Stiffness and Contracture

The elbow joint is particularly prone to developing stiffness due to its high congruency, close continuity of the muscle to the capsule, propensity for comminuted fractures, and unique response to trauma.[8] The incidence of post-traumatic elbow stiffness is usually related to the severity of the injury.

An intra-articular callus may limit motion because the elbow is so congruous. Osteophyte and ectopic calcification may limit flexion/extension. The brachialis muscle, which traverses the elbow joint over the anterior capsule, tears with dislocation. Due to its rich vascularity and large muscle bulk, it is prone to developing scar tissue and ectopic bone during healing. Its rich vascularity also induces contracture of the elbow joint capsule. Half of distal humeral fractures are of the intra-articular T or Y type, and one-half of these are comminuted. These fractures heal poorly and are prone to malunion. The elbow joint, which is tightly congruous, is prone to developing intra-articular adhesions. The three separate articulations may further contribute to the complexity of the fracture, increasing the chance for malunion and scar contracture after healing.

MECHANISMS OF ELBOW STABILITY

Stability against varus/valgus stress and anterior/posterior stability are discussed separately below. The role of different stabilizers also varies in different degrees of elbow flexion and extension. On the whole, the articular congruity and soft tissue constraints contribute roughly equal proportions to elbow stability.

Stability in Valgus

The MCL is the primary stabilizer to valgus stress. The anterior oblique portion of this ligament maintains the stability against valgus stress even when the posterior oblique band is sectioned.

In 90-degree flexion, the medial collateral ligament contributes to 54 percent of the valgus stability. The remainder is provided by the shape of the articular surface and the anterior capsule.[9] The posterior bundle of the MCL provides stability beyond 90 degrees of elbow flexion. In extension, the olecranon is locked in its fossa. Therefore the contribution to valgus stability becomes equally distributed among the MCL, the shape of the articular surfaces, and the anterior capsule.[9]

Stability in Varus

As the lateral ligament complex of the elbow is relatively weak, the capsule and the joint articulation provide the major resistance against varus stress. Morrey and An[9] showed that at 90 degrees of flexion, the radial collateral ligament contributes to only 9 percent of the varus stability. Joint articulation provides 78 percent and the joint capsule 13 percent. In extension, the LCL contributes to 14% of the stability. The remaining 54 percent is provided by joint articulation and 32 percent by the joint capsule. The LCL is usually transected or functionally impaired after the radial head excision. If the LUCL is preserved, varus stability may still be maintained. The anconeus is the main dynamic stabilizer against varus stress.

Anterior-Posterior Stability

Again, the MCL is the major stabilizer here. With intact MCL, excision of 40 to 90 percent of the olecranon (sparing the coronoid insertion of the anterior oblique band of the MCL) does not significantly affect elbow stability.[17] Conversely, excision of the MCL destabilizes the elbow even if the olecranon is intact.

The overall composite stability of the elbow against varus/valgus, rotational, and anteroposterior stress is affected by serial removal of the olecranon, especially when the MCL is affected by removing the distal olecranon.[7] The role of the radial head in elbow stability is more difficult to quantitate. It does provide 15 to 30 percent of the overall resistance to the valgus depending on joint position and mechanism of loading. Anterior instability may be associated with massive elbow trauma, with fracture displacement of the olecranon and collateral ligament rupture.

MECHANISMS OF ELBOW INSTABILITY

Elbow instability can be classified according to the articulations involved, the degree of displacement, the direction of displacement, the chronicity of the injury, and whether fractures are associated.[12]

Importance of the Medial Collateral Ligament

As mentioned above, the MCL is very important for maintenance of valgus stability. It may be injured in acute trauma or chronic overload. Associated injuries include tear of the common flexor pronator origin or lateral ligament complex and fracture of the radial head, all of which contribute to elbow instability.

Traumatic dislocation of the elbow may result from hyperextension. During this injury, the olecranon impinges into the olecranon fossa and hinges open the anterior aspect of the joint, tearing the thin anterior capsule and the anterior bundle of the MCL. When the anterior bundle fails, the trochlea rides superiorly over the top of the coronoid process, resulting in a dislocation. Since the slope of the trochlea is lateral, the dislocation is usually posterior and lateral. The large lateral translational force may further avulse or tear the remaining MCL at its substance or cause a fracture at the medial epicondyle.[19]

Tullos et al.[19] showed that 34 of the 37 elbow dislocations had valgus instability after reduction of the dislocation. All had an anterior bundle MCL tear on exploration. Surgical repair of the MCL results in better function. Therefore they recommended surgical intervention for those elbows that spontaneously redislocate after a reduction. MCL repair can restore valgus stability even if the radial head is also fractured during the dislocation.

However, O'Driscoll[13] believes that the MCL "usually heals following elbow dislocation, perhaps because of the vascularized muscles that surround it and the inherent stability of the reduced joint." If the MCL is functionally incompetent due to healing in a length-

ened position, then the ulnotrochlear joint may be easily disengaged without hyperextension.

Schwab et al.[17] showed that experimentally, posterior and posterolateral dislocation of the elbow cannot be produced without functional disruption of the MCL. However, in clinical practice, the MCL may be intact after a posterior dislocation, and some patients may not give a history of elbow hyperextension.

The Circle Hypothesis and Importance of the Lateral Collateral Ligament Complex

More recently, O'Driscoll et al.[13] proposed the circle hypothesis to explain an alternative mechanism of elbow instability. They observed that elbow dislocation does not necessarily result from hyperextension. Rather, when the outstretched hand attempts to break a fall, axial force is transmitted to the flexed elbow. This, together with the external rotation/supination and valgus moment (because the mechanical axis is medial to the elbow) on the elbow, may induce a posterolateral rotatory subluxation or dislocation of the elbow (Fig. 9-5). The radius and ulnar supinate together and externally rotate as one piece away from the capitellum and the trochlea, with the coronoid pass

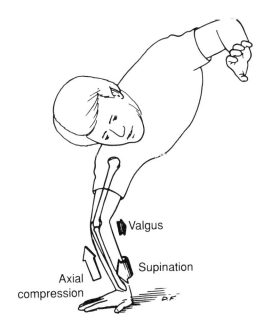

Fig. 9-5. Proposed mechanism of elbow dislocation. (From O'Driscoll,[12] with permission.)

inferior to the trochlea. It is considered to be the most common pattern of elbow dislocation.

The circle of soft tissue from the lateral to the medial side of the elbow may be disrupted in three stages (Fig. 9-6). In stage one, the lateral ulnar collateral ligament is disrupted. This is already sufficient to cause a posterolateral rotatory subluxation of the elbow, which will reduce spontaneously. In stage 2, further force will cause a disruption to the remaining LCL complex as well as the anterior and posterior elbow joint capsule, and an incomplete posterolateral dislocation may result. In stage 3, the MCL is involved. In stage 3A, only the posterior band of the MCL is torn. The elbow pivots around the intact anterior band of the MCL, allowing a posterior dislocation via a posterolateral rotatory mechanism. In the final stage, 3B, the MCL is completely disrupted, and gross varus, valgus, and rotatory instability exist follow reduction.

This mechanism was confirmed by O'Driscoll and colleagues[13] in a cadaveric study. In order to preserve any undisrupted medial soft tissue, O'Driscoll recommended that posterior elbow dislocations be reduced in supination so that the coronoid process may be cleared under the trochlea. After reduction of the dislocation, splintage in full pronation is helpful in recruiting any remaining medial soft tissue as a hinge to provide stability against redislocation. Patients with lateral collateral deficiency will report recurrent snapping, clicking, locking, or sensation of bones "slipping out of the joint" especially when their elbows are supinated and extended. Some are symptomatic during elbow flexion and pronation when the elbow is really reducing from the subluxed supinated extended position. These symptoms usually occur after a subluxation, dislocation, fracture, or surgery of the elbow that has damaged the LUCL. Isolated traumatic LCL complex injury without elbow joint subluxation/dislocation is rare. More commonly, iatrogenic injury to the LUCL can subsequently be seen to release the common extensor tendon for lateral epicondylitis or radial head excision.[9] Morrey found that 25 percent of the failed tennis elbow surgery cases are related to LCL complex insufficiency. Varus injury to the elbow is uncommon.

MECHANISMS OF ELBOW INJURIES

Acute and chronic elbow pain and instability are common in the young athlete. These occur as the sequelae of acute injuries, repetitive injuries, or chronic overuse. Athletes exert their elbows in diverse activities such as catching, throwing, hammering, pushing, and pulling.

Injuries can be sports-specific. Upper extremity macrotrauma with fracture and dislocation may occur in football, wrestling, and ice hockey. Conversely, wear and tear of soft tissues, cartilaginous growth plate, and joint articular surfaces may occur with repeated overuse injuries. Injuries may also be age-specific. In the young and immature, growth plate and cartilaginous injury may result in deformity and functional disability. Above middle age, degeneration, tissue ischemia, and reduced healing potential all contribute to protracted tendinitis.

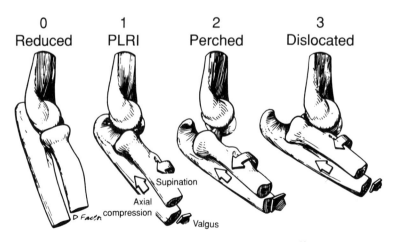

Fig. 9-6. Clinical stages of elbow instability. (From O'Driscoll,[12] with permission.)

Acute stress and chronic overuse involve the ligaments, capsule, muscles, and articular surfaces of the joint. These cause functional impairments in the elbow joint. However, competitive athletes with ligamentous instabilities seldom encounter elbow fractures, unlike their counterparts in the general population. Instability of the elbow is mainly due to valgus stress. Pain, weakness, and recurrent posterior or posterolateral dislocations are sequelae of this instability. In the following sections, we use throwing to illustrate the mechanism of elbow injuries in sports. Specific elbow problems that are unique among young athletes are described in other chapters.

BIOMECHANICS OF THROWING

Four Stages of Throwing

Throwing is divided into four stages[4] (Fig. 9-7):

1. *Wind-up*: this is the initial activity prior to cocking.
2. *Cocking*: the throwing arm proceeds to abduct and rotate externally maximally. Contact of the forefoot divides this stage into early and late phases.
3. *Acceleration*: this stage begins with the end of maximal shoulder external rotation until the ball is released. Valgus strain to the elbow occurs in this phase as the forearm lags behind the trunk and shoulder.
4. *Follow-through*: the forearm proceeds to pronation in this stage.

During the late cocking and acceleration phase of overhead or throwing activities, large valgus tension forces exist in the medial aspect of the elbow with similar large compression forces occurring on the radiocapitellar joint. During this phase, the elbow is flexed between 90 and 120 degrees. The elbow extends to about 25 degrees at ball release. In this range, the elbow is stabilized against valgus force almost solely by the anterior band of the MCL, with little contribution from the bony components.[2,7,11,17]

With improper techniques and mechanics, poor conditioning, poor flexibility, and fatigue, cumulative effects can lead to flexor pronator muscle strain, which allows further stress onto the ulnar collateral ligament. If this force exceeds the tensile strength of the MCL, or if stress is applied at a rate greater than tissue repair, microscopic tears and progressive attenuation leading to rupture of the weakened ligament can occur. This is the overuse syndrome.

Four Stages of Ligamentous Injury

The four stages of ligamentous injury in the overuse syndrome described by Jobe and Nuber[16] are:

1. Edema and inflammation are present, leading to pain, tenderness and swelling.
2. Dissociation of fibers, fibrosis, and scarring occurs. Resolution of symptoms without permanent deformity is expected up to this stage after proper rest and treatment.

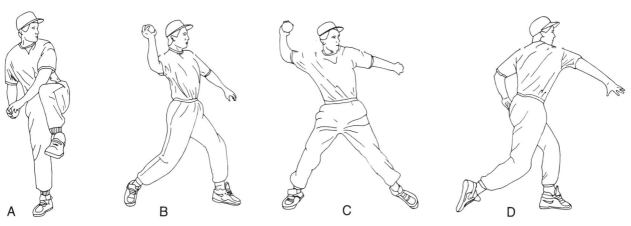

Fig. 9-7. The four stages of throwing. **(A)** Wind-up phase. **(B)** Cocking phase. **(C)** Acceleration phase. **(D)** Follow-through phase.

3. With continued stress and bleeding, calcification of the scarred tissue will lead to joint stiffness. Unequal force distribution may lead to a "stress raiser" within the ligament, which may rupture with minor stress.

4. Ligament becomes attenuated and functionless and may be completely torn. Ligament ossification may lead to pain, stiffness, joint crepitation, and loose body formation.

The patient may report a medial elbow pain, especially during late cocking of the acceleration phase of throwing. Preceding events may include an episode of acute "pop" with sharp pain, gradual onset of pain, or pain following a period of heavy throwing. The ability to throw will be compromised.[3]

Furthermore, incompetency of the MCL results in an increased valgus carrying angle. The medial tip of the olecranon may impinge on the medial wall of the olecranon fossa and produce loose bodies and osteophytes. This accounts for the flexion contracture in professional throwers. With an incompetent MCL and a valgus carrying angle, further valgus stress during throwing produces abnormal compressive stress on the radiocapitellar joint. This joint acts as the secondary stabilizer to valgus stress when the MCL is unstable. A summary of overuse and excessive valgus stress injuries on the elbow is as follows:

1. Articular disturbances: osteophytes, loose bodies, osteochondral defects, and degenerative changes
2. Muscle damages including scarring and ruptures
3. Nerve injuries leading to scarring and nerve entrapment
4. Symptomatic accessory ossicles about the elbow with fragmentation, fracture, or enlargement with impingement
5. In the skeletally immature, epiphyseal and apophyseal hypertrophy, fragmentation, and avulsion

Apart from throwing, few other activities expose the MCL to such stress. This explains why symptomatic elbow instability related to MCL injury rarely occurs in the general population.[15]

Neurologic Injuries in Throwers

Over 40 percent of the patients with MCL insufficiency develop symptoms of ulnar nerve impairment. The ulnar nerve transverses the elbow in the cubital tunnel beneath the medial epicondyle. The cubital tunnel reti-naculum forms the roof of this tunnel. It is the major constraint preventing the subluxation of the ulnar nerve as it passes behind the medial epicondyle. When the elbow is flexed, the retinaculum is tightened, flattening the space for the ulnar nerve, and thus may impinge upon the ulnar nerve. When the retinaculum is deficient, ulnar nerve subluxation occurs. Nerve injuries arise from direct and indirect trauma. Indirect trauma includes traction, friction, and compression (entrapment neuropathy). Medical conditions such as diabetes mellitus, rheumatoid arthritis, hypothyroidism, alcoholism, malnourishment, and renal failure may be predisposing or aggravating factors.

Possible mechanisms for ulnar nerve injury around the elbow in throwers are:

1. *Restriction of ulnar nerve movement:* Normally, the ulnar nerve is free to move medially and longitudinally in its groove. Restriction of this movement (e.g., by scarring and edema after MCL injury) may lead to compressive neuropathy or tethering of the nerve during throwing. Repeated MCL injuries leading to fibrosis, scarring, soft tissue calcification, and ossification further increase this movement restriction. Muscle hypertrophy in the dominant limb of an athlete may have similar effects. In the late stage, ischemic damage to the nerve may occur.

2. *Valgus tensile force on the elbow:* This may injure the ulnar nerve inside the cubital tunnel. It may occur under the following conditions:
   a. The acceleration phase of throwing.
   b. A torn medial collateral ligament complex and malunited medial epicondylar separation causing elbow instability and swelling within the cubital tunnel. The same injury can also produce ulnar nerve instability.
   c. Fixed flexion and valgus deformity of the elbow as a result of macrotrauma or repeated microtrauma in the growing elbow.
   d. Individuals with generalized ligamentous laxity who injure their ulnar nerve by stretching during the valgus stress in forceful throwing. They may also suffer from repeated nerve subluxation during daily activities.

   Tingling, pain, heaviness, and clumsiness of the hand may be noted during and after exertion. If symptoms do not subside with rest or recur after exertion, transposition of the ulnar nerve may be necessary as an effective means of treatment.

CONCLUSIONS

A good understanding of elbow anatomy and biomechanics gives a firm background to plan our management strategy. The elbow joint is structurally stable yet functionally versatile. It allows wide ranges of performance that can be precise, dexterous, and yet powerful and speedy.

Athletes who participate in repetitive high-speed, high-load activities need to be cautioned about the risk of overloading their elbow structurally. Early preventive measures may allow damages to be reversed. Undertreatment may compromise the elbow's future stability and motion. This may ruin an athlete's career and may even affect activities of daily living. Young athletes with immature bones are particularly at risk since their cartilaginous epiphyses are soft. Epiphyseal plate damage may give rise to joint deformities, producing permanent stiffness and malalignment.

Knowing the mechanism of injury allows us to predict the sites where lesions are expected. Knowing the extent of tissue damage allows us to predict the outcome with conservative or operative treatment. Treatment may then be tailored to match the functional demands of the athlete to obtain the optimal result.

The collateral ligament complexes need to be particularly noted. The anterior component of the MCL, which plays a predominant role in elbow stability, must be carefully assessed during operative procedures in order to determine the need to preserve or to repair it. Elbow injuries among throwing athletes are gaining more attention because of the possible long-term sequelae of joint instability, stiffness, and neurologic deficits.

The ulnar nerve is the most common nerve affected in the elbow region during sport activities. Early diagnosis and management is necessary. Simple preventive measures taken by athletes could be effective in avoiding elbow injuries.

REFERENCES

1. Dee R, Ries MD, Hurst LC: Biomechanics of the elbow. p. 515. In Dee R et al. (ed): Principles of Orthopedics Practice. McGraw Hill, New York
2. Hotchkiss RN, Weiland AJ: Valgus stability of the elbow. J Orthop Res 5:372–377, 1987
3. Jobe FW, ElAttrache NS: Diagnosis and treatment of ulnar collateral ligament injuries in athletes. p. 566. In Morrey BF (ed): The Elbow and Its Disorders. 2nd Ed. WB Saunders, Philadelphia, 1993
4. Jobe FW, Moynes, DR, Tibone, JE, Perry J: An EMG analysis of the shoulder in pitching. A special report. Am J Sports Med 12:218–220, 1984
5. Kapandji IA: The Physiology of the Joints. Vol. 1. Edinburgh, Churchill Livingstone, 1982
6. Morrey BF (ed): The Elbow and Its Disorders. 1st Ed. WB Saunders, Philadelphia, 1985
7. Morrey BF: Applied anatomy and biomechanics of the elbow Joint. In: American Academy of Orthopaedic Surgeons, Instructional Course Lectures. Vol. 35. CV Mosby, St. Louis, 1986
8. Morrey BF: Past Traumatic Stiffness: Distraction Arthroplasty. p. 476. In Morrey BF (ed): The Elbow and Its Disorders. 2nd Ed. Philadelphia, WB Saunders, 1993
9. Morrey BF, An KN: Articular and ligamentous contributions to the stability of the elbow joint. Am J Sports Med 11:315–319, 1983
10. Morrey BF, O'Driscoll SW: Lateral collateral ligament injury. p. 515. In Morrey BF (ed): The Elbow and Its Disorders. 2nd Ed. WB Saunders, Philadelphia, 1993
11. Morrey BF, Askew LJ, An KN, Chao EY: A biomechanical study of normal functional elbow motion. J Bone Joint Surg 63A:872–877, 1981
12. O'Driscoll SW: Classification and spectrum of elbow instability: recurrent instability. p. 453. In Morrey BF (ed): The Elbow and Its Disorders. 2nd Ed. WB Saunders, Philadelphia, 1993
13. O'Driscoll SW, Morrey BF, An KN: Intra-articular pressure and capacity of the elbow. Arthroscopy 6:100–103, 1990
14. O'Driscoll SW, Bell DF, Morrey BF: Posterolateral rotatory instability of the elbow. J Bone Joint Surg [Am] 73A:440–446, 1991
15. Ray RD, Johnson RJ and Jameson RM: Rotation of forearm. An experimental study of pronation and supination. J Bone Joint Surg [Am] 33A:993–996, 1951
16. Jobe FW, Nuber G: Throwing injuries of the elbow. Clinic Sports Med 5(4):621–636, 1986
17. Schwab GH, Bennett JB, Woods GM, Tullos HS: Biomechanics of elbow instability: the role of the medial collateral ligament. Clin Orthop 146:42–52, 1980
18. Tillman BH: Contribution to the Function Morphology of Articular Surfaces. George Thieme, Stuttgart, 1978
19. Tullos HS, Bennett J, Shepard D et al: Adult elbow dislocations: mechanism of instability. p. 69. American Academy of Orthopaedic Surgeons, Instructional Course Lectures. Vol. 35. CV Mosby, St. Louis, 1986
20. Yocum LA: The Diagnosis and Non-Operative Treatment of Elbow Problems in the Athlete. Clin in Sports Med 8(3):439–451, 1989

10

Clinical and Radiologic Assessment of Elbow Injuries

MICHAEL HAYES

INTRODUCTION

The elbow joint is frequently injured in athletics, because of direct or indirect trauma or overuse. The elbow joint is arguably the most important in the upper limb, and a satisfactory range of movement (ROM) is essential for day-to-day activity. Injuries to the elbow must be assessed together with function of the component joints of the upper extremity, in particular the shoulder and inferior radioulnar joints.

Sporting injuries are often difficult to manage not only because of the sometimes extraordinary expectations and demands of high-grade athletes but also because of the time frame within which recovery has to be achieved. The problem involves amateur athletes as well. A severe chronic lateral epicondylitis in a 70-year-old widowed golfer may be as distressing from a social, psychological, and functional point of view as the same injury to a person on the professional golf circuit.

The key to successful management is early and accurate diagnosis established by a careful history and examination complemented by the judicious use of an ever-increasing range of radiologic investigations, which are now available in most major centers.

HISTORY

In assessing a patient with a sporting injury, it is important to record demographic data including age, sex, hand dominance, sporting interests and expectations.

Frequently the patient is able to give an accurate history of the injury or, alternatively, highlight variations in training schedule or instances of overtraining that may give a clue to diagnosis.

Specific symptoms such as pain are important to evaluate in detail. Pain associated with a dislocating ulnar nerve may give neuritis-like symptoms associated with activity. Discomfort associated with radiocapitellar degeneration secondary to a long-standing osteochondritic lesion in the lateral humeral condyle may present as a deep, laterally based, aching pain with associated catching and clicking. The pain may be exacerbated by movement or weather change and helped by rest and anti-inflammatory medication. It is important to note whether the patient is experiencing pain at rest and in particular whether night pain is a worrying symptom.

Although the most common causes of elbow problems in the athlete are overuse syndromes such as lateral or medial epicondylitis, conditions such as an osteoid osteoma or even more sinister lesions such as a primary bone tumor must be considered; often the clue to the latter diagnosis is nocturnal pain.

Other symptoms include locking, catching discomfort, weakness, and loss of movement. In addition to determining what factors cause an exacerbation or deterioration of symptoms, it is also important to establish whether any therapeutic measures help to relieve the discomfort. It is important to enquire about types and outcomes of previous treatment. Finally, the history is incomplete without assessing the patient's general health and whether or not previous injuries, illnesses, or surgery have occurred.

EXAMINATION

Examination of the elbow joint complements the history and is carried out systematically with a thorough knowledge of the underlying anatomy. It is important to compare both elbows during the examination and also to examine the shoulders, wrist, and inferior radioulnar joints. Following a routine examination pattern under the headings of observation, palpation, movement, and specific testing helps to eliminate misdiagnosis through errors of omission.

Observation

Contour

The overall appearance of both elbow joints must be examined, looking for evidence of previous surgical or other scars, abnormal swellings (such as an olecranon bursa), or changes in the texture of the skin itself, especially over the lateral epicondyle. Discoloration of the skin and thinning of the subcutaneous tissue indicates previous steroid infiltration.

Midway between the tip of the lateral epicondyle and the olecranon process, a "soft spot" is found where the capsule of the elbow joint is not covered by muscle; at that point, local swelling may indicate the presence of an effusion or synovitis within the elbow joint (Fig. 10-1). Bursal enlargements may occur over the olecranon process or both epicondyles. Acute ligamentous or avulsion injuries or fractures around the elbow joint may cause bruising and swelling.

Deformity

Deformity is defined as the inability to place the arm in a normal anatomic position. In assessing deformity around the elbow joint, it is important to recall that a variation in the "carrying angle" exists between males and females as well as documented changes associated with race.[16] Inability to extend the elbow joint fully is an important clinical finding. This movement is lost initially after any injury to the elbow and is the last to be restored during rehabilitation.

On the other hand, hypermobility of the elbow may indicate that the patient has an underlying related tissue condition such as Marfan syndrome. Valgus deformity of the elbow secondary to nonunited lateral condylar fracture may be associated with a traction neuritis of the ulnar nerve; in addition to the deformity, a surgical scar may be present over the lateral aspect of the elbow. Distally, signs of ulnar nerve damage with wasting of the interossei and a typical "claw hand" picture indicate a long-standing condition.

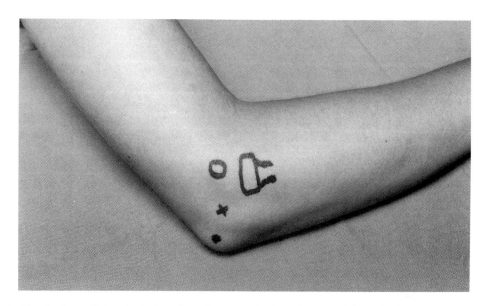

Fig. 10-1. The "soft spot" (marked X) midway between the lateral epicondyle and olecranon process is a site where a joint effusion or synovitis may be palpated.

A varus condition, the "gunstock" deformity, usually indicates an underlying, malunited supracondylar fracture.

Palpation

Many of the structures to be examined are subcutaneous and may be locally tender in the normal individual. Therefore, for an anxious patient who has had a recent injury, it is important to examine the normal elbow, gain the patient's confidence, and then gently examine the injured joint. During the examination, the observer must be conscious of the underlying anatomic structures and must relate the patient's response to the information already gleaned from the clinical history.

In assessing the lateral aspect of the elbow, it is important to commence palpation along the lateral supracondylar ridge and move in a distal direction, paying careful attention to the epicondylar area, radial head, and the distal region where the posterior interosseus nerve passes through the supinator muscle. This point is usually tender in entrapment syndromes of that nerve (Fig. 10-2).

In the interval midway between the lateral epicondyle and olecranon, as previously mentioned, is a point where the intra-articular effusion or synovitis of the elbow joint can be detected. Posteriorly, with the elbow semiflexed, the contents of the olecranon fossa can be palpated; this is another site where synovial proliferation can be detected. In the throwing athlete, tenderness in the region of the olecranon process can indicate an underlying compression injury.

Examination of the medial aspect of the elbow joint is particularly important because the ulnar nerve lies in close proximity to the medial epicondyle and it is important to determine the exact site of tenderness if the observer is to differentiate between a medial epicondylar traction injury or an intrinsic problem involving the ulnar nerve. If the nerve is locally tender, it is essential to assess whether or not the structure is stable in the cubital tunnel; this is often best observed with the patient in a supine position, which allows the clinician to watch the movement of the nerve as the patient actively flexes and extends the elbow (Fig. 10-3). Flexion of the elbow throws the bony prominences of the medial and lateral epicondyles and the olecranon process into prominence; with the joint at 90 degrees, these structures should form an equilateral triangle (Fig. 10-4).

It is important to palpate just above the medial epicondylar area for any evidence of a supracondylar spur, which may correlate with neuritis-like symptoms and suggest entrapment of the median nerve at that level. Temperature changes between the elbow joint and proximal and distal part of the arm are important to

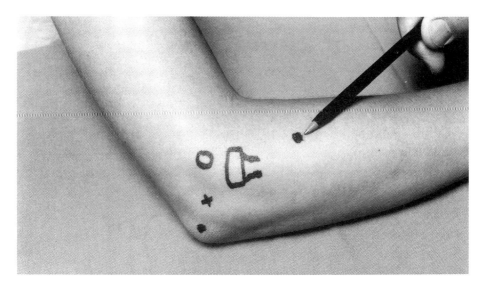

Fig. 10-2. Tenderness over the posterior interosseous nerve as it courses through the supinator muscle is commonly present when the nerve is compressed.

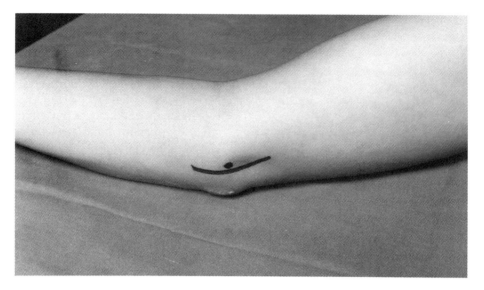

Fig. 10-3. The ulnar nerve can be palpated behind the medial epicondyle as it courses into the forearm.

assess, as such changes may provide a clue to an underlying infective process or synovitis.

Movement

Accurate assessment of the ROM present in the elbow joint is important to record because loss of movement, particularly extension, could give a clue to diagnosis; in addition, careful recording allows assessment of the collected data for both prospective and retrospective studies, as well as for medicolegal purposes.

Both active and passive ranges should be measured and palpation, for crepitus, is important. The range of flexion, although variable, is from 0 to 140 degrees plus or minus 10 degrees; the average range of pronation is 70 degrees and that of supination 85 degrees.[1] In assessing movement of the elbow joint, it is important to exclude movement of the shoulder joint, and mea-

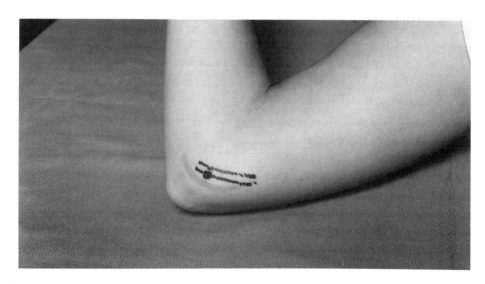

Fig. 10-4. Dislocation of the ulnar nerve when the elbow is flexed is best examined with the patient in the supine position.

surements should be made with the humerus in the vertical position and the elbow by the side.

Strength

Strength is best measured with the elbow by the side in 90 degrees of flexion and neutral rotation. Flexion, extension, supination, and pronation should be assessed and compared with the opposite side. In addition, since a number of nerve entrapment syndromes occur around the elbow joint, careful testing of distal muscle function is important. The method of testing function in the muscles supplied by the median, ulnar, and radial nerves is well documented, but the more specific tests of muscle function supplied by the anterior and posterior interosseous nerves can be overlooked. Anterior interosseous nerve injuries are rare and can be identified by testing function in the flexor pollicus longus muscle, flexor digitorum profundus to the index finger, and pronator quadratus. When an anterior interosseous nerve lesion is present, pinch function between the tip of the thumb and the index finger is altered and results in an abnormal posture, as neither the interphalangeal joint of the thumb nor the distal interphalangeal joint of the index finger can flex; as force is applied, the "joints collapse," and pinch grip relies on ligamentous support.[8]

Although relatively uncommon, entrapment of the posterior interosseous nerve occurs in the athlete and may be associated with chronic lateral epicondylitis. Careful muscle testing reveals normal wrist extension power but weakness of the extensor pollicus longus and extensor digitorum communis muscles.[7] To ensure that the patient understands the tests and applies maximum effort, I first resist flexion of the thumb at the interphalangeal joint and then test extension, once again, comparing the findings in both hands. Even though they have vague complaints of weakness and fatigue, patients are often surprised by the weakness demonstrated between the extensor and flexor muscles.

Neurologic Assessment

Several nerve entrapment syndromes occur around the elbow joint and also careful neurologic testing of power, reflexes, and sensation may reveal a central cause for symptoms, such as a disc lesion. Therefore part of the routine examination of the elbow is to carry out a neurologic assessment.

Reflexes

The biceps, brachioradialis, and triceps reflexes test function of nerve roots C5, C6, and C7, respectively; these should be tested and compared with the opposite side.

Sensation

The ulnar nerve is particularly vulnerable to injury at the elbow joint, and careful testing of the area innervated by the ulnar nerve may help localize the lesion. Injuries to the ulnar nerve proximal to Guyon's canal may result in sensory change over the dorsal aspect of the hand extending into the ring and little fingers. The median nerve can be compressed under a fibrous band arising from the supracondylar process of the humerus; when this condition is suspected, oblique radiographic views of the humerus confirm the diagnosis.

The musculocutaneous nerve can also be involved in an entrapment syndrome at elbow level, since it exits from the arm and continues as the lateral cutaneous nerve of the forearm.[2] The nerve is locally tender as it runs along the side of the biceps tendon and penetrates the brachial fascia just above the elbow crease. Sensory change over the lateral aspect of the forearm is associated and occasionally surgical decompression of the nerve is required.

Accessory Tests

Lateral epicondylitis is probably the most common lesion affecting the elbow in the sporting population. Resisted testing of the wrist extensors may cause pain in the lateral epicondylar region if a tear is present involving the origin of extensor carpi radialus brevis or longus. In addition, the stretch test may be positive. This involves flexing the patient's wrist and fingers and then having the elbow slowly extended. Reproduction of pain indicates a positive test.

INSTABILITY

The elbow joint in extension is stabilized not only by ligamentous and capsular structures but also by the approximation of the olecranon process into the olecranon fossa of the humerus. Collateral ligament stability is tested with the elbow in approximately 15 degrees of flexion, which reduces the stability afforded by bone apposition. The radial collateral ligament is best tested with the forearm in supination and slight flexion, whereas the medial collateral ligament is best assessed with the elbow in slight flexion and supination.[5,16] Recently, O'Driscoll et al.[11,12] described posterolateral instability of the elbow caused by either acute or chronic injury to the lateral band of the ulnar collateral ligament; this condition, which is relatively rare, is demonstrated by the "lateral pivot shift test." A valgus and axial load is applied to the extended elbow with the forearm in supination. Alternatively, the same test can be carried out more easily with the arm over the patient's head, which allows the examiner to apply axial compression and a valgus and supination force (Fig. 10-5). When the test is positive, the humeral head subluxes at approximately 20 to 30 degrees of flexion and reduces when the elbow is further flexed.

RADIOLOGIC ASSESSMENT

Recent technological advances have broadened the number of radiologic investigations now available to assess musculoskeletal injuries. Some more recent techniques, such as computed tomography (CT) scanning, have made previous techniques redundant, but the new investigations require expensive machinery and the final outcome relies on the expertise of the radiologist. The cost of these investigations must be considered; after establishing a working diagnosis based on clinical history and physical examination, the surgeon then needs to consider the radiologic options available to confirm the diagnosis and to help with further management.

Plain Radiographs

Plain radiographs remain the keystone of investigation; in the skeletally immature athlete, views of both elbows may be helpful in assessing whether or not a fracture

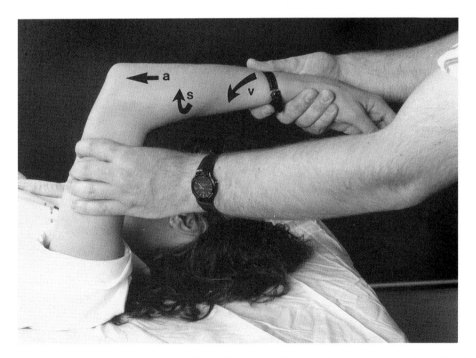

Fig. 10-5. A test for posterolateral instability of the elbow is performed with the arm over the patient's head and the shoulder in external rotation. Axial compression (*a*), supination (*s*), and a valgus force (*v*) is applied to the elbow, which is flexed to approximately 20 to 30 degrees. Further flexion leads to visible and palpable reduction of the subluxation.

is present or, alternatively, whether the radiologic appearances relate to a developing ossific center.

Plain radiographs should include anteroposterior and lateral views; an oblique view may also be extremely helpful in demonstrating injuries to the radial head and neck (Fig. 10-6). In assessing the radiographs, the observer must be acutely aware of variations in soft tissue planes, which may give a clue to diagnosis. Interposed between the capsule and synovium is a layer of fat forming the anterior and posterior fat pads; these may be displaced if a joint effusion is present. The normal anterior fat pad has a tear-drop appearance,

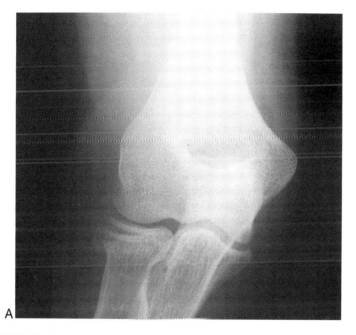

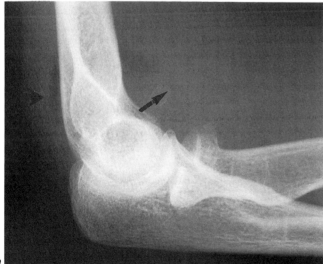

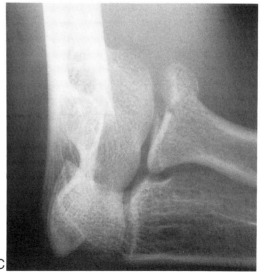

Fig. 10-6. **(A)** Anteroposterior radiograph of the elbow with a fracture of the radial head. **(B)** Lateral radiograph revealing anterior and posterior fat pad signs (*arrows*). **(C)** Oblique view of the radial head revealing the extent of displacement of the fracture fragment.

whereas it assumes the configuration of a ship sail when an effusion is present.[10] When a positive fat sign is seen, careful scrutiny of the radiographs may reveal an unsuspected fracture, for instance, an undisplaced fracture of the radial head. In addition, the presence of a joint effusion may be associated with an unsuspected loose body, particularly if the fragment is predominantly cartilaginous and located in the olecranon fossa. This is a relatively "blind" area on plain radiographic studies, but in a patient presenting with loss of extension on clinical examination and an effusion on radiographs, a loose body in that area should be considered; tomography or CT scanning (depending on the availability of these investigations) often confirm the suspected pathology (Fig. 10-7).

Trispiral Tomography

Trispiral tomography can be useful in determining the extent of an osteochondritic lesion in the lower humerus or, alternatively, helping to locate a loose body. However, CT or magnetic resonance imaging (MRI) give a much clearer anatomic picture; when these facilities are available, they supercede this technique.

Arthrography

Single- or double-contrast elbow arthrography may be helpful in assessing capsular and ligamentous integrity and may also provide valuable information on the synovium and articular surfaces.[4] While the technique may be helpful in assessing acute ligamentous injuries in the athlete, the advent of arthroscopic surgery has not only allowed the surgeon to arrive at a positive diagnosis but also to proceed with treatment such as removal of loose bodies, arthroscopic synovectomy, and so forth. Arthroscopy has the disadvantage of requiring some type of arm block or general anesthesia, but, on the positive side, it eliminates the need for arthrography and thus reduces x-ray radiation.

Computed Tomography

The complex anatomic arrangement of the elbow joint makes assessment of plain radiographs difficult. Subtle fractures may be missed and loose bodies may remain hidden by superimposed bone structures.[6] CT can also be used in the traumatized patient, and detail is not obscured by overlying plaster or fiberglass casts. This investigation has been particularly useful in patients presenting with symptoms of locking, and radiographs may or may not reveal the presence of loose fragments. In addition, at arthroscopy, it is not unusual to find several loose bodies in the elbow joint when a lesser number was expected radiologically. However, a preoperative CT scan helps to delineate the site and number of loose bodies and may help the surgeon decide on patient positioning when carrying out arthroscopic evaluation of the elbow. For instance, if the CT scan shows loose bodies in the posterior compartment but no obvious abnormality anteriorly, then carrying out arthroscopy with the patient in the prone position may be appropriate. CT is also helpful in assessing the extent of more subtle fractures around the elbow; for instance, step deformities of the radial head may be easier to assess, which may help the clinician decide whether or not to proceed with surgical intervention.

CT combined with either single- or double-contrast techniques provides more information than the latter technique alone and in addition may demonstrate cartilaginous lesions not visualized with plain CT scanning.[14] The use of the technique depends to some extent on the availability of elbow arthroscopy, with its attendant requirements and risks.

Bone Scan

Persistent unremitting pain in the elbow is an unusual complaint; when night pain is a component, other lesions such as an osteoid osteoma or even a primary bone tumor need to be considered.[13] In this circumstance, when plain radiographs are not helpful, a nucleotide bone scan may provide positive evidence of increased uptake in the elbow area; having defined the site of the lesion, the original films can be reinspected, other views taken, or, alternatively, more sophisticated assessment using a CT scan or MRI may be indicated.

Ultrasonography

The noninvasive technique of ultrasonography, is useful in assessing lesions around the elbow. An experienced ultrasonographer may be able to demonstrate instability of the ulnar nerve and comment on structural change surrounding the nerve. This may help the clinician differentiate between a medial epicondylitis and ulnar neuritis. Maffulli et al.[9] have analyzed the ultrasonographic images found in a series of tennis

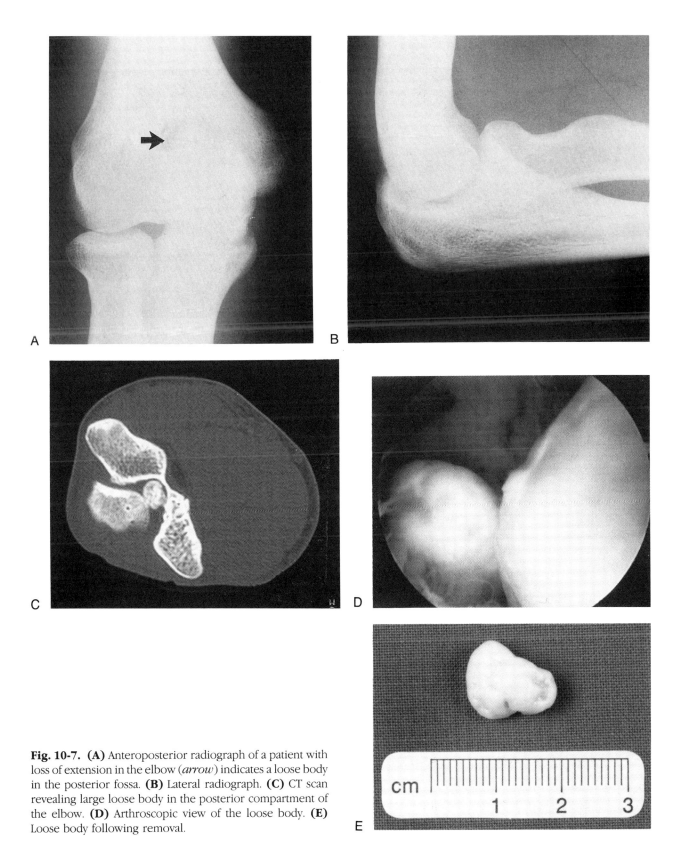

Fig. 10-7. (A) Anteroposterior radiograph of a patient with loss of extension in the elbow (*arrow*) indicates a loose body in the posterior fossa. **(B)** Lateral radiograph. **(C)** CT scan revealing large loose body in the posterior compartment of the elbow. **(D)** Arthroscopic view of the loose body. **(E)** Loose body following removal.

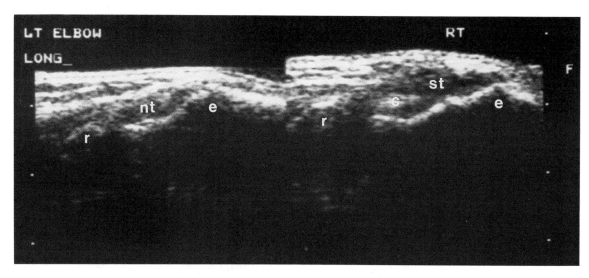

Fig. 10-8. Comparison of the symptomatic right and the symptomatic left elbow in a patient with chronic lateral elbow pain. Region r, radial head: nt, normal tendon: e, epicondyle: st, swollen tendon: c, calcification.

players presenting with symptoms and signs of lateral epicondylitis. They characterize the lesions as follows:

Extratendinous alterations
   Muscular tears
   Bursitis
Pathology of the tendon
   Enthesiopathy
   Tendonitis
   Peritendonitis
   Mixed lesions

Using ultrasonography, lateral elbow pain can be subdivided into one of the above categories and a more logical treatment course undertaken (Fig. 10-8). In addition, it gives the clinician an opportunity of monitoring treatment using a noninvasive and cost-effective technique. However, as with ultrasonography of the shoulder, the examination is observer dependent and very reliant on the assessment of an experienced and interested radiologist.

Magnetic Resonance Imaging

MRI can be used to demonstrate the intra- and extra-articular structures surrounding the elbow. Injuries to the biceps and triceps mechanism have been described,[15] and the findings can be enhanced by the use

of intravenous gadopentetate dimeglumine.[17] Although this investigation does not expose the patient to radiation, it is expensive, and some patients are unable to use it because they have metallic implants or are claustrophobic. Currently the major indication for MRI in the region of the elbow is to determine the type and extent of any bone or soft tissue tumor occurring in the elbow region.

CONCLUSIONS

Normal elbow joint function is critical in many athletic endeavors. The speedy rehabilitation of sports men and women who have elbow injuries depends on a careful clinical history, a thorough and well-recorded physical examination, and the judicious use of an ever-increasing range of radiologic investigations. In using these investigations, the treating surgeon needs to be aware of the shortcomings, risks, and costs of ordering appropriate tests, knowing that careful scrutiny of a well-performed radiographic series may not only confirm the diagnosis but arouse suspicion of significant intra-articular pathology if an effusion is present.

In the future, technology will probably advance to a point at which three-dimensional images are available as a primary screening technique; with the improvement in communication around the world, it may be possible to have case presentations transmitted from center to center throughout the world, thus utilize the knowledge and talents of the international medical profession in an effort to improve diagnosis, treatment, and rehabilitation of patients involved in sport.

REFERENCES

1. American Academy of Orthopaedic Surgeons: Joint Motion: Method of Measuring and Recording. American Academy of Othopaedic Surgeons, Chicago, 1965
2. Bassett FH, Nunley JA: Compression of the musculo cutaneous nerve at the elbow. J Bone Joint Surg [Am] 64A:1050–1052, 1982
3. Bauer M, Jonsson K, Josefsson P, Linden B: Osteochronditis dissecans of the elbow. Clin Orthop 284:156–160, 1992
4. Berquist TH: Diagnostic radiographic techniques of the elbow. p. 92. In Morrey BF (ed): The Elbow and its Disorders. WB Saunders, Philadelphia, 1985
5. Conway JE, Jobe FW, Glousman RE, Pink M: Medial instability of the elbow in throwing athletes. J Bone Joint Surg [Am] 74A:67–83, 1992
6. Franklin PD, Dunlop RW, Whitelaw G et al: Computed tomography of the normal and traumatized elbow. J Comput Assist Tomogr 12:817–823, 1988
7. Kendall HO, Kendall FP: Muscle Testing and Function. Williams & Wilkins, Baltimore, 1949
8. Lister G: The Hand: Diagnosis and Indications. p. 100. Churchill Livingstone, Edinburgh, 1977
9. Maffulli N, Regine MD, Carrillo F et al: Tennis elbow: an ultrasonographic study in tennis players. Br J Sports Med 24:151–155, 1990
10. Newberg AH: The radiographic evaluation of shoulder and elbow pain in the athlete. Clin Sports Med 6:785–809, 1987
11. O'Driscoll SW, Bell DF, Morrey BF: Posterolateral rotatory instability of the elbow. J Bone Joint Surg 73A:440–446, 1991
12. O'Driscoll SW, Morrey BF, Korinec S, An K: Elbow subluxation at dislocation. A spectrum of instability. Clin Orthop 280:186–197, 1992
13. Otsuka NY, Hastings DE, Fornasier VL: Osteoid osteoma of the elbow: a report of six cases. J Hand Surg 17A:458–461, 1992
14. Singson RD, Feldman F, Rosenberg ZS: Elbow joint assessment with double-contrast CT arthrography. Radiology 160:167–173, 1986
15. Tehranzadeh J, Kerr R, Amster J: Magnetic resonance imaging of tendon and ligament abnormalities: Part 1. Spine and upper extremities. Skeletal Radiol 21:1–9, 1992
16. Volz RG, Morrey BF, Morrey BF: The physical examination of the elbow. p. 62. In Morrey BF (ed): The Elbow and its Disorders. 1st Ed. WB Saunders, Philadelphia, 1985
17. Whitten CG, Moore TE, Yuh WTC et al: The use of intravenous gadopentetate dimeglumine in magnetic resonance imaging of synovial lesion. Skeletal Radiol 21:215–218, 1992

11

Surgical Management of Acute and Chronic Elbow Injuries

STUART PATTERSON

INTRODUCTION

For the competitive throwing athlete, an injured elbow frequently means the end of their athletic career.[18,40,88,91,168] The elbow is subjected to joint compressive forces exceeding body weight, as well as significant tensile forces.[69,163] Minor losses of articular congruity, stability, or motion can eliminate the athlete's edge of competitiveness. This chapter reviews the surgical management of those injuries unique or common to athletes. More comprehensive treatises on elbow trauma can be found elsewhere.

LIGAMENT INJURIES
Acute Simple Elbow Dislocations

The incidence of dislocation is highest in the second decade of life and is usually a posterior or posterolateral dislocation of the left elbow.[26,96,99,100,103,113,119,131,146,172,180,183] Associated injuries to the neurovascular structures have been reported, but they are uncommon.[107,118,119,127,146,171,180] Gymnasts, wrestlers, and football players are at particular risk.[11,12,68,167,195]

Elbow dislocations usually result from a fall on the outstretched hand, with the elbow slightly flexed and the forearm either pronated or supinated[96] (Fig. 11-1). Axial load, external rotation, and a valgus moment initiate sequential failure of the soft tissues or skeleton, beginning laterally and ending medially.[50,103,104,160,198]

Josefsson et al.[101–103] demonstrated in their well-documented studies that in most cases, both the medial[138] and lateral ulnar collateral ligaments[161] are avulsed from the humeral origin, frequently accompanied by disruption of the anterior capsule and common extensor and flexor pronator muscle origins. Associated avulsion fractures of the medial and lateral epicondyles and coronoid process are common and are indicators of associated capsuloligamentous disruption.

Valgus stress applied to the reduced elbow may not result in valgus instability,[12,160,163,207] since the medial ulnar collateral ligament (MUCL) anterior bundle can remain intact while the lateral ulnar collateral ligament (LUCL) is torn[145,157,160,163] (Fig. 11-2).

Management

Simple elbow dislocations can usually be managed nonoperatively, since surgical intervention does not improve outcome.[101,102,113] The joint should be reduced only after an appropriate examination and radiologic assessment (Fig. 11-3). Reduction is obtained by gentle longitudinal traction on the fully supinated and slightly flexed elbow.[119,160] If reduction is difficult with neuroleptic agents, it should be done under general anesthesia.[119] Reduction is routinely confirmed by radiographs.

The integrity of the MUCL anterior bundle and LUCL is assessed after reduction, by applying a varus or valgus stress to the elbow flexed 30 degrees[197] (Fig. 11-4). With an intact MUCL anterior bundle and disrupted LUCL, the elbow will be stable through a full range of flexion with the forearm fully pronated, since the elbow is stabilized by the tensioned common extensor muscles, which close the lateral joint space.[10,119,160] In the case of an intact MUCL anterior bundle, the stable, reduced elbow is placed in a hinged brace with the forearm fully pronated and started on immediate active range of motion (ROM).[119]

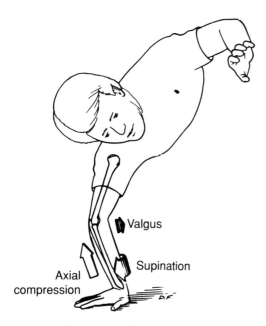

Fig. 11-1. Mechanism of elbow dislocation proposed by O'Driscoll et al. A fall on the outstretched hand, axially loads the slightly flexed elbow, while the body internally rotates on the fixed extremity, applying a valgus moment. (From O'Driscoll et al.,[160] with permission.)

If both the MUCL anterior bundle and LUCL have been completely torn, which is the usual finding, the forearm is placed in a hinged brace in neutral rotation.[119] If the elbow is unstable between 0 and 90 degrees of flexion, an extension block can be built into the hinged brace and motion begun in the stable range.[119] The stability and range of motion of the elbow are evaluated weekly and at 3 weeks; if the elbow is stable, the hinged brace is discontinued after 3 weeks and active motion continued.[119] Night-time extension splinting is often used when a flexion contracture is present. Mehlhoff et al.[131] demonstrated that immobilization of the elbow for less than 2 weeks always resulted in a good or excellent outcome, while immobilization for 4 weeks or longer always yielded a fair or poor result. This is supported by the findings of others.[96,172]

The incidence of symptomatic heterotopic ossification following a simple elbow dislocation is less than 3 percent and is not a significant factor.[26,60,96,99,101–103,105,113,118,131,146,172,203] Some authors have postulated that heterotopic ossification occurs secondary to the initiation of early elbow motion, in particular, passive motion.[122] However, no evidence supports this hypothesis.[32] Nevertheless, passive stretching is not required acutely and should not be introduced.

The long-term results of simple elbow dislocations are generally very good, with loss of full extension being the most common finding.[99,102] Symptomatic instability is quite uncommon.[99,102] The unstable elbow, in which a reduction cannot be maintained, is managed by surgical stabilization, as discussed in the next section.[208]

Complex Dislocations of the Elbow

Elbow fracture-dislocations are difficult to manage.[219] These elbows are grossly unstable, due to loss of both the primary and secondary joint stabilizers.[83,104,137,141,188,207,208] In the skeletally immature athlete, the medial epicondyle is often avulsed, whereas in the adult, the MUCL anterior bundle is torn.[167,188,207] Fractures of the articular surfaces and the presence of osteochondral loose bodies increase the risk of posttraumatic arthritis.[32,104] The fractures commonly encountered in association with elbow dislocations include the following:

1. Radial head and neck
2. Coronoid process of the ulna
3. Olecranon

The greater the comminution of the radial head, the more extensive the injury to the capsuloligamentous complex circumferentially.[96] The circle concept of stability has been used to explain injury patterns seen in the elbow[160] (Fig. 11-5). The presence of a comminuted fracture of the radial head (Mason type 3)[128] should direct the physician to exclude an injury to the MUCL anterior bundle,[207,208] as well as the possibility of a co-existing disruption of the forearm interosseous membrane and distal radioulnar joint[20,53,55] (Fig. 11-6). Failure to recognize the Essex-Lopresti injury can result in chronic wrist and elbow pain.[53,55] Large-fragment coronoid fractures (Regan type 3)[176] are highly correlated with loss of reduction,[20,104] as are Mason type 3 radial head fractures.[104,208,219]

Management

Following appropriate examination and radiologic assessment, consideration should be given to joint reduc-

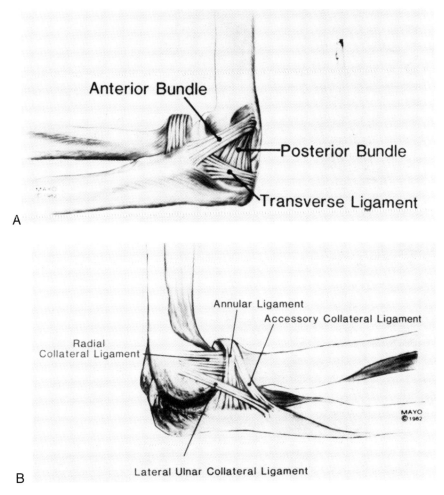

Fig. 11-2. The medial and lateral ligamentous constraints of the elbow. **(A)** The medial ulnar collateral ligament consists of three portions, a transverse ligament, a posterior bundle, and the major stabilizer, the anterior bundle. **(B)** The lateral ligamentous complex consists of the radial collateral ligament, the annular ligament, the accessory collateral ligament, and the lateral ulnar collateral ligament (LUCL). The LUCL is the primary stabilizer on the lateral side of the elbow. (By permission of the Mayo Foundation.)

tion. These injuries should be reduced under general anesthesia for the following reasons:

1. A minimally displaced fracture of the radial head may be converted to a grossly displaced fracture if the reduction is not accomplished with ease.
2. Elbow flexion and forearm rotation can be assessed to exclude a mechanical block to motion.
3. Elbow stability can be assessed.
4. If indicated, reconstructive surgery can be undertaken.

The elbow should be reduced as for simple dislocation and examined under an image intensifier (Fig. 11-7). The joint should be scrutinized to exclude the presence of an osteochondral loose body. The following findings would constitute indications to proceed with operative management:

1. Inability to obtain or maintain a closed reduction of the elbow joint[208]
2. A displaced articular fracture[74,189]
3. An osteochondral loose body[91]

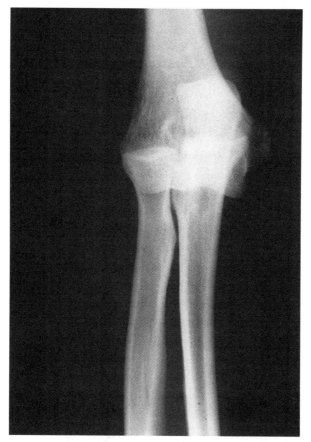

A

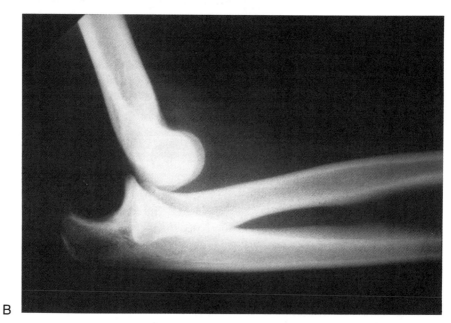

B

Fig. 11-3. A typical simple posterior dislocation of the elbow. **(A)** AP view. **(B)** Lateral view.

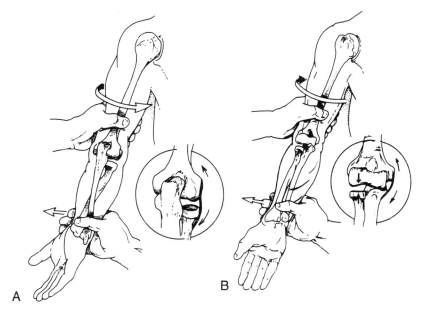

Fig. 11-4. Examination of the elbow for stability. **(A)** Lateral stability is assessed by applying a varus stress to the elbow, with the shoulder maximally internally rotated and the elbow flexed 30 degrees. **(B)** Medial stability is assessed by applying a valgus stress to the elbow with the shoulder maximally externally rotated and the elbow flexed 30 degrees. (From Regan and Morrey,[177] with permission.)

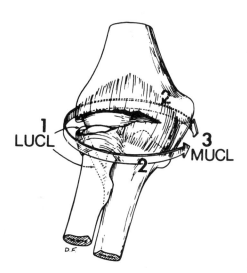

Fig. 11-5. The circle concept of capsuloligamentous failure. Stage 1, lateral collateral ligament torn; stage 2, antero/posterior capsule disrupted; stage 3, medial collateral ligament torn (3A posterior portion only and 3B complete). (From O'Driscoll et al.,[160] with permission.)

4. A mechanical block to motion
5. A vascular injury[127]

The goal of reconstructive surgery is to achieve a congruous and stable elbow reduction, such that the elbow can be rehabilitated in the same manner as a simple elbow dislocation. Reconstruction is directed to the primary and secondary stabilizers of the elbow joint.[137,138,141,207,208] Occasioanlly, augmentation of the disrupted collateral ligaments may be required with autogenous tendon. A surgical approach is used, which allows safe circumferential access to the elbow joint, causes minimal additional damage to the soft tissues, and allows early mobilization of the extremity. The elbow is exposed through a posterior, midline approach, avoiding injury to the medial antebrachial cutaneous nerve (MABCN).[173] The ulnar nerve is usually transposed anteriorly into a subcutaneous position.[52] If repair or reconstruction of the MUCL anterior bundle is required, the flexor carpi ulnaris (FCU) is elevated extraperiosteally from the proximal ulna and distal humerus, preserving all ulnar nerve motor branches. Usually the flexor-pronator origin is completely disrupted with the MUCL anterior bundle avulsed from the humeral insertion.

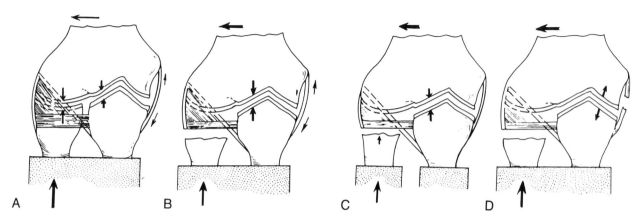

Fig. 11-6. Factors associated with elbow stability. **(A)** Elbow stability is dependent on the integrity of the joint's primary (ligaments) and secondary (bony) constraints. **(B)** In the presence of an intact medial collateral ligament, loss of the radial head does not cause elbow instability. **(C)** Disruption of the interosseous membrane and distal radioulnar joint, in association with a radial head fracture, will result in proximal migration of the radius. **(D)** Valgus instability will occur if a fracture of the radial head is associated with disruption of the anterior bundle of the medial collateral ligament. (From Morrey,[135] with permission.)

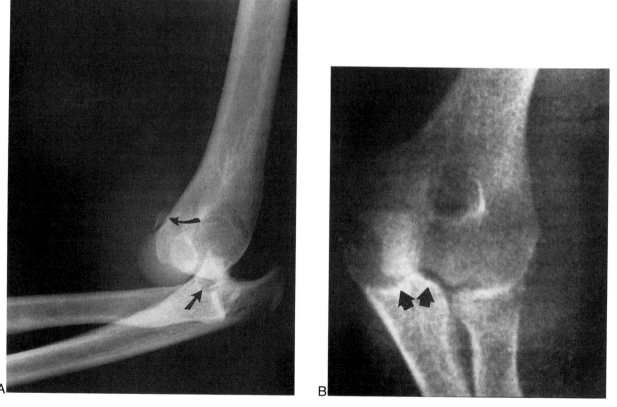

Fig. 11-7. Fracture dislocation of the elbow. **(A)** Lateral view showing a coronoid fracture (*arrow down*) and an associated radial head fracture (*arrow up*). **(B)** Intraoperative valgus stress view, demonstrating medial instability of the elbow, due to complete rupture of the medial collateral ligament.

To obtain elbow stability, an associated coronoid fracture may require stabilization.[74,176,189] This is achieved through the posteromedial approach by further dissection of the FCU off the anterior, proximal ulna, thus exposing the anterior aspect of the ulna and coronoid process. A type 3 coronoid fracture may be repaired with screw fixation, whereas type 1 or 2 coronoid fractures are repaired by a suture technique, with drill holes placed through the ulna.[74]

The MUCL anterior bundle is repaired with drill holes placed through the medial epicondylar insertion of the anterior bundle of the MUCL.[207,208] A #1 nonabsorbable suture is woven through the anterior bundle of the MUCL anterior bundle; then, with the elbow reduced in 30 degrees of flexion and neutral forearm rotation, the suture is brought through the humeral drill holes and tied over the posterior aspect of the medial epicondyle[40] (Fig. 11-11B).

The disrupted LUCL, or radial head fracture, is approached between the anconeus and extensor carpi ulnaris (ECU). The fracture of the radial head or capitellum is reconstructed using AO or Herbert screws.[64,104,108,129] If the radial head is not reconstructible, it may be replaced with a Silastic[37,50,113,166,201,207,208] or metallic implant (see Radial Head Fracture).[75]

Drill holes are placed through the isometric insertion of the avulsed LUCL, and this is repaired back to the lateral epicondyle.[145] The flexor-pronator and common extensor origins are repaired back to the epicondyles and olecranon. The wound is closed over a suction drain and a posterior splint is applied with the elbow in 90 degrees of flexion for 24 hours.

Postoperative Management and Rehabilitation

Unless contraindications exist, all patients are started on indomethacin 25 mg tid PO for 6 weeks,[60] since the incidence of heterotopic ossification can be as high as 20 percent.[60,203] Twenty-four hours after surgery, a hinged brace with a 30-degree extension block is fitted and active ROM is initiated.[108,207] Immobilization of the elbow is associated with a poor outcome, especially if continued longer than 4 weeks.[32]

The brace is discontinued between 4 and 6 weeks, active motion is continued, and a program of gentle, passive stretching is instituted after 6 weeks. A nighttime resting extension splint is used for up to 6 months. Gentle isometric strengthening is introduced at 9 weeks, but no resisted strengthening is undertaken until 12 weeks after surgery. Persistent elbow contractures are treated by turnbuckle splinting. The active ROM of the elbow will continue to improve up to 12 months following the date of injury.

Acute Rupture of the Medial Ulnar Collateral Ligament

Acute, isolated tears of the MUCL anterior bundle are uncommon.[20,40,90,94,92,93,96,111,117,154,205,207] This injury occurs in athletes, particularly baseball pitchers and javelin throwers.[20,40,94,132,215] The injury results from an acute valgus stress of the partially flexed elbow, with application of a tensile load to the MUCL anterior bundle that exceeds its tensile strength.[96] The athlete experiences acute pain over the medial aspect of the elbow, often associated with a snap or pop, followed by ecchymosis, swelling, and ulnar nerve paresthesiae.[23,54,111,154]

Tenderness and swelling is found over the MUCL anterior bundle and pain with valgus stress or full extension of the elbow.[96,111,154,207] A palpable defect in the flexor-pronator origin may be noted.[154] Plain radiographs may demonstrate an avulsion fracture from the medial epicondyle.[96] Stress views will show medial joint space opening, and an arthrogram will demonstrate medial joint line dye extravasation.[20,96,111,207] Magnetic resonance imaging (MRI) may show disruption of the ligament.

Management

The general recommendation has been to repair the acute ligament tear associated with instability and manage the partial tear without instability, nonoperatively.[40,90,111,154] The partial tear is treated by initial rest for 2 to 4 weeks. Application of ice may be beneficial during the inflammatory phase of healing, along with nonsteroidal anti-inflammatory drugs (NSAIDs). Steroid injections are not recommended.[45,93,155] Active ROM is begun at approximately 3 weeks, strengthening at 8 weeks, and a throwing program at 12 weeks. Return to normal activities would be anticipated at 6 months. If the MUCL anterior bundle is completely ruptured, or if no improvement is seen after 6 months of nonoperative management, surgery should be considered.[93] The surgical procedure and the postoperative rehabilitation are described in the section on chronic MUCL instability.

Chronic Medial Ulnar Collateral Ligament Instability

Repetitive valgus stress to the elbow that exceeds the tensile strength of the MUCL anterior bundle will result in ligament failure.[21,90,91,92] If the ligament is not rested and allowed to heal, attenuation, lengthening, calcification, and ossification, with instability, will occur.[40,90,91,92] This is seen in the throwing athlete, especially baseball pitchers and javelin throwers.[21,91,194] Baseball pitchers complain of pain during the late cocking, acceleration, and release phases of pitching, when the most severe valgus strain occurs[40,45,48,92,165,194,205] (Fig. 11-8).

Examination may reveal tenderness along the anterior bundle of the MUCL anterior bundle, and pain with medial instability may be elicited by applying a valgus stress to the elbow flexed 30 degrees. Some athletes will experience symptoms of ulnar nerve irritation.[21,40] If insufficiency exists in the MUCL anterior bundle, impingement may occur between the posteromedial aspect of the olecranon and the olecranon fossa, producing pain and tenderness along the posteromedial ulnohumeral joint line (valgus-extension overload).[8]

Plain radiographs may demonstrate loose bodies at the olecranon tip, MUCL anterior bundle calcification, or ossification (Fig. 11-9), and a gravity, or manual stress radiograph may demonstrate medial joint line opening[21,207] (Fig. 11-10). MRI has not proved to be a helpful investigation. Inability to demonstrate objective evidence of medial instability does not preclude the presence of MUCL anterior bundle insufficiency, and the diagnosis of medial instability may be made solely on the basis of an athlete's history.[54]

Management

Avoidance of throwing for up to 12 weeks should be encouraged. A NSAID and physical modalities may be used.[93] Inability to return to normal throwing activities, despite adequate nonoperative management, is an indication for operative reconstruction.[91–94] The supine patient is positioned with the affected extremity abducted and externally rotated on an arm table. The extremity is prepared to allow for harvesting of the palmaris longus tendon, which has a strength similar to the MUCL anterior bundle.[178] If this is unavailable, a strip of the Achilles tendon, plantaris tendon, or a long toe extensor tendon may be utilized.[92] A posteromedial incision, adjacent to the olecranon, places the incision in a cutaneous internervous plane, sparing branches of the MABCN.[173] The ulnar nerve is not handled, or transposed, unless symptoms of ulnar neuropathy exist. Elattrache and Jobe[54] have reported a modified approach, in which the flexor-pronator origin is exposed and split between the FCU and the flexor carpi radialis, exposing the MUCL anterior bundle. The flexor-pronator origin is not detached unless an ulnar nerve transposition is to be undertaken.[54]

When the MUCL anterior bundle has been acutely ruptured, the joint is immediately visualized after splitting the flexor musculature.[40] Occasionally the flexor-pronator origin may be avulsed. In a chronic injury, the ligament is split longitudinally and the joint inspected. Loose bodies are removed and calcification or ossification in the ligament are excised. Osteophytes on the posteromedial margin of the olecranon are excised through a separate posteromedial arthrotomy.[40]

When the MUCL anterior bundle has an acute tear, the ligament may be avulsed from its insertion on the ulna, or from its insertion on the medial epicondyle.[40,96] The ligament should be repaired by placing a nonabsorbable 1 suture through the ligament in Bunnell fashion and securing it to bone through drill holes placed at the point of insertion of the MUCL anterior bundle (Fig. 11-11).

With a chronic, attenuated ligament tear, augmentation should be undertaken. Two vertically oriented, convergent 3.2-mm drill holes are created 1 cm apart at the level of the coronoid tubercle, on the anteromedial aspect of the coronoid process, which corresponds to

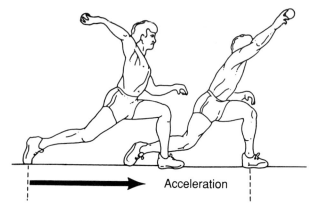

Acceleration

Fig. 11-8. The acceleration phase of a baseball pitcher. Note that the pitcher's body is ahead of the throwing arm initially: opening the body. (From Conway et al.,[40] with permission.)

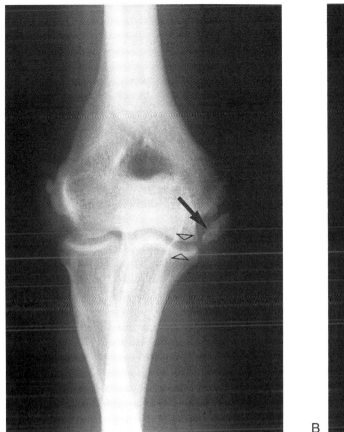
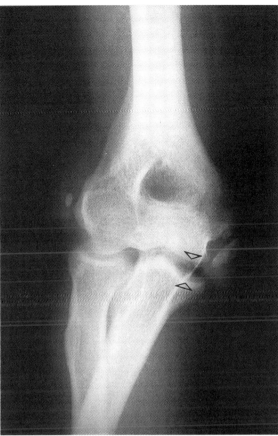

A

B

Fig. 11-9. Medial instability of the elbow. **(A)** Plain film of an elbow, demonstrating ossification at the humeral insertions of the medial and lateral collateral ligaments (*arrow*), and a normal medial joint space (*arrowhead*). **(B)** Valgus stress film demonstrating medial joint space opening (*arrows*), indicative of an incompetent medial collateral ligament.

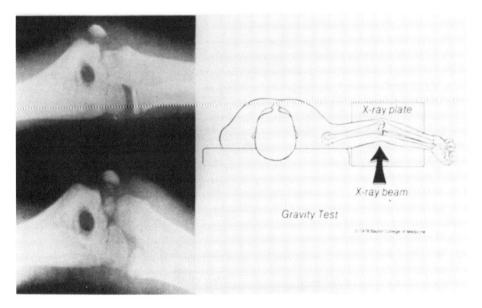

Fig. 11-10. A gravity stress radiograph may also document the presence of medial elbow instability. (From Schwab et al.,[188] with permission.)

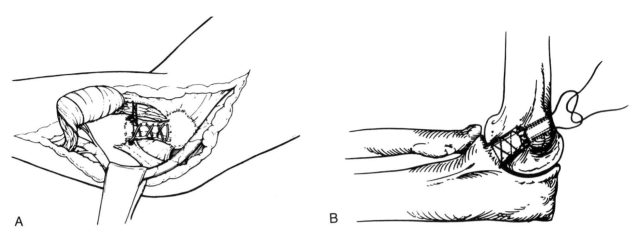

Fig. 11-11. Avulsion of the medial collateral ligament. **(A)** Avulsion of the medial collateral ligament from the ulna is repaired with a Bunnell-type suture through drill holes in the ulna. **(B)** Avulsion of the medial collateral ligament from the medial epicondyle is repaired with a Bunnell-type suture through drill holes in the medial epicondyle. (From Conway et al.,[40] with permission.)

the insertion of the anterior bundle. A second group of divergent 3.2-mm drill holes are made through the medial epicondyle, beginning anteriorly at the origin of the anterior bundle, such that they exit posteriorly, anterior to the intermuscular septum and ulnar nerve (Fig. 11-12A). The isometry of these drill holes can be confirmed by placing a suture through the holes and then moving the elbow, ensuring constant tension on the suture. The tendon graft, which should be at least

15 cm long, is passed through the drill holes in a figure-of-eight fashion, with the graft ends placed within the bony tunnel (Fig. 11-12B). With the forearm fully supinated, the elbow in neutral valgus/varus, and 45 degrees of flexion, the ligament is maximally tensioned and sutured to itself, and any remaining MUCL anterior bundle, using a nonabsorbable #1 suture. The graft should not abrade or impinge on the margins of the joint. The split in the flexor origin is closed with an

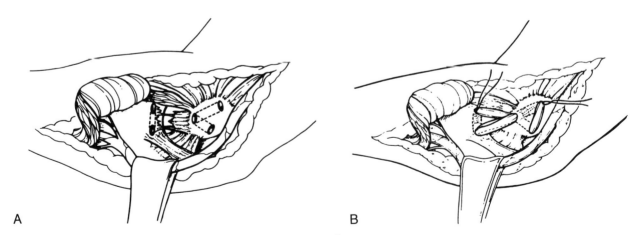

Fig. 11-12. Reconstruction of the medial ulnar collateral ligament with anterior transposition of the ulnar nerve. **(A)** Drill holes are placed at the humeral and ulnar insertions of the anterior bundle. The ulnar nerve is gently retracted posteriorly. **(B)** The tendon graft is passed through the bone tunnels in a figure-of-eight fashion, such that the tendon ends are buried in the bone. (From Conway et al.,[40] with permission.)

absorbable 2–0 suture, and the skin is closed with a 4–0 subcuticular suture. A long-arm splint is applied with the elbow at 90 degrees of flexion and in neutral rotation.

Postoperative Management and Rehabilitation

Postoperative management is as described by Jobe and Elattrache.[93] Immediate hand, wrist, and shoulder motion is initiated. The patient is given a soft ball to squeeze to maintain flexor-pronator strength. Between 10 and 14 days, the splint is removed and active elbow motion begun. Between 4 and 6 weeks, wrist and elbow strengthening is initiated, starting with isometric exercises and progressing through isotonic, isokinetic, and resisted strengthening. After 3 to 4 months, a throwing program is initiated for the throwing athlete, incorporating a short toss. At approximately 5 months, the baseball pitcher is allowed a 60-foot toss with no wind-up. At 6 months, he is allowed to pitch from the mound at 50 percent of his normal speed, and at 8 months at 75 percent of his normal speed. Around 1 year following surgery, he is allowed to pitch at full speed but is limited to one to two innings at each outing. Thereafter, the number of innings at each outing is increased such that he is back to full competition at approximately 18 months.[92] A loss of elbow extension should be anticipated. This may be as much as 25 degrees but does not preclude an excellent result.[40] Development of pain or swelling over the reconstructed ligament dictates a period of rest from throwing until the symptoms subside. To avoid a relapse, a gradual return to throwing is allowed.[92]

The results of surgery are excellent,[21] provided that no previous surgery has been undertaken.[40] Elattrache and Jobe[54] reported an 80 percent good or excellent result, with 68 percent of the athletes returning to their previous level of competition.

Posterolateral Rotatory Instability of the Elbow

Osborne and Cotterill[162] described the clinical and pathologic findings of posterolateral rotatory instability (PLRI), as well as the surgical management. Isolated injury of the LUCL was reported by Johansson,[96] O'Driscoll and Morrey[139,145,157] have described a clinical test that is pathognomonic of PLRI and also their technique to reconstruct the LUCL.

Johansson[96] felt that the injury resulted from adduction of the flexed elbow. He reported two cases in which the injury occurred when the arm was fully internally rotated behind the back and then forced cranially. The most likely mechanism of injury occurs when a valgus, external rotational moment is applied to the axially loaded, slightly flexed elbow, which results in failure of the posterolateral complex, with or without elbow dislocation (Fig. 11-13).[160,164] The MUCL anterior bundle remains intact, and the elbow will be stable to valgus stress if the forearm is fully pronated.

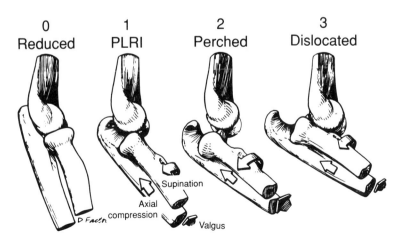

Fig. 11-13. Postulated stages of posterolateral dislocation of the elbow, illustrating forces responsible for displacement. (From O'Driscoll et al.,[160] with permission.)

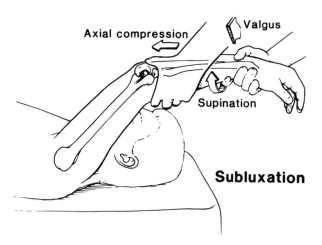

Fig. 11-14. Posterolateral rotatory instability of the elbow. The patient is examined supine with the upper extremity beside the patient's head. With the shoulder maximally externally rotated and the forearm maximally supinated, a valgus stress is applied to the axially loaded elbow, while it is slowly flexed and extended. Posterolateral subluxation is noted visibly and palpably. (From O'Driscoll et al.,[157] with permission.)

Recurrent subluxation may result in degenerative arthritis, with formation of loose bodies. A history of previous elbow injury or dislocation is followed by symptoms of instability. A sensation of the elbow "giving way" when subjected to an axial load, or "popping"

with elbow movement, particularly with the forearm supinated, may be reported. Pain occurs over the lateral aspect of the elbow, and a mistaken diagnosis of lateral epicondylitis may be entertained. Limited elbow extension and crepitus with motion may be found. The pathognomonic finding is a positive lateral pivot-shift sign, as described by O'Driscoll et al.[139,157] (Fig. 11-14). This may be positive in the conscious patient but is usually easier to demonstrate in the anesthetized individual. Radiographs are often normal.

Management

Symptomatic chronic PLRI is best managed by surgical intervention. Osborne and Cotterill[163] divided the extensor origin and opened the joint posterior to the LUCL. The lateral humerus is scarified and two transverse drill holes are placed as close to the articular margins as possible. The posterolateral capsule is then sutured to the bone, obliterating any capsular redundancy. The elbow is immobilized in about 40 degrees of flexion for 4 weeks and then active motion is begun. They reported 100 percent success in eight patients treated by this method.

Nestor and colleagues[145] approach the elbow through a Kocher incision (Fig. 11-15). The common extensor origin and anconeus are elevated off the lateral capsuloligamentous complex. The joint is opened

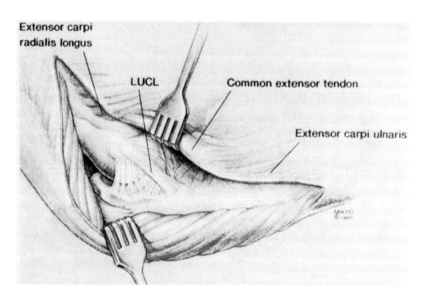

Fig. 11-15. The posterolateral approach to the elbow is utilized for reconstruction or repair of the lateral collateral ligament (LUCL). (From Nestor et al.,[145] with permission.)

longitudinally, loose bodies extracted, and the radiocapitellar articulation inspected for degenerative changes. The capsule is tightened with plication sutures. If an intact LUCL is lax, a Bunnell-type suture is placed through it and sutured to the anatomic insertion of the LUCL (Fig. 11-16).

Should the LUCL be deficient, it can be augmented with an autogenous tendon graft. Two 3.2-mm drill holes are placed 1 cm apart immediately posterior to the tubercle of the supinator crest. A suture is placed through the ulnar drill holes and the two free ends held against the lateral epicondylar insertion of the LUCL (Fig. 11-17). The elbow is placed through a range of motion to ensure that constant tension is maintained on the suture. This confirms the isometric insertion and the anterior 3.2-mm drill hole is placed at this point, with two divergent posterior drill holes being created. The graft is passed through the drill holes in a figure-of-eight fashion. With the elbow in full pronation and flexed 30 degrees, the tendon is sutured at maximal

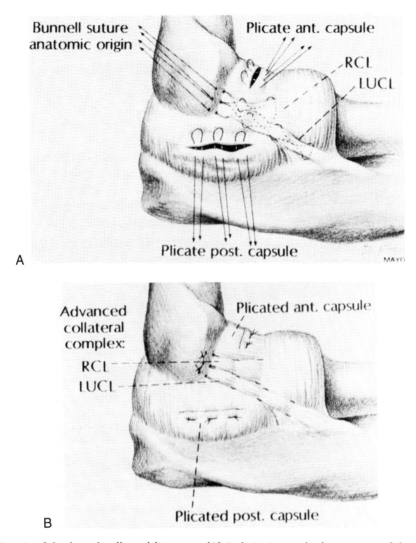

Fig. 11-16. Repair of the lateral collateral ligament. **(A)** Imbrication and advancement of the lateral collateral ligament (LUCL) and radial collateral ligament (RCL) is performed first. Anterior and posterior capsular plication is then undertaken. **(B)** The sutures through the collateral ligaments are tied, followed by the plicating sutures in the anterior and posterior capsule. (From Nestor et al.,[145] with permission.)

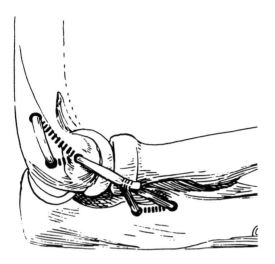

Fig. 11-17. Reconstruction of the lateral collateral ligament. The tendon graft is placed through drill holes in the lateral epicondyle and lateral aspect of the ulna (supinator crest), such that there are three tendon strands crossing the joint. (From Nestor et al.,[145] with permission.)

tension to itself (Fig. 11-1). The tendon is not allowed to abrade against any of the bony margins. The capsular plication sutures are tied last to achieve maximum tension (Fig. 11-16). The elbow is then examined to ensure that the instability has been eliminated. With the elbow at 90-degree flexion and in full pronation, a posterior plaster splint is applied.

Postoperative Management and Rehabilitation

The elbow is immobilized in a cast for 4 weeks with the joint in 90-degree flexion and the forearm fully pronated.[145] A cast-brace with a 30-degree extension block is then worn for 6 weeks.[139] After 10 weeks, the extension block is removed and the brace worn for an additional 4 to 6 weeks. Following removal of the brace, a graduated program of motion, strengthening, and endurance is instituted. The goal is to return the athlete to full activities at 12 months.[139] For the throwing athlete, the rehabilitation program would be identical to the short toss, long toss program previously described following reconstruction of the MUCL anterior bundle.

Using this technique, Nestor and colleagues[145] reported 64 percent good, or excellent results and 36 percent fair or poor results. Previous surgery was associated with a fair or poor outcome.

INTRA-ARTICULAR FRACTURES

Radial Head Fractures

A fall on the outstretched, pronated hand is the usual cause of a radial head fracture.[97] Radial head fractures constitute one of the commonest elbow injuries.[97,167] Athletes who place high demands on the elbow will not tolerate an incongruous radial head; therefore operative intervention is more frequent in athletes than in the general population.

Management

The athlete with a radial head fracture should be carefully examined for associated injuries, including an elbow dislocation, an olecranon fracture, a MUCL anterior bundle tear, carpal injuries, and the Essex-Lopresti injury[53,55] (Fig. 11-18). Radiographs of the elbow and both wrists should be requested routinely. The elbow should be aspirated and injected with local anesthetic to assess the range of motion. A block to motion is an indication for surgical intervention.

Undisplaced (Mason type 1) fractures may be managed by aspiration of the acute hemarthrosis and immediate active motion.[129] Night-time extension splinting in supination is used for 6 weeks. A minimally displaced (Mason type 2) fracture, without a mechanical block to elbow flexion, extension, and forearm rotation, may be treated nonoperatively, as for a Mason type 1 fracture.[129] Fractures displaced 2 mm or more, with or without a block to motion, should undergo open reduction and internal fixation.[65,108]

Whenever possible, the displaced radial head fracture should be reduced and internally fixed to allow immediate active ROM, to prevent joint stiffness,[65,108] and to avoid proximal migration of the radius.[64,97] A simple, displaced wedge fracture may be approached either through a posterolateral Kocher incision or through a simple lateral extensor-splinting approach.[108]

The comminuted fracture is best exposed by an osteotomy of the lateral epicondyle with distal reflection of the common extensor origin.[64,65] This provides excellent exposure, preserves the LUCL, and decreases the risk of injury to the posterior interosseous nerve (PIN).[65,185] The epicondyle is reattached with one or two 3.5-mm AO cortical screws. Fixation of the radial head with either mini-AO, Herbert, or cannulated Whipple-Herbert screws is preferred.[64,65,129]

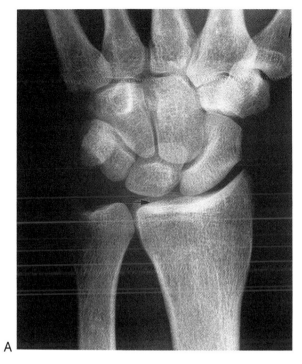
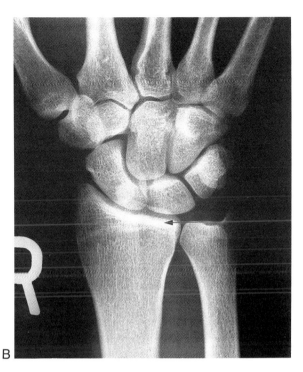

Fig. 11-18. Essex-Lopresti injury. Standard PA wrist views of a patient with a comminuted radial head fracture and wrist pain. The ulnar plus variance is clearly seen on the left, compared with the normal right side. **(A)** Left wrist. **(B)** Right wrist for normal side comparison.

Absorbable pins may be used for small fragments (Fig. 11-19).

If the fracture is not reconstructable, a decision between excision and replacement arthroplasty has to be made. If disruption of the interosseous membrane exists, a metallic implant should be inserted,[75] as Silastic implants will not resist the normal axial loading.[37,84] Resection of the radial head without replacement following an Essex-Lopresti injury may result in proximal migration of the radius, with the development of wrist and elbow pain[53,84,97] (Fig. 11-20).

In the presence of an intact interosseous membrane, and a stable wrist and elbow joint, simple excision is preferred. Bennett and colleagues[20,207,208] recommend replacement arthroplasty of the comminuted radial head fracture, when the MUCL anterior bundle has been repaired. Should the surgeon elect to preserve the radial head, despite indications to excise it, evidence suggests that late excision will not affect the final outcome.[31,32]

Postoperative Management and Rehabilitation

The day following surgery, active ROM is begun.[65] Night-time splinting in maximum extension is encouraged for at least 6 weeks. Passive stretching is allowed after 6 weeks, with introduction of isometric strengthening and resisted strengthening at 9 weeks. Return to athletic throwing activities at 3 to 4 months is anticipated after an isolated radial head fracture.

Olecranon Fractures

The olecranon may fracture as a result of direct trauma or a fall on the outstretched hand, or secondary to repetitive stress from throwing.[85]

Management

Fractures displaced less than 2 mm may be treated in a removal resting splint, with the elbow in 90 degrees of flexion for 3 weeks.[33] Gentle active motion is begun

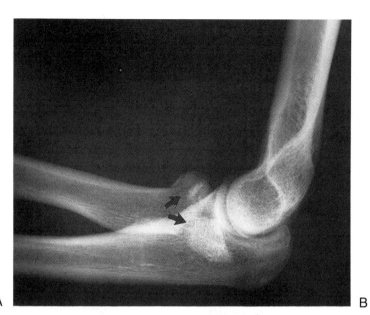
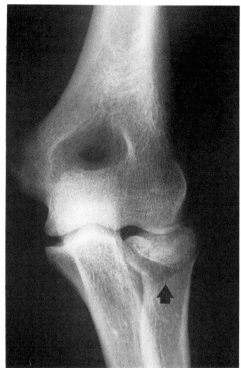
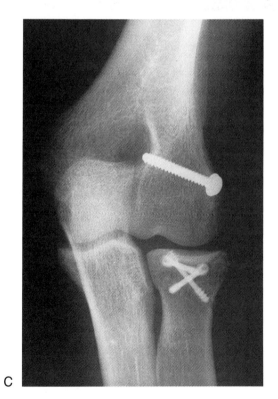
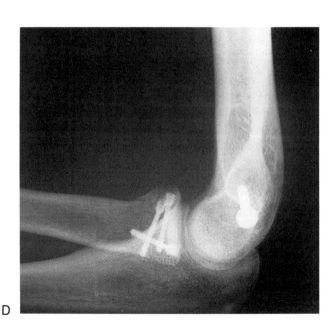

Fig. 11-19. A comminuted radial head fracture (Mason type 3). **(A)** Preoperative lateral view. Comminuted fragments of fractured radial head (*arrows*). **(B)** Preoperative AP view. Comminuted fragments of fractured radial head (*arrows*). **(C)** Postoperative AP view. Open reduction and internal fixation with Herbert screws. Lateral epicondylar osteotomy to obtain exposure is internally fixed with a 3.5-mm compression screw. **(D)** Postoperative lateral view.

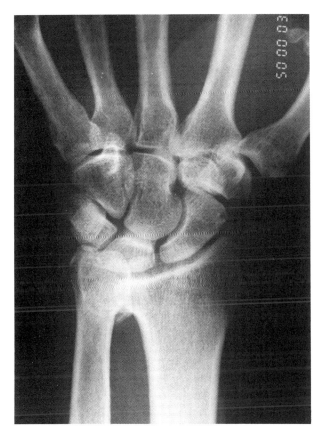

Fig. 11-20. Essex-Lopresti injury. Following resection of a comminuted radial head fracture, this patient presented 8 years later with a history of chronic wrist and elbow pain. Proximal migration of the radius is evident on this film.

[204,206,215,220] In adolescents, the injury occurs through the olecranon physis and may go on to non-union.[204,220] The fracture occurs as a result of repetitive throwing.[19,156,204,220] If the player presents early, union can be anticipated when the elbow is rested or immobilized for 3 weeks.[45] Failure to respond to rest and immobilization is an indication for open reduction, internal fixation, and bone grafting.[45,85]

Postoperative Management and Rehabilitation

The goal of surgery is to achieve stable fixation such that active motion can be initiated immediately postoperatively. A sling may be worn temporarily but should be discarded within 2 weeks. Night-time extension splinting may be required. Strengthening is begun at 6 weeks, when fracture union is present

TENDON AVULSIONS
Distal Biceps Brachii Avulsion

Rupture of the distal insertion of the biceps brachii is uncommon.[4,9,13,27,28,56,123,134,140,214] It occurs as a result of a forceful eccentric contraction.[4,56,123,214] All ruptures

at 3 weeks with unrestricted motion at 6 weeks (Fig. 11-21). Displaced fractures require open reduction and internal fixation.[12] Simple transverse fractures are fixed either with a double-twist tension band technique, or an AO one-third tubular plate.[61,82,144] For the tension band technique, the wire loops should be placed anterior to the longitudinal Kirschner wires or AO screw.[182] Distal oblique, or comminuted fractures, should be fixed with a 3.5 mm pelvic reconstruction plate, or a one-third tubular plate,[33,61,82,86] especially if a Regan type 3 coronoid fracture is present,[176] associated with elbow instability (Fig. 11-22). Comminuted proximal fractures, which are not amenable to internal fixation, may be treated by excision and repair of the triceps to the ulna.[19,33,63,188]

Stress fractures are uncommon but have been described in both adolescents and adults.[14,19,85,112,132,156,]

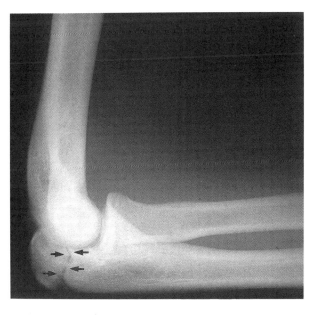

Fig. 11-21. An olecranon fracture displaced less than 2 mm. This is a stable fracture pattern due to the integrity of the overlying fascia of the triceps, anconeus, and flexor carpi ulnaris and can be managed nonoperatively.

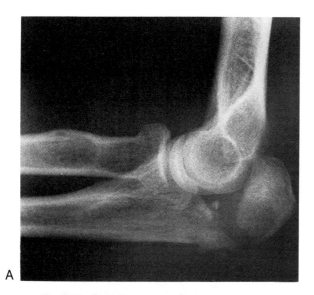

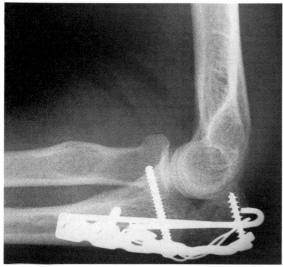

Fig. 11-22. A comminuted fracture of the olecranon, requiring internal fixation using a 3.5-mm pelvic reconstruction plate combined with a tension band wire technique. **(A)** Preoperative appearance. Note the impaction of the articular surface, which is a contraindication for tension band fixation alone. **(B)** Postoperative appearance. It is imperative to restore the normal coronoid-olecranon relationship.

reported have been in men and usually involve the dominant extremity.[137] Kannus and Józsa[106] have demonstrated that ruptures only occur in degenerative tendons. The patient experiences sudden, severe, antecu-

bital pain, followed by swelling, ecchymosis, and weakness of elbow flexion and forearm supination.[134,214] Proximal retraction of the biceps is noted, with the absence of a palpable tendon. Partial rupture of the tendon has been described.[27]

Repair of the biceps tendon to the radial tuberosity will restore strength and endurance.[4,123,140,153] Failure to repair the biceps will result in an 86 percent loss in supination endurance, a 55 percent loss in supination strength, a 21 percent loss in elbow flexion endurance, and a 36 percent loss in elbow flexion strength.[13]

Management

Repair of the biceps tendon may be achieved either by a single-incision anterior approach[123] or by a two-incision Boyd and Anderson approach,[28,214] modified to avoid a radioulnar synostosis[56] (Fig. 11-23). The technique described by Morrey[134] is preferred. An anterior Henry approach is used to expose the biceps tendon and tuberosity. The tendon is identified, trimmed, and two #1 nonabsorbable Bunnell-type sutures are placed through it.

A curved Kelly forcep is directed posteriorly between the radius and ulna until the posterior skin is tented. The skin is incised and the muscle bluntly split to expose the tuberosity. A burr is used to create an aperture in the tuberosity. With the elbow flexed 90 degrees and fully supinated, the tendon is brought into the radius and the sutures brought through three drill holes and tied posteriorly.

Postoperative Management and Rehabilitation

The elbow is immobilized in an above-elbow cast in 90 degrees of flexion and full supination for 6 weeks.[214] Alternatively, the elbow is immobilized in a cast for 3 weeks and then placed in a dynamic splint for 3 weeks, as described by Morrey (preferred technique).[134] Following removal of the cast, a graduated and supervised program of elbow motion, strengthening, and endurance is instituted. An excellent functional result can be anticipated.[214]

Distal Triceps Brachii Avulsion

Rupture of the distal insertion of the triceps brachii muscle is rare[57,164,191,202,211] and accounts for 1.3 percent of all closed upper extremity tendon disruptions.[9] It

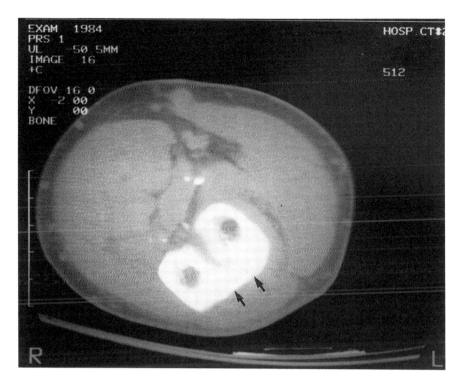

Fig. 11-23. Proximal radioulnar synostosis, following repair of a distal biceps tendon avulsion.

occurs as a result of a violent eccentric contraction, especially in weightlifters.[77,81]

Patients complain of pain at the insertion, with difficulty extending the elbow. Swelling, tenderness, and a palpable defect proximal to the olecranon are found. Inability to extend against gravity or resistance is noted. Viegas[211] described a modification of the Thompson test, to confirm the diagnosis. Radiographs may demonstrate a small olecranon avulsion in 75 percent of cases[202] (Fig. 11-24). Tears may be partial or complete, and it is generally recommended that complete tears be repaired.[57]

Management

Surgical repair of the avulsed triceps tendon to the olecranon, using a nonabsorbable #5 suture is preferred, followed by 3 weeks of immobilization at 60 degrees of flexion.[202] Active ROM is then allowed with a program of strengthening and endurance, initiated at 6 weeks. Excellent results have been reported using this technique.[202]

TENDINITIS

Lateral Epicondylitis

The etiology and management of lateral epicondylitis continue to be sources of controversy.[38,69,70,78,114,136,148,213] Although commonly called tennis elbow, most affected individuals do not play tennis. Between 23 and 50 percent of tennis players have been reported to develop symptoms of lateral epicondylitis.[41,150,168,169] The wrist extensors are active in all three tennis strokes (serve, forehand, backhand), which explains why this condition occurs in tennis players.[142] Affected individuals are usually between 40 and 50 years of age, and the dominant extremity is usually affected.[90]

Evidence shows that this is a chronic, degenerative condition of the common extensor origin and not an inflammatory condition.[38,42,149,175,187,209] Injury may occur due to direct trauma or, more usually, due to cumulative microtrauma.[91,110,147] Repetitive use that exceeds the tensile strength of the collagen fibers causes tendon

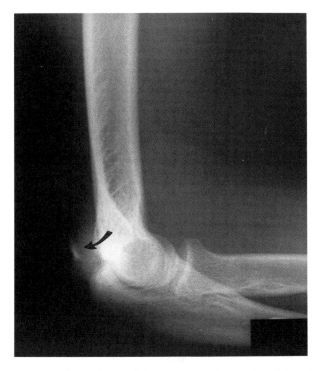

Fig. 11-24. Avulsion of the triceps tendon with a flake of bone (*arrow*) from the olecranon.

failure.[42,149,151] Continued use prevents tendon repair, with the formation of granulation tissue.[151,187]

The extensor carpi radialis brevis (ECRB) is most frequently affected, but the extensor carpi radialis longus (ECRL) and extensor digitorum communis (EDC) may also be involved.[22,41,90,148] PIN may be compressed by the ECRB aponeurosis, resulting in an associated radial tunnel syndrome.[136] The ECRB is intimately related to the ECRL, EDC, supinator, annular ligament and elbow capsule. Therefore injury to the origin of the ECRB may involve these adjacent structures.[30,187,209] In tennis players, the racket head and handle size, string tension, and frame material have all been implicated.[72,87,114,170,213] Priest et al.[169] have shown that the factors responsible for tennis elbow are increased age, increased frequency of play, increased number of years of play, and superior playing ability. The backhand stroke appears to be the most common stroke responsible for the initiation and maintenance of lateral epicondylitis.[147]

The patient will complain of lateral elbow pain, often radiating distally to the dorsoradial wrist and proximally to the shoulder. Pain is intensified by manual activities, especially those involving forearm pronation, wrist extension, and gripping or pinching.[70] Tenderness is always present over the common extensor origin, just anterior to the lateral epicondyle. Evidence for a radial tunnel syndrome should be sought. Inability to extend the elbow fully, secondary to pain, may be noted. Resisted wrist extension and gripping, with the forearm fully extended and pronated, will cause lateral elbow pain.[44]

The diagnosis may be confirmed by compressing the ECRB muscle belly with the examiner's thumb, while asking the patient to squeeze the examiner's fingers. This should alleviate the pain in a fashion analogous to a counterforce brace. Injection of 3 ml 1 percent lidocaine into the area of tenderness over the lateral epicondyle will eliminate the usual pain.[136]

Radiographs undertaken to exclude unsuspected elbow joint pathology may demonstrate calcification over the lateral epicondyle.[12,70,147,210] Bone scans, ultrasonography, and MRI are rarely helpful. Lateral epicondylitis should be differentiated from radial tunnel syndrome, posterolateral instability of the elbow, anconeus compartment syndrome, radiocapitellar arthritis, and cervical radiculopathy.[1,133,136,150]

Management

Approximately 90 percent of patients will respond satisfactorily to nonsurgical intervention.[42,110,151,152] Icing, avoidance of provocative activities (not absolute rest), NSAIDs,[152,184] and air-splint counterforce bracing,[71,196] may all be useful.[150] Local corticosteroid injection is utilized on no more than three occasions.[36,41,44,90,110,150,216] High-voltage galvanic stimulation has been recommended.[90,152] Ultrasonography,[25] common extensor stretching, strengthening, and reconditioning are introduced as soon as pain allows.[24,66,114,216]

Tennis players may benefit from a change in racquet handle size,[22] racquet material, head size, string tension, and stroke mechanics.[22,72,87,114,147,149,150,170,213] Adelsberg[3] does not recommend changing the racquet handle size, based on an electromyographic (EMG) analysis. A lower incidence of tennis elbow has been reported in those players who use two-handed strokes,[22] which may be useful in treatment and prevention.[22,169,216] Prematch stretching and warm-up should be emphasized.

Approximately 90 percent of players will recover without surgical intervention.[90] Disabling symptoms and failure to respond to adequate nonsurgical management after 6 to 12 months are indications for surgery.[42,90,170]

An 8-cm longitudinal incision is made, extending distally from the lateral epicondyle, between the ECRL and EDC, to expose the ECRB deep to the EDC and ECRL.[114,148] The degenerated ECRB tendon origin is excised completely, including the deep aponeurosis fascia overlying the PIN[148,151] (Fig. 11-25). If degenerative tissue is seen in the EDC and ECRL origins, this is excised, preserving the LUCL. The lateral epicondyle is debrided back to bleeding bone.[151] The ECRL and EDC are sutured to one another with absorbable suture, and the skin is closed.[151] If a radial tunnel syndrome is also present, the PIN is completely decompressed, utilizing the same incision.

Percutaneous release of the extensor origin has been described,[16] but this is not recommended due to the potential risk of injury to the LUCL.[139,162]

Postoperative Management and Rehabilitation

The day after surgery, active elbow, wrist, and hand motion is begun,[66] with the rehabilitation following the same guidelines as those described in the section on nonoperative management. Recovery can take between 3 to 6 months, with return to athletic activities after 6 months.

Medial Epicondylitis

Medial epicondylitis is seven to ten times less common than lateral epicondylitis.[41,42] The pathology is similar in that degeneration of the flexor-pronator origin exists, secondary to overuse or trauma.[35,42,148] The area between the pronator teres and the flexor carpi radialis (FCR) is usually involved.[42,149,150] Patients are usually between 40 and 50 years of age.[210] This condition is seen in throwing athletes, golfers, and racquet sports players.[147,168,210,224]

Pain is experienced over the medial epicondyle and may radiate distally along the anteromedial forearm

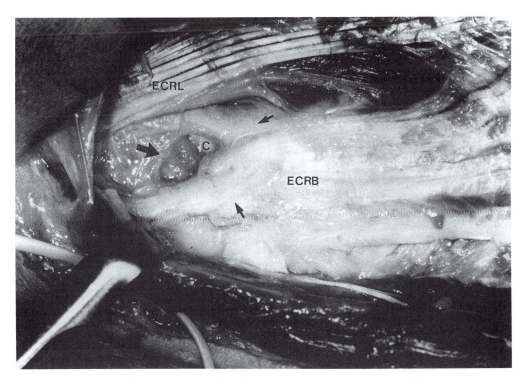

Fig. 11-25. A severe case of lateral epicondylitis, demonstrating complete rupture of the extensor carpi radialis brevis tendon from its origin (*small arrows*). The underlying capsule is also disrupted with exposure of the joint (*large arrow*). ECRL, extensor carpi radialis longus; ECRB, extensor carpi radialis brevis; C, capitellum.

into the hand and wrist. Activity increases the pain. The tennis serve and baseball pitch are provocative activities.[48,168] Cubital tunnel syndrome is a frequent associated finding.[149,150,210] Tenderness is noted over the flexor-pronator origin. Gripping or resisted wrist palmar flexion, with the elbow fully extended and supinated, will cause increased pain. Counterforce pressure over the flexor-pronator muscles may diminish pain during provocative testing. Local anesthetic infiltration into the flexor-pronator origin will alleviate the pain.

Radiographs taken to exclude intra-articular pathology may demonstrate medial epicondylar calcification.[210] Bone scans, MRI, and ultrasonography are not usually helpful. Medial epicondylar pain should be differentiated from MUCL anterior bundle insufficiency, ulnar neuropathy, pronator teres syndrome, and the valgus-extension overload syndrome.

Management

Nonoperative management is similar to that for lateral epicondylitis.[42,45,224] Approximately 90 percent of patients will recover without surgery. If 6 to 12 months of adequate nonsurgical management, fail to produce a response and if disabling symptoms are present, surgery is indicated.

A posteromedial incision, avoiding the medial antebrachial cutaneous nerve, is utilized. The flexor-pronator origin is elevated anterior to the ulnar nerve, and degenerative tissue is debrided.[149,210] The medial epicondyle is scarified and the flexor-pronator origin is anatomically reattached (Fig. 11-26).

Postoperative Management and Rehabilitation

Twenty-four hours postoperatively, active elbow, wrist, and hand motion is encouraged. Strengthening is begun after 6 weeks, with a return to sport after 4 months. Vangsness and Jobe[210] have reported good to excellent surgical results in 97 percent of patients, while Nirschl[148] has reported complete pain relief for both medial and lateral epicondylitis in 85 percent of cases.

Triceps Tendinitis

Triceps tendinitis is the least common tendonitis of the elbow.[149,150] It is seen predominantly in the throwing sports.[150] It is best treated nonoperatively in a manner similar to treatment of medial and lateral epicondylitis.

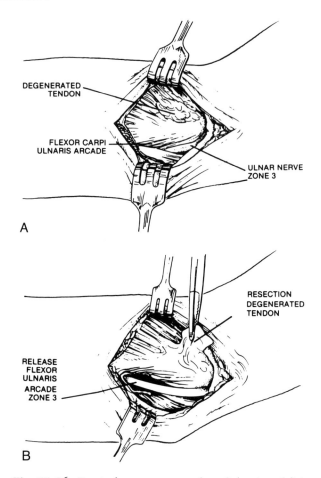

Fig. 11-26. Surgical management of medial epicondylitis. **(A)** Degenerative tissue is usually found at the origins of the pronator teres and flexor carpi radialis. **(B)** Excision of the pathologic tissue with preservation of all normal tissue. (From Nirschl,[150] with permission.)

Rarely, surgical intervention is required; degenerative tissue is found at the insertion of the triceps to the olecranon. This is excised with repair of the triceps back to the olecranon.[149] Postoperative management consists of a graduated program of active ROM, followed by isometric and resisted strengthening.[149]

THE MEDIAL STRESS SYNDROME

Repetitive forceful valgus stress applied to the elbow is responsible for the medial stress syndrome.[8,62,73,88,90,109,194,205] The features described include:

1. Valgus-extension overload[8,221,222]
2. Loose body formation[6,8,17,20,109,194]
3. MUCL anterior bundle injury[93]
4. Osteochondritis dissecans of the capitellum[6,8,90]
5. Medial epicondylitis[210]
6. Ulnar neuropathy[95]
7. Elbow flexion contractures and an increased elbow carrying angle[88,90,109]

Some of these topics are described in separate sections. Since repetitive, forceful valgus stress is the cause of injury, whether it be to the pitcher or javelin thrower, this can be managed by technique modification.[5,6,8,132] In the overhand throw, the extremity trails behind the body (opening the body less), and it is the rapid arm acceleration from this position that applies valgus stress to the elbow.[90,109,205] Valgus stress can be reduced by "opening the body less,"[90] meaning that the arm is brought through with the body.[121] Side-arm pitches, or throws, have also been implicated, and more vertical deliveries, especially for javelin throwers, are preferred.[5,121,132] Proper conditioning and warm-up appear to prevent injury.[90,205] Reduction in the number and force of the throws will reduce the likelihood of injury.[73,90,193]

Valgus-Extension Overload

Wilson and colleagues[221,222] drew attention to posteromedial ulnohumeral impingement, secondary to attenuation of the MUCL anterior bundle. Hypertrophy of the humerus and narrowing of the olecranon fossa contribute to impingement.[98,109] This results in marginal "kissing osteophytes" with loose body formation,[109] causing elbow locking or loss of extension[8] (Fig. 11-27). When a posteromedial osteophyte is present, surgery is the most effective treatment.[221]

Management

This condition is usually managed arthroscopically; this treatment is not discussed in detail in this chapter. The elbow is approached through a posterolateral incision.[221] The joint is debrided of loose bodies and, using an osteotome, the osteophyte at the olecranon tip is excised, followed by removal of the medial osteophyte.[8,221] Postoperatively, the elbow is actively mobilized,[221] with a good result anticipated.[8] Return to pitching activities is allowed at about 8 weeks.[8]

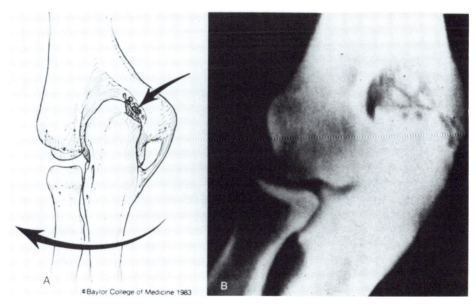

© Baylor College of Medicine 1983

Fig. 11-27. Valgus-extension overload. **(A)** Valgus displacement of the elbow with laxity of the medial collateral ligament results in posteromedial ulnohumeral impingement and loose body formation. **(B)** Radiographic appearance of loose bodies in the olecranon fossa.

NERVE INJURY SYNDROMES

Most of the nerve injury syndromes occur in throwing[17,47,79,80,91,132] and racquet sports.[79,80,192,223] However, they may be seen in swimming,[79,80] weightlifting,[43] gymnastics,[79,80,91] or wrestling.[79,80] The ulnar nerve is the most commonly affected nerve at the elbow.[80] Although nerve injuries are discussed separately in this section, co-existent pathology may also require surgical correction, for example, chronic MUCL anterior bundle insufficiency with ulnar neuropathy (seen in 40 percent of patients), or lateral epicondylitis with radial tunnel syndrome.[93]

Ulnar Neuropathy

Ulnar neuropathy may be due to traction, compression, or friction.[58,90,91,95,124] Symptoms are aggravated by elbow flexion and wrist extension.[218] Baseball pitchers, racquet sports players, and weightlifters are more commonly affected.[47,90]

Valgus overload of the elbow, seen predominantly in baseball pitchers (termed the *medial stress syndrome*), may present with ulnar neuropathy as part of the symptom complex. Hypertrophy of the FCU and a type IB cubital tunnel retinaculum (CTR) may cause compression[158] (Fig. 11-28). This is a pathologically thick CTR

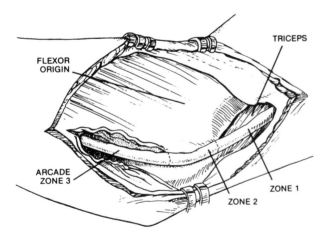

Fig. 11-28. Ulnar nerve compression at the elbow. According to Nirschl, compression of the ulnar nerve is most commonly encountered in zone 3, due to hypertrophy of the flexor carpi ulnaris muscle. (From Nirschl,[150] with permission.)

that becomes taut, compressing the nerve between 90 and 120 degrees of flexion.[158] Recurrent injury to the MUCL may result in scar formation, calcification, and ossification with resultant ulnar nerve compression.[17,18,90] The secondary joint changes that occur, including bony hypertrophy, osteophyte formation, and elbow flexion contracture, may also contribute to nerve injury.[90,109] Attenuation of the MUCL anterior bundle, with valgus instability and an increased carrying angle, will result in traction on the ulnar nerve during throwing activities.[91] Deficiency of the CTR, present in 16.2 percent of people, allows anterior subluxation of the ulnar nerve with elbow flexion.[39,159] As a result of friction, inflammation occurs, causing pain and limiting activities.[91]

The athlete presents with the typical features of ulnar neuropathy.[95] Pain over the cubital tunnel, radiating distally along the medial border of the forearm, especially when throwing, is common.[47,95] A painful pop may occur with a subluxating ulnar nerve when doing a bench-press or during rapid flexion of the elbow, for example, during a tennis serve.[91] Paresthesiae, numbness, clumsiness, or heaviness of the hand may be experienced.[90,91] Palpation of the nerve may elicit tenderness with a markedly positive Tinel's sign.[91] Subluxation may be evident. An elbow flexion test may reproduce the usual symptoms of paresthesiae in the ring and small fingers.[34,174,212] Two-point discrimination may be altered. Alteration of sensation over the dorsoulnar aspect of the hand should be sought to differentiate the proximally compressed nerve from entrapment in Guyon's canal. Wasting of the intrinsics is a late sign and signifies a poor prognosis.[2,59] The FCU and flexor digitorum profundus are rarely affected.[91]

The differential diagnosis includes cervical radiculopathy, thoracic outlet syndrome, compression in Guyon's canal, brachial neuritis, and a Pancoast tumor.[2,91] In addition, medial elbow pain may be secondary to deficiency of the MUCL, posteromedial ulnohumeral impingement, loose bodies, or medial epicondylitis. Nirschl[149] noted that 60 percent of patients operated on for medial epicondylitis will have symptoms of ulnar nerve dysfunction.

Radiographs of the elbow are helpful in diagnosing intra-articular causes of medial elbow pain. Electrodiagnostic tests are frequently normal in the early stages when treatment is most effective.[90,91] Treatment should therefore be largely directed by the clinical findings.

Management

The early neuropathy or acute injury is treated by resting the elbow.[91] A night-time splint in 30-degree flexion is often useful.[46,49,124,190] NSAIDs are used infrequently, and steroid injections should not be used.[47,91] Most athletes with a symptomatic ulnar nerve will require surgery.[47,90,95]

A procedure that only decompresses the ulnar nerve is inadequate for the throwing athlete, since the tension applied to the nerve, when the elbow is flexed, remains unaltered.[91] Epicondylectomy risks injuring the MUCL anterior bundle and should not be performed.[159] Although subcutaneous anterior transposition has been recommended,[52,200] submuscular transposition is preferred, as it places the nerve in a protected, well-vascularized bed.[47,59,67,90,95,115] Division and repair of the flexor-pronator origin has not affected function in high-caliber throwing athletes.[47,95]

Internal neurolysis has not been shown to improve outcome and should not be performed.[91,125,126,130]

A longitudinal incision is placed posteriorly, immediately medial to the ulna, and carried proximally in the midline of the arm. This ensures that the incision lies in a cutaneous internervous plane, with decreased risk to the medial antebrachial cutaneous nerve[173] (Fig. 11-29). The ulnar nerve is identified and dissected free with its vessels. The CTR is divided along with the aponeurosis between the two heads of the FCU. The intermuscular septum is resected to the level of the arcade of Struthers[7,59,116] (Fig. 11-29). The FCU is elevated from both the ulna and the medial epicondyle, preserving the ulnar nerve motor branches.[116] The MUCL lies immediately beneath the FCU and is protected. The flexor-pronator origin is released from the medial epicondyle, leaving a tendinous cuff on the epicondyle for later reattachment.[116] The ulnar nerve is transposed anteriorly onto the brachialis muscle,

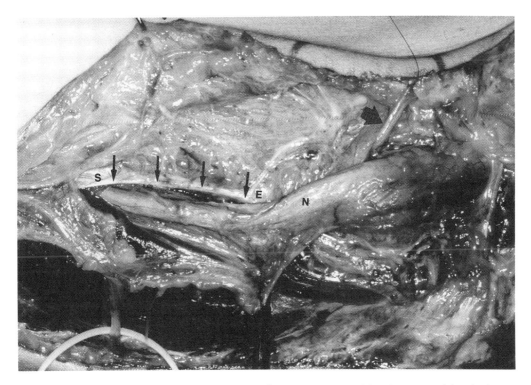

Fig. 11-29. At revision of a failed anterior subcutaneous ulnar nerve transposition, it was noted that the intermuscular septum had been left intact (*small arrow*). Note the nerve constriction at the epicondyle and that there was a neuroma of a branch of the medial antebrachial cutaneous nerve (*large arrow*). N, ulnar nerve; E, Medial epicondyle; S, medial intermuscular septum.

deep to the flexor-pronator musculature (Fig. 11-30).[115] The flexor-pronator origin, including the FCU, is sutured back to the ulna and medial epicondyle with #1 absorbable sutures. With the nerve under direct vision, all sutures are tied together (Fig. 11-30). The arm is immobilized in a long-arm splint with the elbow flexed to 90 degrees.

Postoperative Management and Rehabilitation

The following day, the drain and splint are removed. Immediate active ROM is begun, to allow nerve excursion and to avoid epineurial scarring. Strengthening is initiated at 6 weeks, and a short-toss, long-toss program is begun at 8 weeks in the throwing athlete. Return to full competition should be anticipated at approximately 4 to 6 months.[47,67,91,95]

Musculocutaneous Nerve Compression

Bassett and Nunley[15] described 11 patients with acute or chronic compression of the lateral antebrachial cutaneous nerve by the biceps aponeurosis and tendon. One of these patients was a swimmer, and three were tennis players. All presented with pain in the anterolateral elbow, mimicking lateral epicondylitis. Burning dysesthesia along the radial aspect of the volar forearm was noted in those with acute onset. Repeated forearm pronation and supination accentuated the pain in those with chronic symptoms. Four patients responded to nonoperative treatment, including NSAIDs and rest, while the remaining seven patients were relieved of their symptoms by excision of a triangular wedge of the biceps tendon.

Pronator Teres Syndrome

Repetitive activities such as rowing, weight training, tennis, and throwing have been implicated in pronator teres syndrome.[76] Compression occurs as a result of pronator teres hypertrophy, a fibrous band within the pronator teres, thickening of the lacertus fibrosis, or a tight fibrous arch of the flexor digitorum superficialis.[76] Symptoms are usually vague and consist of proximal forearm aching, especially with vigorous activity.[76] Clumsiness, weakness, and a loss of dexterity may be described. Paresthesiae are generally mild and do not usually occur at night, differentiating this condition from carpal tunnel syndrome.[76]

Symptoms may be provoked by resistance to forearm pronation and supination, elbow flexion, and long finger flexion.[76] The most reliable findings are tenderness over the proximal forearm associated with a positive pronator compression test.[76] Motor strength and sensory testing are usually normal. Carpal tunnel syndrome may co-exist and should be differentiated. Electrodiagnostic studies are positive in approximately 15 to 20 percent of patients.[76]

Management

Initial management is directed at avoidance of repetitive activity, splinting of the elbow in 90 degrees of flexion and neutral rotation, and the use of NSAIDs. Failure of nonoperative treatment is an indication for surgical exploration and decompression of the nerve by division of the offending structures. This is a difficult diagnosis; however, in well-selected cases, good results can be expected in 78 percent of cases treated surgically.[76]

Radial Tunnel Syndrome

The diagnosis of radial tunnel syndrome has been disputed since the first description by Roles and Maudsley.[181] The literature and personal experience indicate that the syndrome does exist but that it is uncommon and overdiagnosed.[51,89,120,179,217] It may occur in isolation or in conjunction with lateral epicondylitis.[89,179] Sanders[186] suggests that these two conditions overlap, due to the relationship between the common extensor origin and PIN; he has proposed a unified theory.

The PIN may be compressed by the

1. Fibrous bands at the radial head
2. Radial recurrent vessels[120]
3. Tendinous margin of the ECRB[120,143]
4. Arcade of Frohse[120,217]
5. Distal edge of the supinator[120,199]

The patient will present with chronic, vague aching in the proximal lateral forearm.[143] The pain may radiate proximally and distally to the dorsoradial aspect of the wrist.[51] Pain is aggravated by repetitive forearm rotation. Unilateral tenderness is found over the radial tunnel. No muscle weakness or wasting is found.

The diagnosis needs to be differentiated from cervical radiculopathy, lateral epicondylitis, anconeus com-

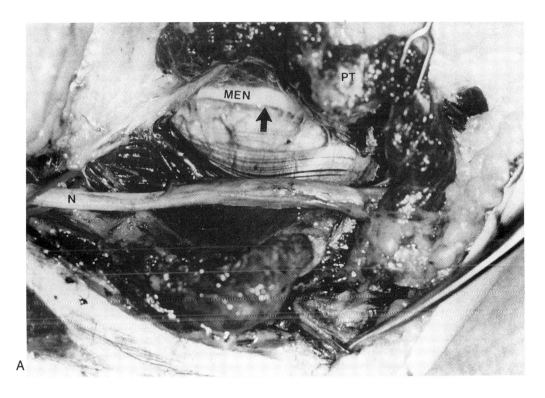

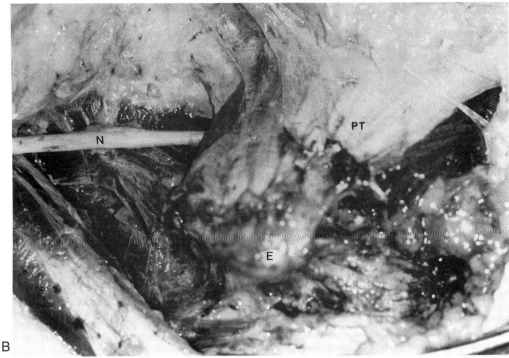

Fig. 11-30. Anterior submuscular transposition of the ulnar nerve. **(A)** The ulnar nerve is shown lying on the brachialis muscle with the median nerve lying adjacent to it, on the deep surface of the flexor-pronator musculature (*arrow*). MEN, median nerve; N, ulnar nerve; PT, flexor-pronator musculature. **(B)** Following transposition, the ulnar nerve is shown passing deep to the flexor-pronator origin, in a straight line, with no residual areas of compression. E, epicondyle; N, ulnar nerve; PT, flexor-pronator musculature.

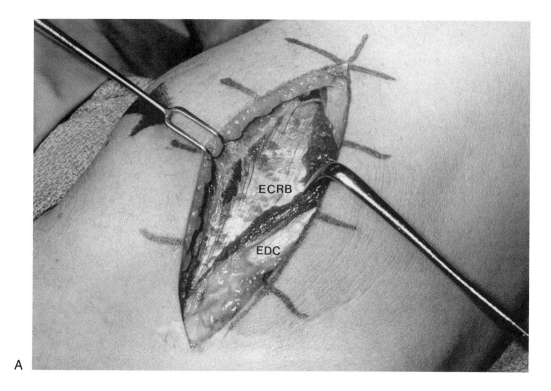

A

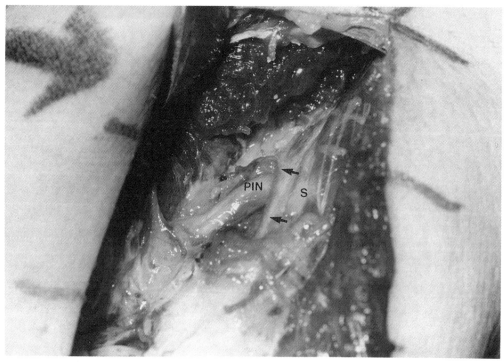

B

Fig. 11-31. The surgical approach to the posterior interosseous nerve and lateral epicondylar origin of the extensor carpi radialis brevis (ECRB). **(A)** The ECRB tendon is exposed deep to the extensor carpi radialis longus and extensor digitorum communis through an intermuscular splitting incision. ECRB, extensor carpi radialis brevis; EDC, extensor digitorum communis. **(B)** The posterior interosseous nerve (PIN) is shown passing deep to the arcade of Frohse (*arrow*) and supinator muscle (*S*). (*Figure continues.*)

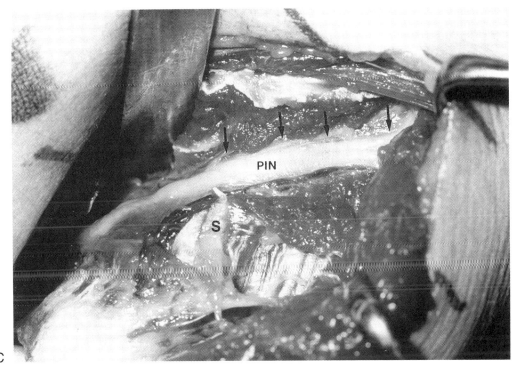

Fig. 11-31 (*Continued*). **(C)** The entire PIN has been decompressed from the proximal margin of the supinator (*S*), to its distal edge (*arrow*).

partment syndrome, radiocapitellar arthrosis, and posterolateral rotatory instability of the elbow.[136] Numerous provocative tests have been described to differentiate between radial tunnel syndrome and lateral epicondylitis, but these are unreliable.[51] Electrodiagnostic testing is usually normal.[136,179,217] The two most useful findings are discrete tenderness over the PIN and elimination of the usual pain by injecting 5 ml of 1 percent lidocaine into the radial tunnel.[136,179] Accurate placement of local anesthetic is confirmed by the development of a PIN palsy.

Management

Nonoperative management is usually unsuccessful. Surgical decompression provides good-to-excellent results in about 50 percent of patients.[89,179] The surgical approach is described in the section on lateral epicondylitis (Fig. 11-31). Postoperative management and rehabilitation are identical to that used following release of the common extensor origin.

REFERENCES

1. Abrahamsson S-O, Sollerman C, Söderberg T et al: Lateral elbow pain caused by anconeus compartment syndrome: a case report. Acta Orthop Scand 58:589–591, 1987
2. Adelaar RS, Foster WC, McDowell C: The treatment of the cubital tunnel syndrome. J Hand Surg 9A:90–95, 1984
3. Adelsberg S: The tennis stroke: an EMG analysis of selected muscles with rackets of increasing grip size. Am J Sports Med 14:139–142, 1986
4. Agins HJ, Chess JL, Hoekstra DV, Teitge RA: Rupture of the distal insertion of the biceps brachii tendon. Clin Orthop 234:34–38, 1988
5. Albright JA, Jokl P, Shaw R, Albright JP: Clinical study of baseball pitchers: correlation of injury to the throwing arm with method of delivery. Am J Sports Med 6:15–21, 1978
6. Allman FL: Overuse injury in the throwing sports. p. 417. In Torg JS, Welsh PR, Shepard RJ (eds): Current Therapy in Sports Medicine. Vol. 2. BC Decker, Philadelphia, 1990

7. Al-Qattan MM, Murray KA: The arcade of Struthers: an anatomical study. J Hand Surg 16B:311–314, 1991

8. Andrews JR: Bony injuries about the elbow in the throwing athlete. p. 323. In: American Academy of Orthopaedic Surgeons Instructional Course Lectures, Vol. 34. CV Mosby, St. Louis, 1985

9. Anzel SH, Covey KW, Weiner AD, Lipscomb PR: Disruption of muscles and tendons. Surgery 45:406–414, 1959

10. Arnold JA, Nasca RJ, Nelson CL: Supracondylar fractures of the humerus. The role of dynamic factors in prevention of deformity. J Bone Joint Surg [Am] 59A:589–595, 1977

11. Aronen JG: Problems of the upper extremity in gymnastics. Clin Sports Med 4:61–71, 1985

12. Badgley CE, Hayes JT: Athletic injuries to the elbow, forearm, wrist and hand. Am J Surg 98:432–446, 1959

13. Baker BE, Bierwagen D: Rupture of the distal tendon of the biceps brachii. Operative versus non-operative treatment. J Bone Joint Surg [Am] 67A:414–417, 1985

14. Barnes DA, Tullos HS: An analysis of 100 symptomatic baseball players. Am J Sports Med 6:62–67, 1978

15. Bassett FH, Nunley JA: Compression of the musculocutaneous nerve at the elbow. J Bone Joint Surg [Am] 64A:1050–1052, 1982

16. Baumgard SH, Schwartz DR: Percutaneous release of the epicondylar muscles for humeral epicondylitis. Am J Sports Med 10:233–236, 1982

17. Bennett GE: Shoulder and elbow lesions of the professional baseball pitcher. JAMA 117:510–514, 1941

18. Bennett GE: Shoulder and elbow lesions distinctive of baseball players. Ann Surg 126:107–110, 1947

19. Bennett GE: Elbow and shoulder lesions of baseball players. Am J Surg 98:484–492, 1959

20. Bennett JB, Tullos HS: Acute injuries to the elbow. p. 319. In Nicholas JA, Hershmann EB (eds): The Upper Extremity in Sports Medicine. CV Mosby, St. Louis, 1990

21. Bennett JB, Green MS, Tullos HS: Surgical management of chronic medial elbow instability. Clin Orthop 278:62–68, 1992

22. Bernhang AM, Dehner W, Fogarty C: Tennis elbow: a biomechanical approach. J Sports Med 2:235–260, 1974

23. Biles JG, Grana WA: Ruptured ulnar collateral ligament. Orthopedics 10:1595–1596, 1987

24. Binder AI, Hazleman BL: Lateral humeral epicondylitis—a study of natural history and the effect of conservative therapy. Br J Rheumatol 22:73–76, 1983

25. Binder A, Hodge G, Greenwood AM et al: Is therapeutic ultrasound effective in treating soft tissue lesions? BMJ 290:512–514, 1985

26. Borris LC, Lassen MR, Christensen CS: Elbow dislocation in children and adults. A long-term follow-up of conservatively treated patients. Acta Orthop Scand 58:649–651, 1987

27. Bourne MH, Morrey BF: Partial rupture of the distal biceps tendon. Clin Orthop 271:143–148, 1991

28. Boyd HB, Anderson LD: A method for reinsertion of the distal biceps brachii tendon. J Bone Joint Surg [Am] 43A(7):1041–1043, 1961

29. Boyd HB, McLeod AC: Tennis elbow. J Bone Joint Surg [Am] 55A:1183–1187, 1973

30. Briggs CA, Elliott BG: Lateral epicondylitis. A review of structures associated with tennis elbow. Anat Clin 7:149–153, 1985

31. Broberg MA, Morrey BF: Results of delayed excision of the radial head after fracture. J Bone Joint Surg [Am] 68A:669–674, 1986

32. Broberg MA, Morrey BF: Results of treatment of fracture-dislocations of the elbow. Clin Orthop 216:109–119, 1987

33. Browner BD, Jupiter JB, Levine AM, Trafton PG: Trauma to the adult elbow and fractures of the distal humerus. p. 1125. In Jupiter JB, Mehne DK (eds): Skeletal Trauma. WB Saunders, Philadelphia, 1992

34. Buehler MJ, Thayer DT: The elbow flexion test. A clinical test for the cubital tunnel syndrome. Clin Orthop 233:213–216, 1988

35. Cabrera JM, McCue FC: Nonosseous athletic injuries of the elbow, forearm, and hand. Clin Sports Med 5:681–700, 1986

36. Calvert PT, Allum RL, Macpherson IS, Bentley G: Simple lateral release in treatment of tennis elbow. J R Soc Med 78:912–915, 1985

37. Carn RM, Medige J, Curtain D, Koenig A: Silicone rubber replacement of the severely fractured radial head. Clin Orthop 209:259–269, 1986

38. Chard MD, Hazleman BL: Tennis elbow—a reappraisal. Br J Rheumatol 28:186–190, 1989

39. Childress HM: Recurrent ulnar-nerve dislocation at the elbow. Clin Orthop 108:168–173, 1975

40. Conway JE, Jobe FW, Glousman RE, Pink M: Medial instability of the elbow in throwing athletes. Treatment by repair or reconstruction of the ulnar collateral ligament. J Bone Joint Surg [Am] 74A:67–83, 1992

41. Coonrad RW: Tennis elbow. p. 94. In: American Academy of Orthopaedic Surgeons, Instructional Course Lectures. Vol. 35. CV Mosby, St. Louis, 1986

42. Coonrad RW, Hooper WR: Tennis elbow: its course, natural history, conservative and surgical management. J Bone Joint Surg [Am] 55A:1177–1182, 1973

43. Dangles CJ, Bilos ZJ: Ulnar nerve neuritis in a world champion weightlifter. Am J Sports Med 8:443–445, 1980

44. Day BH, Govindasamy N, Patnaik R: Corticosteroid injections in the treatment of tennis elbow. Practitioner 220:459–462, 1978

45. DeHaven KE, Evarts CM: Throwing injuries of the elbow in athletes. Orthop Clin North Am 4:801–808, 1973

46. Dellon AL: Review of treatment results for ulnar nerve entrapment at the elbow. J Hand Surg 14A:688–700, 1989

47. Del Pizzo W, Jobe FW, Norwood L: Ulnar nerve entrapment syndrome in baseball players. Am J Sports Med 5:182–185, 1977

48. DiGiovine NM, Jobe FW, Pink M, Perry J: An electromyographic analysis of the upper extremity in pitching. J Shoulder Elbow Surg 1:15–25, 1992

49. Dimond ML, Lister GD: Cubital tunnel syndrome treated by long-arm splintage, abstracted. J Hand Surg 10A:430, 1985

50. Dürig M, Müller W, Rüedi TP, Gauer EF: The operative treatment of elbow dislocation in the adult. J Bone Joint Surg [Am] 61A:239–244, 1979

51. Eaton CJ, Lister GD: Radial nerve compression. Hand Clin 8:345–357, 1992

52. Eaton RG, Crowe JF, Parkes JC: Anterior transposition of the ulnar nerve using a non-compressing fasciodermal sling. J Bone Joint Surg [Am] 62A:820–825, 1980

53. Edwards GS, Jupiter JB: Radial head fractures with acute distal radioulnar dislocation. Essex-Lopresti revisited. Clin Orthop 234:61–69, 1988

54. Elattrache NS, Jobe FW: Ulnar collateral ligament injury in the athlete. Instructional Course Lecture, presented at the American Academy of Orthopaedic Surgeons 60th Annual Meeting, San Francisco, 1993

55. Essex-Lopresti P: Fractures of the radial head with distal radio-ulnar dislocation. J Bone Joint Surg [Br] 33B:244–247, 1951

56. Failla JM, Amadio PC, Morrey BF, Beckenbaugh RD: Proximal radioulnar synostosis after repair of distal biceps brachii rupture by the two-incision technique. Report of four cases. Clin Orthop 253:133–136, 1990

57. Farrar EL, Lippert FG: Avulsion of the triceps tendon. Clin Orthop 161:242–246, 1981

58. Feindel W, Stratford J: Cubital tunnel compression in tardy ulnar palsy. Can Med Assoc J 78:351–353, 1958

59. Foster RJ, Edshage S: Factors related to the outcome of surgically managed compressive ulnar neuropathy at the elbow level. J Hand Surg 6:181–192, 1981

60. Frassica FJ, Coventry MB, Morrey BF: Ectopic ossification about the elbow. p. 505. In: The Elbow and Its Disorders. WB Saunders, Philadelphia, 1993

61. Fyfe IS, Mossad MM, Holdsworth BJ: Methods of fixation of olecranon fractures. An experimental mechanical study. J Bone Joint Surg [Br] 67B:367–372, 1985

62. Gainor BJ, Piotrowski G, Puhl J et al: The throw: biomechanics and acute injury. Am J Sports Med 8:114–118, 1980

63. Gartsman GM, Sculco TP, Otis JC: Operative treatment of olecranon fractures. Excision or open reduction with internal fixation. J Bone Joint Surg [Am] 63A:718–721, 1981

64. Geel CW, Palmer AK: Radial head fractures and their effect on the distal radioulnar joint. A rationale for treatment. Clin Orthop 275:79–84, 1992

65. Geel CW, Palmer AK, Ruedi T, Leutenegger AF: Internal fixation of proximal radial head fractures. J Orthop Trauma 4:270–274, 1990

66. Gellman H: Tennis elbow (lateral epicondylitis). Orthop Clin North Am 23:75–82, 1992

67. Glousman RE: Ulnar nerve problems in the athlete's elbow. Clin Sports Med 9:365–377, 1990

68. Goldberg MJ: Gymnastic injuries. Orthop Clin North Am 11:717–726, 1980

69. Goldberg EJ, Abraham E, Siegel I: The surgical treatment of chronic lateral humeral epicondylitis by common extensor release. Clin Orthop 233:208–212, 1988

70. Goldie I: Epicondylitis lateralis humeri (epicondylalgia or tennis elbow): a pathogenetical study. Acta Chir Scand, suppl. 339:1–119, 1964

71. Groppel JL, Nirschl RP: A mechanical and electromyographical analysis of the effects of various joint counterforce braces on the tennis player. Am J Sports Med 14:195–200, 1986

72. Gruchow HW, Pelletier D: An epidemiologic study of tennis elbow. Incidence, recurrence, and effectiveness of prevention strategies. Am J Sports Med 7:234–238, 1979

73. Hang Y-S, Lippert FG, Spolek GA et al: Biomechanical study of the pitching elbow. Int Orthop 3:217–223, 1979

74. Hanks GA, Kottmeier SA: Isolated fracture of the coronoid process of the ulna: a case report and review of the literature. J Orthop Trauma 4:193–196, 1990

75. Harrington IJ, Tountas AA: Replacement of the radial head in the treatment of unstable elbow fractures. Injury 12:405–412, 1981

76. Hartz CR, Linscheid RL, Gramse RR, Daube JR: The pronator teres syndrome: compressive neuropathy of the median nerve. J Bone Joint Surg [Am] 63A:885–890, 1981

77. Herrick RT, Herrick S: Ruptured triceps in a powerlifter presenting as cubital tunnel syndrome. Am J Sports Med 15:514–516, 1987

78. Heyse-Moore GH: Resistant tennis elbow. J Hand Surg 9B:64–66, 1984

79. Hirasawa Y: Injuries to peripheral nerve in sports. Semin Orthop 3:240–250, 1988

80. Hirasawa Y, Sakakida K: Sports and peripheral nerve injury. Am J Sports Med 11:420–426, 1983

81. Holder SF, Grana WA: Complete triceps tendon avulsion. Orthopedics 9:1581–1582, 1986

82. Horner SR, Sadasivan KK, Lipka JM, Saha S: Analysis

of mechanical factors affecting fixation of olecranon fractures. Orthopedics 12:1469–1472, 1989

83. Hotchkiss RN, Weiland AJ: Valgus stability of the elbow. J Orthop Res 5:372–377, 1987

84. Hotchkiss RN, An K-N, Sowa DT, et al: An anatomic and mechanical study of the interosseous membrane of the forearm: pathomechanics of proximal migration of the radius. J Hand Surg 14A:256–261, 1989

85. Hulkko A, Orava S, Nikula P: Stress fractures of the olecranon in javelin throwers. Int J Sports Med 7:210–213, 1986

86. Hume MC, Wiss DA: Olecranon fractures. A clinical and radiographic comparison of tension band wiring and plate fixation. Clin Orthop 285:229–235, 1992

87. Ilfeld FW: Can stroke modification relieve tennis elbow? Clin Orthop 276:182–186, 1992

88. Indelicato PA, Jobe FW, Kerlan RK et al: Correctable elbow lesions in professional baseball players: a review of 25 cases. Am J Sports Med 7:72–75, 1979

89. Jalovaara P, Lindholm RV: Decompression of the posterior interosseous nerve for tennis elbow. Arch Orthop Trauma Surg 108:243–245, 1989

90. Jobe FW, Nuber G: Throwing injuries of the elbow. Clin Sports Med 5:621–637, 1986

91. Jobe FW, Bradley JP: Ulnar neuritis and ulnar collateral ligament instabilities in overarm throwers. p. 419. In Torg JS, Welsh PR, Shephard RJ (eds): Current Therapy in Sports Medicine. Vol. 2. BC Decker, Philadelphia, 1990

92. Jobe FW, Kvitne RS: Reconstruction of the ulnar collateral ligament of the elbow. Techn Orthop 6:39–42, 1991

93. Jobe FW, Elattrache NS: Diagnosis and treatment of ulnar collateral ligament injuries in athletes. p. 566. In Morrey BF (ed): The Elbow and Its Disorders. WB Saunders, Philadelphia, 1993

94. Jobe FW, Stark H, Lombardo SJ: Reconstruction of the ulnar collateral ligament in athletes. J Bone Joint Surg [Am] 68A:1158–1163, 1986

95. Jobe FW, Fanton GS, Elattrache NS: Ulnar nerve injury. p. 560. In Torg JS, Welsh PR, Shepard RJ (eds): The Elbow and Its Disorders. WB Saunders, Philadelphia, 1993

96. Johansson O: Capsular and ligament injuries of the elbow joint. A clinical and arthrographic study. Acta Chir Scand, suppl. 287:1–159, 1962

97. Johnston GW: A follow-up of one hundred cases of fracture of the head of the radius with a review of the literature. Ulster Med J 31:51–56, 1962

98. Jones HH, Priest JD, Hayes WC et al: Humeral hypertrophy in response to exercise. J Bone Joint Surg [Am] 59A:204–208, 1977

99. Josefsson PO, Nilsson BE: Incidence of elbow dislocation. Acta Orthop Scand 57:537–538, 1986

100. Josefsson PO, Johnell O, Gentz C-F: Long-term sequelae of simple dislocation of the elbow. J Bone Joint Surg [Am] 66A:927–930, 1984

101. Josefsson PO, Gentz C-F, Johnell O, Wendeberg B: Surgical versus non-surgical treatment of ligamentous injuries following dislocation of the elbow joint. A prospective randomized study. J Bone Joint Surg [Am] 69A:605–608, 1987

102. Josefsson PO, Gentz C-F, Johnell O, Wendeberg B: Surgical versus nonsurgical treatment of ligamentous injuries following dislocations of the elbow joint. Clin Orthop 214:165–169, 1987

103. Josefsson PO, Johnell O, Wendeberg B: Ligamentous injuries in dislocations of the elbow joint. Clin Orthop 221:221–225, 1987

104. Josefsson PO, Gentz C-F, Johnell O, Wendeberg B: Dislocations of the elbow and intraarticular fractures. Clin Orthop 246;126–130, 1989

105. Jupiter JB: Heterotopic ossification about the elbow. p. 41. In: American Academy of Orthopaedic Surgeons, Instructional Course Lectures. Vol. 40. American College of Orthopaedic Surgeons, 1991

106. Kannus P, Józsa L: Histopathological changes preceding spontaneous rupture of a tendon. J Bone Joint Surg [Am] 73A:1507–1525, 1991

107. Kerin R: Elbow dislocation and its association with vascular disruption. J Bone Joint Surg [Am] 51A:756–758, 1969

108. King GJW, Evans DC, Kellam JF: Open reduction and internal fixation of radial head fractures. J Orthop Trauma 5:21–28, 1991

109. King J, Brelsford HJ, Tullos HS: Analysis of the pitching arm of the professional baseball pitcher. Clin Orthop 67:116–123, 1969

110. Kivi P: The etiology and conservative treatment of humeral epicondylitis. Scand J Rehabil Med 15:37–41, 1982

111. Kuroda S, Sakamaki K: Ulnar collateral ligament tears of the elbow joint. Clin Orthop 208:266–271, 1986

112. Kvidera DJ, Pedegana LR: Stress fracture of the olecranon. Orthop Rev 12:113–116, 1983

113. Lansinger O, Karlsson J, Körner L, Mare K: Dislocation of the elbow joint. Arch Orthop Traumatic Surg 102:183–186, 1984

114. Leach RE, Miller JK: Lateral and medial epicondylitis of the elbow. Clin Sports Med 6:259–272, 1987

115. Learmonth JR: A technique for transplanting the ulnar nerve. Surg Gynecol Obstet 75:792–793, 1942

116. Leffert RD: Anterior submuscular transposition of the ulnar nerves by the Learmonth technique. J Hand Surg 7:147–155, 1982

117. Lesin BE, Balfour GW: Acute rupture of the medial collateral ligament of the elbow requiring reconstruction. J Bone Joint Surg [Am] 68A:1278–1280, 1986

118. Linscheid RL, Wheeler DK: Elbow dislocations. JAMA 194:1171–1176, 1965
119. Linscheid RL, O'Driscoll SW: Elbow dislocations. p. 441. In Morrey BF (ed): The Elbow and Its Disorders. WB Saunders, Philadelphia, 1993
120. Lister GD, Belsole RB, Kleinert HE: The radial tunnel syndrome. J Hand Surg 4:52–59, 1979
121. Loomer RL: Elbow injuries in athletes. Can J Appl Sports Sci 7:164–166, 1982
122. Loomis LK: Reduction and after-treatment of posterior dislocation of the elbow with special attention to the brachialis muscle and myositis ossificans. Am J Surg 63:56–60, 1944
123. Louis DS, Hankin FM, Eckenrode JF et al: Distal biceps brachii tendon avulsion. A simplified method of operative repair. Am J Sports Med 14:234–236, 1986
124. Lundborg G: Surgical treatment for ulnar nerve entrapment at the elbow. J Hand Surg 17B:245–247, 1992
125. Mackinnon SE, Dellon AL: Evaluation of microsurgical internal neurolysis in a primate median nerve model of chronic nerve compression. J Hand Surg 13A:345–351, 1988
126. Mackinnon SE, McCabe S, Murray JF et al: Internal neurolysis fails to improve the results of primary carpal tunnel decompression. J Hand Surg 16A:211–218, 1991
127. Mains DB, Freeark RJ: Report on compound dislocation of the elbow with entrapment of the brachial artery. Clin Orthop 106:180–185, 1975
128. Mason ML: Some observations on fractures of the head of the radius with a review of one hundred cases. Br J Surg 42:123–132, 1954
129. McArthur RA: Herbert screw fixation of fracture of the head of the radius. Clin Orthop 224:79–87, 1987
130. McPherson SA, Meals RA: Cubital tunnel syndrome. Orthop Clin North Am 23:111–123, 1992
131. Mehlhoff TL, Noble PC, Bennett JB, Tullos HS: Simple dislocation of the elbow in the adult. Results after closed treatment. J Bone Joint Surg [Am] 70A:244–249, 1988
132. Miller JF: Javelin thrower's elbow. J Bone Joint Surg [Br] 42B:788–792, 1960
133. Morrey BF: Reoperation for failed surgical treatment of refractory lateral epicondylitis. J Shoulder Elbow Surg 1:47–55, 1992
134. Morrey BF: Tendon injuries about the elbow. p. 492. In: The Elbow and Its Disorders. WB Saunders, Philadelphia, 1993
135. Morrey BF: Radial head fracture. p. 395. In: The Elbow and Its Disorders. WB Saunders, Philadelphia, 1993
136. Morrey BF: Surgical failure of the tennis elbow. p. 553. In: The Elbow and Its Disorders. WB Saunders, Philadelphia, 1993
137. Morrey BF, An K-N: Articular and ligamentous contribu-
tions to the stability of the elbow joint. Am J Sports Med 11:315–319, 1983
138. Morrey BF, An K-N: Functional anatomy of the ligaments of the elbow. Clin Orthop 201:84–90, 1985
139. Morrey BF, O'Driscoll SW: Lateral collateral ligament injury. p. 573. In: The Elbow and Its Disorders. WB Saunders, Philadelphia, 1993
140. Morrey BF, Askew LJ, An K-N, Dobyns JH: Rupture of the distal tendon of the biceps brachii. A biomechanical study. J Bone Joint Surg [Am] 67A:418–421, 1985
141. Morrey BF, Tanaka S, An K-N: Valgus stability of the elbow. A definition of primary and secondary constraints. Clin Orthop 265:187–195, 1991
142. Morris M, Jobe FW, Perry J et al: Electromyographic analysis of elbow function in tennis players. Am J Sports Med 17:241–247, 1989
143. Moss SH, Switzer HE: Radial tunnel syndrome: a spectrum of clinical presentations. J Hand Surg 8:414–420, 1983
144. Murphy DF, Greene WB, Gilbert JA, Dameron TB: Displaced olecranon fractures in adults. Biomechanical analysis of fixation methods. Clin Orthop 224:210–214, 1987
145. Nestor BJ, O'Driscoll SW, Morrey BF: Ligamentous reconstruction for posterolateral rotatory instability of the elbow. J Bone Joint Surg [Am] 74A:1235–1241, 1992
146. Neviaser JS, Wickstrom JK: Dislocation of the elbow: a retrospective study of 115 patients. South Med J 70:172–173, 1977
147. Nirschl RP: The etiology and treatment of tennis elbow. J Sports Med 2:308–323, 1975
148. Nirschl RP: Soft-tissue injuries about the elbow. Clin Sports Med 5:637–652, 1986
149. Nirschl RP: Prevention and treatment of elbow and shoulder injuries in the tennis player. Clin Sports Med 7:289–308, 1988
150. Nirschl RP: Muscle and tendon trauma: tennis elbow. p. 537. In Morrey BF (ed): The Elbow and Its Disorders. WB Saunders, Philadelphia, 1993
151. Nirschl RP, Pettrone FA: Tennis elbow. The surgical treatment of lateral epicondylitis. J Bone Joint Surg 61A:832–839, 1979
152. Nirschl RP, Sobel J: Conservative treatment of tennis elbow. Physician Sports Med 9:43–54, 1981
153. Norman WH: Repair of avulsion of insertion of biceps brachii tendon. Clin Orthop 193:189–194, 1985
154. Norwood LA, Shook JA, Andrews JR: Acute medial elbow ruptures. Am J Sports Med 9:16–19, 1981
155. Noyes FR, Grood ES, Nussbaum NS, Cooper SM: Effect of intra-articular corticosteroids on ligament properties. A biomechanical and histological study in Rhesus knees. Clin Orthop 123:197–209, 1977
156. Nuber GW, Diment MT: Olecranon stress fractures in

throwers. A report of two cases and a review of the literature. Clin Orthop 278:58–61, 1992

157. O'Driscoll SW, Bell DF, Morrey BF: Posterolateral rotatory instability of the elbow. J Bone Joint Surg [Am] 73A:440–446, 1991

158. O'Driscoll SW, Horii E, Carmichael SW, Morrey BF: The cubital tunnel and ulnar neuropathy. J Bone Joint Surg [Br] 73B:613–617, 1991

159. O'Driscoll SW, Jaloszynski R, Morrey BF, An K-N: Origin of the medial ulnar collateral ligament. J Hand Surg 17A:164–168, 1992

160. O'Driscoll SW, Morrey BF, Korinek S, An K-N: Elbow subluxation and dislocation. A spectrum of instability. Clin Orthop 280:186–197, 1992

161. O'Driscoll SW, Horii E, Morrey BF, Carmichael SW: Anatomy of the ulnar part of the lateral collateral ligament of the elbow. Clin Anat 5:296–303, 1992

162. O'Neil J, Sarkar K, Uhthoff HK: A retrospective study of surgically treated cases of tennis elbow. Acta Orthop Belg 46:189–196, 1980

163. Osborne G, Cotterill P: Recurrent dislocation of the elbow. J Bone Joint Surg [Br] 48B:340–346, 1966

164. Pantazopoulos T, Exarchou E, Stavrou Z, Hartofilakidis-Garofalidis G: Avulsion of the triceps tendon. J Trauma 15:827–829, 1975

165. Pappas AM, Zawicki RM, Sullivan TJ: Biomechanics of baseball pitching. A preliminary report. Am J Sports Med 13:216–222, 1985

166. Pribyl CR, Kester MA, Cook SD et al: The effect of the radial head and prosthetic radial head replacement on resisting valgus stress at the elbow. Orthopedics 9:723–726, 1986

167. Priest JD, Weise DJ: Elbow injury in women's gymnastics. Am J Sports Med 9:288–295, 1981

168. Priest JD, Jones HH, Nagel DA: Elbow injuries in highly skilled tennis players. J Sports Med 2:137–149, 1974

169. Priest JD, Braden V, Goodwin Gerberich S: The elbow and tennis, Part 1: an analysis of players with and without pain. Physician Sports Med 8:81–91, 1980

170. Priest JD, Braden V, Goodwin Gerberich S: The elbow and tennis, Part 2: a study of players with pain. Physician Sports Med 8:77–85, 1980

171. Pritchard DJ, Linscheid RL, Svien HJ: Intra-articular median nerve entrapment with dislocation of the elbow. Clin Orthop 90:100–103, 1973

172. Protzman RR: Dislocation of the elbow joint. J Bone Joint Surg 60:539–541, 1978

173. Race CM, Saldana MJ: Anatomic course of the medial cutaneous nerves of the arm. J Hand Surg 16A:48–52, 1991

174. Rayan GM, Jensen C, Duke J: Elbow flexion test in the normal population. J Hand Surg 17A:86–89, 1992

175. Regan W, Morrey BF: Microscopic pathology of lateral epicondylitis. Presented at the Canadian Orthopaedic Association 44th Annual Meeting, Toronto, 1989

176. Regan W, Morrey B: Fractures of the coronoid process of the ulna. J Bone Joint Surg [Am] 71A:1348–1354, 1989

177. Regan WD, Morrey BF: The physical examination of the elbow. p. 83. In: The Elbow and Its Disorders. WB Saunders, Philadelphia, 1993

178. Regan WD, Korinek SL, Morrey BF, An K-N: Biomechanical study of ligaments around the elbow joint. Clin Orthop 271:170–179, 1991

179. Ritts GD, Wood MB, Linscheid RL: Radial tunnel syndrome. A ten year surgical experience. Clin Orthop 219:201–205, 1987

180. Roberts PH: Dislocation of the elbow. Br J Surg 56:806–815, 1969

181. Roles NC, Maudsley RH: Radial tunnel syndrome. Resistant tennis elbow as a nerve entrapment. J Bone Joint Surg [Br] 54B:499–508, 1972

182. Rowland SA, Burkhart SS: Tension band wiring of olecranon fractures. A modification of the AO technique. Clin Orthop 277:238–242, 1992

183. Royle SG: Posterior dislocation of the elbow. Clin Orthop 269:201–204, 1991

184. Saartok T, Eriksson E: Randomized trial of oral naproxen or local injection of betamethasone in lateral epicondylitis of the humerus. Orthopedics 9:191–194, 1986

185. Sanders RA, French HG: Open reduction and internal fixation of comminuted radial head fractures. Am J Sports Med 14:130–135, 1986

186. Sanders WE: Lateral epicondylitis and radial tunnel syndrome: a unified theory. Presented at the 43rd Annual Meeting of the American Society for Surgery of the Hand, Baltimore, 1990

187. Sarkar K, Uhthoff HK: Ultrastructure of the common extensor tendon in tennis elbow. Virchows Arch [A] 386:317–330, 1980

188. Schwab GH, Bennett JB, Woods GW, Tullos HS: Biomechanics of elbow instability: the role of the medial collateral ligament. Clin Orthop 146:42–52, 1980

189. Selesnick FH, Dolitsky B, Haskell SS: Fracture of the coronoid process requiring open reduction with internal fixation. J Bone Joint Surg [Am] 66A:1304–1306, 1984

190. Seror P: Treatment of ulnar nerve palsy at the elbow with a night splint. J Bone Joint Surg 75B:322–327, 1993

191. Sherman OH, Snyder SJ, Fox JM: Triceps tendon avulsion in a professional body builder. Am J Sports Med 12:328–329, 1984

192. Sicuranza MJ, McCue FC: Compressive neuropathies in the upper extremity of athletes. Hand Clin 8:263–273, 1992

193. Sisto DJ, Jobe FW, Moynes DR, Antonelli DJ: An electromyographic analysis of the elbow in pitching. Am J Sports Med 15:260–263, 1987

194. Slocum DB: Classification of elbow injuries from baseball pitching. Texas Med 64:48–53, 1968
195. Snook GA: Injuries in women's gymnastics. Am J Sports Med 7:242–244, 1979
196. Snyder-Mackler L, Epler M: Effect of standard and Aircast tennis elbow bands on integrated electromyography of forearm extensor musculature proximal to the bands. Am J Sports Med 17:278–281, 1989
197. Sojbjerg JO, Ovesen J, Nielsen S: Experimental elbow instability after transection of the medial collateral ligament. Clin Orthop 218:186–190, 1987
198. Sojbjerg JO, Helmig P, Kjærsgaard-Anderson P: Dislocation of the elbow: an experimental study of the ligamentous injuries. Orthopedics 12:461–463, 1989
199. Sponseller PD, Engber WD: Double-entrapment radial tunnel syndrome. J Hand Surg 8:420–423, 1983
200. Stuffer M, Jungwirth W, Hussl H, Schmutzhardt E: Subcutaneous or submuscular anterior transposition of the ulnar nerve? J Hand Surg 17B:248–250, 1991
201. Swanson AB, Jaeger SH, La Rochelle D: Comminuted fractures of the radial head. J Bone Joint Surg [Am] 63-A:1039–1049, 1981
202. Tarsney FF: Rupture and avulsion of the triceps. Clin Orthop 83:177–183, 1972
203. Thompson HC, Garcia A: Myositis ossificans: aftermath of elbow injuries. Clin Orthop 50:129–134, 1967
204. Torg JS, Moyer RA: Non-union of a stress fracture through the olecranon epiphyseal plate observed in an adolescent baseball pitcher. J Bone Joint Surg [Am] 59A:264–265, 1977
205. Tullos HS, King JW: Throwing mechanism in sports. Orthop Clin North Am 4:709–720, 1973
206. Tullos HS, Erwin WD, Woods GW et al: Unusual lesions of the pitching arm. Clin Orthop 88:169–182, 1972
207. Tullos HS, Schwab G, Bennett JB, Woods GW: Factors influencing elbow instability. p. 185. In: American Academy of Orthopaedic Surgeons, Instructional Course Lectures. Vol. 30. CV Mosby, St. Louis, 1981
208. Tullos HS, Bennett J, Shepard D et al: Adult elbow dislocations: mechanism of instability. p. 69. In: American Academy of Orthopaedic Surgeons, Instructional Course Lectures. Vol. 35. CV Mosby, St. Louis, 1986
209. Uhthoff HK, Sarkar K: A re-appraisal of tennis elbow. Acta Orthop Belg 46:74–82, 1980
210. Vangsness CT, Jobe FW: Surgical treatment of medial epicondylitis: results in 35 elbows. J Bone Joint Surg [Br] 73B:409–411, 1991
211. Viegas SF: Avulsion of the triceps tendon. Orthop Rev 19:533–536, 1990
212. Wadsworth TG: The external compression syndrome of the ulnar nerve at the cubital tunnel. Clin Orthop 124:189–204, 1977
213. Wadsworth TG: Tennis elbow: conservative, surgical, and manipulative treatment. BMJ 294:621–624, 1987
214. Ware HE, Nairn DS: Repair of the ruptured distal tendon of the biceps brachii. J Hand Surg 17B:99–101, 1992
215. Waris W: Elbow injuries of javelin-throwers. Acta Chir Scand 93:563–575, 1946
216. Warren RF: Tennis elbow (epicondylitis). Epidemiology and conservative treatment. p. 233. In: American Academy of Orthopaedic Surgeons: Symposium on Upper Extremity Injuries in Athletes. CV Mosby, St. Louis, 1986
217. Werner C-O: Lateral elbow pain and posterior interosseous nerve entrapment. Acta Orthop Scand, suppl. 174:1–62, 1979
218. Werner C-O, Ohlin P, Elmqvist D: Pressures recorded in ulnar neuropathy. Acta Orthop Scand 56:404–406, 1985
219. Wheeler DK, Linscheid RL: Fracture-dislocations of the elbow. Clin Orthop 50:95–106, 1967.
220. Wilkerson RD, Johns JC: Nonunion of an olecranon stress fracture in an adolescent gymnast. A case report. Am J Sports Med 18:432–434, 1990
221. Wilson FD: Valgus extension overload in pitching elbow. p. 431. In Torg JS, Welsh PR, Shepard RJ (eds): Current Therapy in Sports Medicine. Vol. 2. BC Decker, Toronto, 1990
222. Wilson FD, Andrews JR, Blackburn TA, McCluskey G: Valgus extension overload in the pitching elbow. Am J Sports Med 11:83–88, 1983
223. Wojtys EM, Smith PA, Hankin FM: A cause of ulnar neuropathy in a baseball pitcher. A case report. Am J Sports Med 14:422–424, 1986
224. Wright CS: Overuse syndromes. p. 425. In Torg JS, Welsh PR, Shepard RJ (eds): Current Therapy in Sports Medicine. Vol. 2. BC Decker, Toronto, 1990

12

Arthroscopy of the Elbow

JAMES R. ANDREWS
LAURA A. TIMMERMAN
KEVIN E. WILK

INTRODUCTION

Injuries to the elbow in throwing and racquet sports are seen in athletes of all ages. These injuries can be caused by an acute macrotrauma such as a fracture or dislocation, or (more commonly) they can be secondary to a repetitive microtrauma, including tendinitis, ligament attenuation, and degenerative changes of the joint.[4,8,16] The evaluation and treatment of many elbow conditions is straightforward, but at times the clinical diagnosis is unclear.[17] In addition, with traditional treatments such as immobilization and open surgical procedures, the elbow has the propensity to develop contractures and resultant loss of range of motion (ROM).

The advantages of arthroscopy (namely, minimal dissection and faster rehabilitation) have been well demonstrated in treatment of disorders of the shoulder and the knee. The development of arthroscopy of the elbow has been a major advance in treating elbow disorders in athletes.[2,3,12,23] Initially the arthroscope was used primarily in a diagnostic fashion, but as arthroscopic surgical techniques have become further refined, the indications for operative elbow arthroscopy have increased.[2–4,6,7,9,12,17,20,23] However, due to the close proximity of neurovascular structures and the size constraints of the elbow joint, elbow arthroscopy is a difficult procedure and its widespread use has been concurrently limited.

INDICATIONS AND CONTRAINDICATIONS

Elbow arthroscopy is useful for diagnosis and removal of loose bodies[6]; evaluation and treatment of osteochondritis dissecans of the capitellum and chondomalacia of the radial head[12,23]; excision of bony spurs from the coronoid and posterior olecranon[1–4]; lysis of adhesions in post-traumatic elbow joints[2,9]; partial synovectomy and excision of fibrotic bands[7]; treatment of septic arthritis; debridement of osteoarthritic joints[2,9]; evaluation of the ulnar collateral ligament and the medial stability of the elbow[28]; and evaluation of the painful elbow when the diagnosis is ambiguous.[17]

Contraindications to elbow arthroscopy include bony ankylosis and severe fibrous ankylosis, which make introduction of the arthroscope into the joint difficult.[3] A relative contraindication would be an acute injury to the elbow that produces both swelling, obscures external landmarks, and capsular tears with resultant extravasation of fluid and danger of compartment syndrome.

SURGICAL TECHNIQUE
General Set-up

The patient is usually given a general anesthetic to provide complete muscle relaxation and avoid any intraoperative patient discomfort, but an axillary block has been used.[22] For ease of set-up and anesthetic reasons we prefer the patient to be in a supine position on a standard operating table, although the prone position has been utilized with success.[22]

The hand is placed in a prefabricated wrist gauntlet, and the affected arm is suspended from an overhead arthroscopic shoulder holder using a counterweight (usually 5 lb) and pulley system (Fig. 12-1). If a concur-

rent open procedure on the elbow is anticipated, sterile finger traps can be used to suspend the arm after preparation and drape. The arm is positioned so that it hangs freely off the side of the table with the elbow in 90 degrees of flexion and the shoulder in 90 degrees of abduction and neutral rotation. A tourniquet is used to improve visualization by providing hemostasis. The arm and hand are then prepared and draped in a sterile

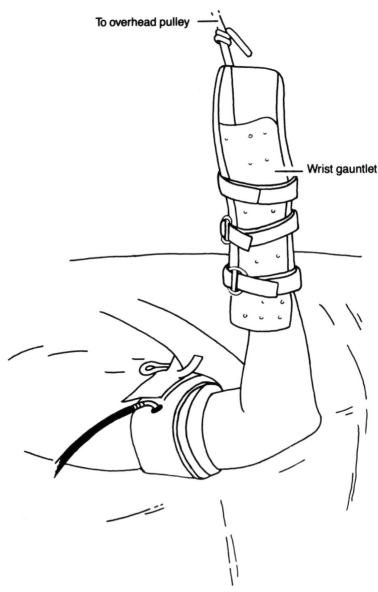

To overhead pulley

Wrist gauntlet

Fig. 12-1. Patient positioning and set-up for elbow arthroscopy. The arm is suspended to allow the elbow to hang freely off the side of the table.

fashion. The surgeon and assistant are seated on rolling stools with the elbow at chest level, allowing a comfortable working height for the surgeon's arms. This allows access to both the medial and lateral sides of the elbow, and the forearm can be easily moved. The viewing monitor is directly across the surgeon on the opposite side of the patient.

The 4.0-mm, 30-degree and the 2.7-mm, 30-degree arthroscopes are routinely used. Occasionally the 4.0-mm, 70-degree arthroscope is useful in evaluating the tight medial side of the joint. A one-piece immersible video-arthroscope unit is recommended to prevent fogging during the procedure. The standard arthroscopy instruments are used, including graspers and motorized debriders. Small osteotomes should be available for bony work.

Prior to inflation of the torniquet the anatomic landmarks and portals are delineated with a marking pen. This is important because with swelling and joint distension previous easily identified anatomic structures can become obscured and difficult to locate. Medially the ulnar nerve is palpated and its subcutaneous route marked. The medial and lateral epicondyles, radial head, and olecranon tip are all outlined. The appropriate portals are then measured and marked.

Portals

The portals used in elbow arthroscopy include the direct lateral, anterolateral, anteromedial, posterolateral, and straight posterior. It is important to understand the location, anatomy about the portal, and visualization possible with each portal.

The *anterolateral portal* is located distal and anterior to the lateral epicondyle at the level of the radial head-capitellar articulation. The puncture is made just anterior to the radial head, which can be palpated by pronating and supinating the forearm (Fig. 12-2). It is approximately 3 cm distal and 1 cm anterior to the

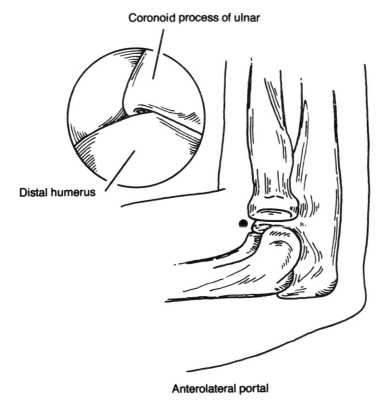

Coronoid process of ulnar

Distal humerus

Anterolateral portal

Fig. 12-2. The anterolateral portal is located just anterior to the radial head, approximately 3 cm distal and 1 cm anterior to the lateral epicondyle.

lateral epicondyle, but these measurements depend on the size of the patient. This portal traverses the extensor carpi radialis brevis and is in close proximity to the radial nerve.[4] It is always made after the joint is distended with approximately 30 ml of fluid injected through a spinal needle placed in the soft spot. With joint distension the nerve displaces 11 mm from the portal, compared with 4 mm without distension.[14] It is important when making this portal that the instruments be directed toward the center of the joint and that the capsule be "trapped" behind the radial head. This prevents the trocar from being directed too much in the lateral-medial plane toward the neurovascular structures. This portal is used as the initial viewing portal, and it allows visualization of the medial joint, including the coronoid, the ulnohumeral articulation, and the medial capsule. Usually only a small portion of the radial head is seen.

The *anteromedial portal* is located approximately 2 cm distal and 2 cm anterior to the medial epicondyle (Fig. 12-3). This portal traverses the tendinous portion of the pronator teres and the radial aspect of the flexor digitorum superficialis. Cadaver studies show that this portal comes within 1 cm of the median nerve and brachial artery[4]; again, joint distension displaces the median nerve from 4 to 14 mm, and the brachial artery from 9 to 17 mm from the portal.[14] Through this portal the radial head and capitellum are visualized best; by withdrawing the arthroscope slightly the coronoid process is visualized. This portal is not used in patients with a previous ulnar nerve transfer.

The *direct lateral portal* is located between the lateral epicondyle, radial head, and olecranon tip (Fig. 12-4). This portal corresponds to the lateral soft spot of the elbow, which is often used for elbow aspirations. As described above, the elbow joint is initally distended with fluid via a spinal needle in the soft spot. Through this portal the lateral aspect of the radial head, capitellum, and olecranon are visualized, as is the lateral capsule. It is the pathway to the posterior compartment of the elbow, by following the lateral olecranon-humeral articulation the posterior compartment can be entered easily, allowing direct visualization using a spinal needle to make the posterior portal. This portal is relatively safe; only the skin and anconeus muscle are traversed, but consequently the soft tissue plane is thin and it is easy to pull out of the joint with the arthroscope and instruments.

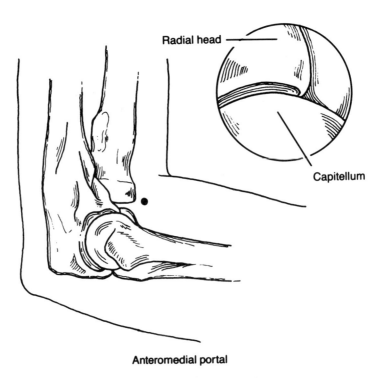

Radial head

Capitellum

Anteromedial portal

Fig. 12-3. The anteromedial portal is located approximately 2 cm distal and 2 cm anterior to the medial epicondyle.

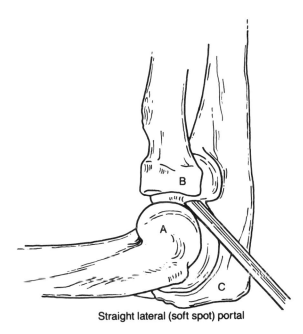

Straight lateral (soft spot) portal

Fig. 12-4. The direct lateral portal is located between the lateral epicondyle, radial head, and olecranon tip, in the soft spot of the elbow joint.

The two posterior portals are established by straightening the elbow to approximately 40 degrees of flexion. This relaxes the triceps muscle and allows distension of the posterior elbow joint. The *posterolateral portal* is located 3 cm proximal to the olecranon tip and just posterior and superior to the lateral epicondyle, along the lateral epicondylar ridge, just lateral to the border of the triceps tendon (Fig. 12-5). This portal is best made under direct visualization from the lateral portal with the aid of a spinal needle.

Once the posterolateral portal is established, a second posterior portal can be used as an operative portal. It is called the *straight posterior portal*. This is placed 2 cm medial to the posterolateral portal, with a triceps splitting incision in line with the muscle fibers. Medial displacement of this portal should be avoided secondary to danger to the ulnar nerve; cadaveric dissections demonstrate that this portal comes within 1.8 cm of the ulnar nerve.[4]

Procedure

As with any arthroscopic procedure, a systematic and reproducible method for examination of the joint should be employed. The tourniquet is inflated. An 18-gauge spinal needle is inserted into the soft spot, or direct lateral portal, and the joint is distended with approximately 30 to 40 ml of saline solution. Entry into the joint is confirmed by free backflow of saline. The anterolateral portal site is noted and a spinal needle placed in the direction of the portal; backflow of saline is confirmed. Remembering the angle of this needle, a small 5 to 6-mm incision with an #11 blade is made through the skin only, followed by dissection to the capsular level with a small hemostat (to avoid damage to the lateral antebrachial cutaneous nerve). The blunt obturator is then used to enter the joint. Backflow of saline is again confirmed, and the distension is maintained via the soft spot spinal needle. The arthroscope is then inserted into the sheath. We use a pump system to maintain flow and sense pressure through the arthroscopic sheath. If a pump system is not utilized, the flow is initially placed through the arthroscope, and then once the anteromedial portal is established, a flow cannula can be placed. Once a portal is established, the cannulas should be kept in the joint to limit extravasation of fluid and provide easy access to return to the portal.

Inspection of the anterior compartment begins with the coronoid. The coronoid can develop large osteophytes, which cause impingement in flexion; loose bodies or fractures of the coronoid can also be detected. The coronoid fossa or the radial fossa of the humerus (or both) are visualized; this area can become filled in with scar tissue or bony osteophytes and can block full flexion. The medial capsule is seen. The ulnohumeral articulation is visualized. Medial instability is reflected by an opening in the ulnohumeral joint as valgus stress at 70 degrees of flexion to the elbow is applied. The ulnar collateral ligament is intimately associated with the medial capsule, but cadaveric studies we have done show that only the most anterior portion of the ligament is actually visualized arthroscopically.[28]

The anteromedial portal is established under direct visualization from the arthroscope in the anterolateral portal. An 18-gauge spinal needle is inserted just anterior to the medial epicondyle toward the center of the joint, deep to the antecubital structures. The skin incision and trocar insertion is performed in the same manner as above, to avoid damage to the medial antebrachial cutaneous nerve. Via this portal the radial head and capitellum are noted. Flow can be maintained in this portal as the straight lateral portal is made.

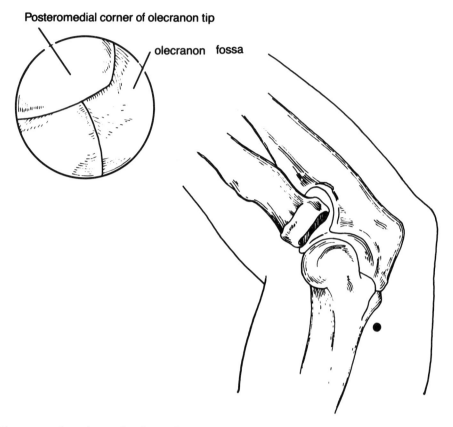

Posteromedial corner of olecranon tip

olecranon fossa

Fig. 12-5. The posterolateral portal is located 3 cm proximal to the olecranon tip just medial to the lateral epicondylar ridge. The straight posterior portal is established approximately 2 cm medial, in a triceps splitting incision, to the posterolateral portal.

Once the viewing of the anterior compartment is completed, the straight lateral portal is made by a small incision over the needle in the soft spot portal. The small 2.7-mm sheath and trocar are then introduced. The smaller arthroscope is usually used in this lateral compartment because the space is constrained, but in larger individuals the smaller arthroscope is not always necessary. With the arthroscope the articulation of the radial head, humerus, and olecranon is seen. By pronating and supinating the forearm the radial head is visualized. Debridement of lateral capsular scar tissue and other operative procedures can be performed by making an accessory lateral portal and working with the instruments in a parallel fashion. This accessory portal is made approximately 1 cm anterior and slightly distal to the straight lateral portal. By sweeping the arthroscope from anterior to posterior the articulation of the olecranon and trochlear groove is seen. In the center

of the olecranon a small area of absent articular cartilage is seen that appears to be an erosion. We believe that this is a normal finding because we have seen it in children. It represents the scarification of the apophyseal line of the olecranon. In addition, loose bodies and areas of traumatic chondromalacia can be seen in this location. The posterior joint is entered by following the curve of the olecranon.

The posterior compartment is inspected last. While viewing the posterior joint from the direct lateral portal, an 18-gauge spinal needle is introduced from the location of the posterolateral portal, just medial to the lateral epicondylar ridge. Once properly positioned, a #11 blade can be used to cut directly on the needle, so the blade is visualized with the arthroscope. The trocar is then introduced, and, once the sheath is visualized in the joint, the 4.0-mm arthroscope with the inflow is switched, thus setting up the posterolateral portal. It is important to make sure the sheath is in the joint completely to prevent extravasation of fluid posteriorly, which can extend externally into the olecranon bursa and compress the joint space. From the posterolateral portal the olecranon fossa, tip of the olecranon, and posterior trochlea are visible. The posterior bundle of the ulnar collateral ligament can be seen by looking around the corner of the humerus in the ulnar gutter.

If a second working posterior portal is necessary, it can be established under arthroscopic visualization. This is the straight posterior portal. A spinal needle is used to confirm that it will reach the operative area, and a #11 knife blade can then be used to make a triceps fiber splitting incision. The operating instruments, including a motorized resector, graspers, and small osteotomes can be introduced through this portal. Care should be taken when using motorized instruments posteriorly: the ulnar nerve is vulnerable because it is only separated from the joint by a thin layer of capsule.

At the completion of the procedure the tourniquet is deflated. Through the arthroscopic sheath a small Hemovac drain is placed into the joint. The portals are left open for drainage, or closed, depending on surgeon preference. A soft bulky dressing is then placed.

MECHANISMS OF INJURY IN SPORTS

Sporting activities that involve the elbow usually place a valgus stress across the elbow joint.[1,8,13] Slocum[25] classified throwing injuries into medial tension, lateral compression, and extension overload injuries The combination of these forces is referred to as *valgus extension overload of the elbow*[1] (Fig. 12-6). The term *valgus extension overload* is used in reference to the throwing motion, but the mechanism of injury can be related to many sports activities. In the cocking and acceleration phase (just prior to ball release) of the overhead throwing motion, maximum force is placed across the medial side soft tissues, with concurrent lateral joint compression.[5] During the deceleration phase (after release) the elbow is in maximum extension (approximately 15 degrees of flexion) with contraction of the triceps and resulting posterior compression.[5] The nature of injuries seen about the elbow

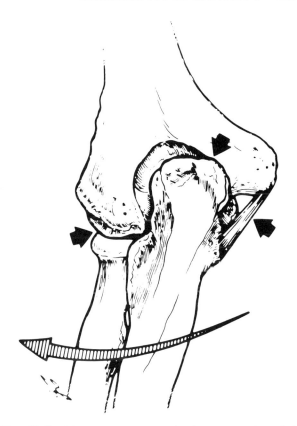

Fig. 12-6. Valgus extension overload consists of medial tension on the ulnar collateral ligament, with lateral compression of the radiocapitellar joint, and posteromedial impingement of the olecranon tip on the trochlea (*arrows*). A "kissing" lesion of the trochlea may result, as well as formation of posteromedial osteophytes on the olecranon.

depends on the age of the athlete. In the skeletally immature, osteochondritis of the capitellum from compression and medial epicondyle traction apophysitis from valgus stress are commonly seen.[11,19] Posteriorly the skeletally immature athlete can suffer from olecranon traction apophysitis,[11,19] an avulsion fracture of the olecranon,[5] or a stress fracture through the olecranon epiphyseal plate.[21,29] In the older player soft tissue changes are more prominent medially, including ulnar collateral ligament strain and flexor-pronator muscle tendinitis.[5] Laterally, degenerative changes of the joint are seen, as is extensor muscle tendinitis. Extension overload results in osteophyte formation at the tip of the olecranon with fibrous tissue deposition in the olecranon fossa and loose body formation; the valgus stress results in abutment of the medial aspect of the olecranon process against the medial olecranon fossa with formation of posterior medial osteophytes.[1]

Tennis players suffer from valgus extension overload-type injuries caused by the overhead serving motion; they can also develop lateral pathology including lateral epicondylitis, a lateral fibrotic band of tissue within the capsule, and lateral radial head chondromalacia.

Golf injuries are also associated with overload-type phenomena. In the right elbow of a right-handed golfer medial epicondylitis is seen; lateral epicondylitis can affect either elbow. Radiocapitellar chondromalacia, posterior spur formation with valgus extension overload, and loose body formation can all occur. In the older athlete posterior impingement is seen.

In gymnastics the elbow becomes a weight-bearing joint, with extensive shear and compressive forces across the radiocapitellar joint.[12] Gymnasts are most often skeletally immature, with this force directed across an area undergoing endochondral ossification at a period of development when the vascular supply is limited.

TREATMENT OF SPECIFIC CONDITIONS
Loose Bodies

Symptomatic loose bodies are a common form of elbow pathology in the athlete. We have noticed that preoperative computed tomography (CT) arthrograms are frequently negative in symptomatic patients who are found to have a loose body subsequently at surgery. Osteocartilaginous loose bodies are usually the result of osteochondritic lesions of the capitellum or they are fragmented off the posterior impingement of the olecranon and trochlea. Arthroscopic removal of loose bodies from the elbow joint has been shown in several studies to be beneficial, especially in the elbow free of degenerative changes.[2,6,9,17]

A complete inspection of the elbow joint is necessary when searching for loose bodies; at arthroscopy, defects from the anterior portion of the elbow are frequently found posteriorly. If one loose body is found, a careful exploration for additional loose bodies should be undertaken. It is generally easier to remove a loose body anteriorly through the anterolateral portal rather than the anteromedial portal because of less interposed soft tissue. If a loose body is found that is too large to remove through the arthroscopic portal, it can be removed either in a piecemeal fashion with the debrider, or by breaking it up in several pieces with a clamp.

Posterior Impingement

A common source of pain in the throwing elbow is posteromedial osteophytes on the olecranon with secondary chondromalacia (or a kissing lesion) of the trochlea at the area of impingement.[1,25,31] Such patients have pain with forced extension, and they may lack full extension. Ulnar nerve symptoms can also develop secondary to the close relationship of the nerve.

This condition is easily diagnosed through the posterolateral portal (Fig. 12-7), and removal of the offending olecranon osteophyte can be accomplished with an osteotome and motorized burr introduced through the straight lateral portal. It is important to remove the posteromedial corner of the olecranon completely to prevent further impingement. The area of chondromalacia on the trochlea may be debrided

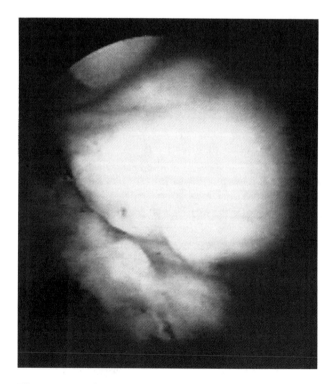

Fig. 12-7. Arthroscopic view through the posterolateral portal of a posteromedial olecranon osteophyte.

to stimulate bleeding and fibrocartilage formation. Removal of the posteromedial osteophyte may result in increased medial instability secondary to the loss of part of the bony structure (bony stabilizer), with a resultant increase in the load across the ulnar collateral ligament. This can be associated with an increase in the preloading of this ligament; we have just recently become aware of this potential problem.

An uncommon, but frequently misdiagnosed, source of posterior pain in the throwing athlete is a stress fracture of the olecranon.[5] Olecranon stress fractures are seen in the middle and proximal portion of the ulna. The skeletally immature athlete can have a delayed union through the olecranon epiphyseal plate,[21,29] which normally closes around age 16 in males.[19] In the athlete, this delayed union can persist unilaterally into the middle of the third decade of life secondary to the repeated stress of throwing, or a stress fracture can occur in this same location in the older athlete. Clinically, lateral tenderness is usually present at the site of the fracture. It may require open reduction with internal fixation. This stress fracture can be seen at arthroscopy via the direct lateral portal with opening of the fracture site detected.

Lateral Compression

During throwing, the valgus moment about the elbow causes lateral compression of the bony structures; osteochondrosis of the capitellum and chondromalacia of the radial head can result.[1] The straight lateral portal is used to view the capitellum; a second straight lateral portal can be used for instrumentation. Jackson et al.[12] described treatment of osteochondritic lesions in the young female gymnast's elbow using a combination of arthroscopy and a small arthrotomy to curette and drill the lesions, and to remove the loose bodies. Although they found that the arthroscope was valuable in assessment and managment of the condition, the clinical results were guarded. Ruch and Poehling[23] recently described use of the arthroscope in treatment of osteochondrosis of the capitellum, with removal of the loose body and debridement of the defect performed arthroscopically. We have found that simple arthroscopic debridement of the defect, instead of attempting reattachment of the lesion, has worked best in our hands.

A consistent finding in athletes with persistent lateral elbow pain that fails the usual conservative treatment course is a condition first described by Clarke[7] as a lateral plica of the elbow. A thickening of a lateral synovial fringe becomes fibrotic and can cause impingement between the radial head and the capitellum. A large amount of hypertrophied synovium, without fibrosis, can also cause lateral pain. This is especially common in tennis players. A corresponding kissing lesion of the radial head seen under the band is found, much like the medial plica of the knee and the associated changes seen on the medial femoral condyle. Clinical symptoms in these patients include locking and catching with lateral joint pain. Excision of the band, or hypertrophied synovium, usually results in relief of the symptoms, although some of these patients also have a concurrent lateral epicondylitis.

Medial Tension

The medial soft tissues of the elbow are subject to tremendous tension with throwing. The ulnar collateral ligament is the primary stabilizer of the elbow joint to valgus stress from 20 to 120 degrees of flexion, and with repeated forces this ligament can become attenuated, or tear.[10,15,26] The greatest degree of instability after sectioning the ulnar collateral ligament is seen at 70 degrees of flexion, which corresponds to the position of elbow flexion in the throwing motion that is subject to the greatest valgus stress.[26] Detection of the resulting medial instability can often be difficult clinically.[7] It may be that it is a dynamic instability that requires the high forces of throwing to become symptomatic. Although magnetic resonance imaging, stress radiographs, and CT arthrogram studies have been helpful, they are at times inconclusive.

The medial capsule is easily visualized through the anterolateral portal, and with an assistant who stabilizes the humerus and applies a valgus force to the 70-degree flexed elbow, medial instability can be detected by noting the degree of opening between the articulation of the ulna and humerus medially. In normal elbows no opening in this joint exists, or only the trace of one; in elbows with ulnar collateral ligament tears, 3 mm or more of opening can be seen (Fig. 12-8). With a large amount of opening the arthroscope can be placed in between the articulation of the ulna and humerus with direct visualization of the tear. The ulnar collateral ligament is very taut over the medial joint and is intimately associated with the medial capsule; consequently, it is quite difficult to visualize this liga-

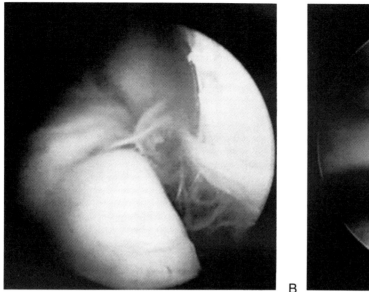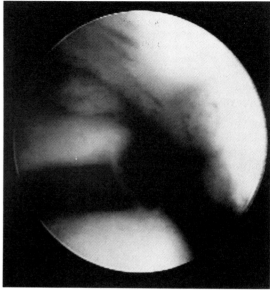

Fig. 12-8. (A) Arthroscopic view through the anterolateral portal of the ulnohumeral joint without stress applied. **(B)** The same view of the ulnohumeral joint as stress is applied to the 70-degree flexed elbow. Note the increase in joint space between the ulna and humerus, indicating medial instability of the elbow.

ment directly. Cadaveric studies we have done show that only the most anterior portion of the ligament is visualized, and if a large tear is seen medially, it involves the anteromedial capsule as well as the ulnar collateral ligament.[28] The nature of the medial wall can be detected; for example, patients with an ulnar collateral ligament pathology fequently have synovitis and inflammation of the medial capsule. This view is enhanced with a 70-degree arthroscope placed in the anterolateral portal.[28] Posteriorly, medial inflammation can be noted, but only the posterior half of the posterior bundle can be seen arthroscopically. Despite these limitations, the arthroscope is a useful adjuvant in evaluation of medial instability.

Anterior Lesions

Hypertrophy of the coronoid process can occur in response to the distraction forced during the deceleration phase of throwing, and with repetitive elbow flexion the osteophytes can impinge in the coronoid fossa and radial fossa causing chondromalacia and loose body formation.[1] With trauma to the elbow joint, anterior capsular contractures can form, and both the coronoid fossa and radial fossa of the humerus can fill

in with scar tissue, limiting full extension. This area of the elbow can be easily visualized through the anterolateral and anteromedial portals. The scar tissue can be resected using a full radius resector; care must be taken anteriorly because of the close proximity of the neurovascular structures. An osteotome or burr can be used on the coronoid, with a burr used to re-form the coronoid fossa, as well as the radial fossa.

REHABILITATION AFTER ELBOW ARTHROSCOPY

Early and diligent rehabilitation is critical in obtaining satisfactory results after elbow arthroscopy. The primary goal of the initial phase of rehabilitation is regaining full elbow extension.[30] The program begins on the first postoperative day (Table 12-1). The drain is pulled; the dressing is removed; and Steri-Strips are applied to the portal sites. The patient begins early ROM of the wrist without weights and gripping therapeutic putty. By the third postoperative day 1 lb of resistance is added to the program. The hand-held weight produces a passive extension stretch and is an extremely effective exercise designed to obtain full

Table 12-1. Postoperative Rehabilitative Protocol
for Elbow Arthroscopy

I. Initial phase (week 1). Goal: attain full wrist and elbow ROM, decrease swelling, decrease pain, retard muscle atrophy
   A. Day of surgery
      Begin gently moving elbow in bulky dressing
   B. Postop days 1–2
      1. Remove bulky dressing; replace with elastic bandages.
      2. Start postop hand, wrist, and elbow exercises immediately.
        a. Putty/grip strengthening
        b. Wrist flexor stretching
        c. Wrist extensor stretching
        d. Wrist curls
        e. Reverse wrist curls
        f. Neutral wrist curls
        g. Pronation/supination
        h. A/AAROM elbow extension/flexion
   C. Postop days 3–7
      1. Begin PROM elbow extension/flexion
      2. Begin PRE exercises with 1-lb weight
        a. Wrist curls
        b. Reverse wrist curls
        c. Neutral wrist curls
        d. Pronation/supination
        e. Broomstick roll-up
II. Intermediate phase (weeks 2–4). Goal: improve muscular strength and endurance; normalize joint arthrokinematics
   A. Week 2: ROM exercises (overpressure into extension)
      1. Addition of biceps curl and triceps extension
      2. Continue to progress PRE weight and repetitions as tolerable
   B. Week 3
      1. Initiate biceps and triceps eccentric exercise program
      2. Initiate rotator cuff exercise program
        a. External rotators
        b. Internal rotators
        c. Deltoid
        d. Supraspinatus
        e. Scapulothoracic strengthening
III. Advanced phase (weeks 4–8). Goal: preparation of athlete for return to functional activities
   A. Criteria to progress to advanced phase:
      1. Full nonpainful ROM
      2. No pain or tenderness
      3. Isokinetic test that fulfills criteria to throw
      4. Satisfactory clinical examination
   B. Weeks 3–6
      1. Continue maintenance program, emphasizing muscular strength, endurance, and flexibility
      2. Initiate interval throwing program, phase I

elbow extension. On the fourth through seventh day passive ROM of the elbow is added to the routine.

Once the patient has achieved nearly full ROM and has minimal swelling and tenderness, strengthening exercises are added to the program. On days 10 through 14 progressive resistance exercises are added, and the weights are increased to a maximum of 5 lb. After reaching the 5-lb limit, repetitions should be increased rather than weight. It is important to address the shoulder as well, with emphasis on strengthening the rotator cuff musculature. Once the patient has achieved strength, in approximately 70 percent of the contralateral side, advanced strengthening exercises can be added, including plyometrics and high-speed energy strengthening.[30] Ice, high-voltage pulsed galvanic stimulation, transcutaneous neuromuscular stimulation, and other modalities are used to diminish pain and inflammation.

The ultimate goal of rehabilitation is to return the athlete to sport as rapidly as possible. Criteria that must be met include: (1) full, nonpainful ROM; (2) no pain or tenderness on clinical examination; and (3) good muscular strength, power, and endurance.[30] Once these guidelines are met, the athlete is allowed to return to activity through a planned interval program that permits a gradual return to full performance level.

COMPLICATIONS

As we have stressed throughout this chapter, direct damage to the neurovascular structures about the elbow is a very real possibility with elbow arthroscopy. Cases of damage to the radial nerve secondary to arthroscopy have been reported.[14,18] In over 450 cases of elbow arthroscopy, we have had one case of nerve damage; an ulnar nerve neuropraxia occurred with debridement of synovium along the medial gutter in the posterior compartment. In order to avoid these complications, we attempt to minimize the risk by carefully delineating the surface anatomy, placing portals under arthroscopic visualization, and making incisions only through the skin.

As with all operative procedures, infection is a potential complication. Prophylactic antibiotics are used, and careful sterile technique is necessary. Although we have not seen a case of septic arthritis, we have had one case of cellulitis involving the olecranon bursa that required incision and drainage. Occasionally, the posterior portals will have persistent drainage, but this has resolved without complication.

With arthroscopy there is always the danger of neurovascular compromise and compartment syndrome from the extravasation of fluid. Once a portal is established but no longer used, we advise keeping a cannula with a blunt trocar in place. This minimizes the extravasation of fluid into the soft tissues and allows return to these portals without further traumatizing the soft tissues. We constantly watch the degree of swelling and are prepared to abandon the procedure if necessary. We know of one outside case of volar forearm compartment syndrome secondary to the extravasation of saline that required acute surgical decompression. The amount of time spent in various compartments should be limited, for example, if one knows that posterior pathology is present, then the time in the anterior compartment should be limited to allow for adequate treatment posteriorly. Injection of local anesthetic into the elbow joint and portals is contraindicated because a confusing transient postoperative nerve palsy may develop.[2] A careful postoperative neurovascular assessment is of obvious importance.

CONCLUSIONS

The development of elbow arthroscopy over the last decade has offered tremendous advantages in the treatment of injuries in the athlete's elbow. With its minimally invasive nature, improved visualization of intra-articular pathology, and ability to allow early aggressive rehabilitation, the benefits in treating sports-related injuries to the elbow are obvious. However, the technique is complex, and serious potential complications may result if careful operative technique is not observed. In the proper hands elbow arthroscopy is a formidable treatment modality for disorders about the elbow.

REFERENCES

1. Andrews JR: Bony injuries about the elbow in the throwing athlete. In: American Academy of Orthopaedic Surgeons, Instructional Course Lectures. Vol. 34. CV Mosby, St Louis, MO, 1985
2. Andrews JR, Carson WG: Arthroscopy of the elbow. Arthroscopy 1:97–107, 1985
3. Andrews JR, Miller RH: Arthroscopic surgery of the elbow. p. 1571. In Chapman MW (ed): Operative Orthopaedics. 1st Ed. Vol. 3. JB Lippincott, Philadelphia, 1988
4. Andrews JR, St Pierre RK, Carson WG: Arthroscopy of the elbow. Clin Sports Med 5:653–662, 1986
5. Andrews JR, Schemmel SP, Whiteside JA: Evaluation, treatment, and prevention of elbow injuries in throwing athletes. In Nicholas JA, Hershman EB (eds): The Upper Extremity in Sports Medicine. CV Mosby, St Louis, 1990
6. Boe S: Arthroscopy of the elbow. Diagnosis and extraction of loose bodies. Acta Orthop Scand 57:52–53, 1986
7. Clarke RP: Symptomatic lateral synovial fringe (plica) of the elbow joint. Arthroscopy 4:112–116, 1988
8. Conway JE, Jobe FW, Glousman RE, Pink M: Medial instability of the elbow in throwing athletes. J Bone Joint Surg [Am] 74A:67–83, 1992
9. Guhl JF: Arthroscopy and arthroscopic surgery of the elbow. Orthopedics 8:1290–1296, 1985
10. Hotchkiss RN, Weiland AJ: Valgus stability of the elbow. J Orthop Res 5:372, 1987
11. Ireland ML, Andrews JR: Shoulder and elbow injuries in the young athlete. Clin Sports Med 7:473–493, 1988
12. Jackson DW, Silvino N, Reiman P: Osteochondritis in the female gymnast's elbow. Arthroscopy 5:129–136, 1989
13. Jobe FW, Stark A, Lombardo SJ: Reconstruction of the ulnar collateral ligament in athletes. J Bone Joint Surg [Am] 68A:1158, 1986
14. Lynch GJ, Meyers JF, Whipple TL, Caspari RB: Neurovascular anatomy and elbow arthroscopy; inherent risks. Arthroscopy 2:190–197, 1986
15. Morrey BF, An KN: Articular and ligamentous contributions to the stability of the elbow joint. Am J Sports Med 11:315–319, 1983
16. Norwood LA, Shook JA, Andrews JR: Acute medial elbow ruptures. Am J Sports Med 9:16, 1981
17. O'Driscoll SW, Morrey BF: Arthroscopy of the elbow. J Bone Joint Surg [Am] 74A:84–94, 1992
18. Papillion JD, Neff RS, Shall LM: Compression neuropathy of the radial nerve as a complication of elbow arthroscopy: a case report and review of the literature. Arthroscopy 4:284–286, 1988
19. Pappas AM: Elbow problems associated with baseball during childhood and adolescence. Clin Orthop 164:30–41, 1982
20. Parisien JS: Arthroscopic surgery of the elbow. Bull Hosp Joint Dis Orthop Inst 48:149–158, 1988
21. Pavlov H, Torg JS, Jacobs B, Vigorita V: Nonunion of olecranon epiphysis: two cases in adolescent baseball pitchers. AJR 136:819–820, 1981
22. Poehling GG, Whipple TL, Sisco L, Goldman B: Elbow arthroscopy: a new technique. Arthroscopy 5:222–224, 1989
23. Ruch DS, Poehling GG: Arthroscopic treatment of Panner's disease. Clin Sports Med 10:629–636, 1991
24. Schwab GH, Bennett JB, Woods GW, Tullos HS: Biomechanics of elbow instability: the role of the medial collateral ligament. Clin Orthop 146:42, 1980
25. Slocum DB: Classification of elbow injuries from baseball pitching. Texas Med 64:48–53, 1968
26. Sojbjerg JO, Ovensen J, Neilsen S: Experimental elbow

instability after transection of the medial collateral ligament. Clin Orthop 218:186, 1987

27. Thomas AM, Fast A, Shapiro D: Radial nerve damage as a complication of elbow arthroscopy. Clin Ortop 215:130–131, 1987

28. Timmerman LA, Andrews JR: Histology and arthroscopic anatomy of the ulnar collateral ligament of the elbow. Am J Sports Med 22(5):667–673, 1994

29. Torg JS, Moyer RA: Non-union of a stress fracture through the olecranon epiphyseal plate observed in an adolescent baseball pitcher. J Bone Joint Surg [Am] 59A:264–265, 1977

30. Wilk KE, Arrigo CL, Andrews JR: Rehabilitation of the elbow in the throwing athlete. J Orthop Sports Phys Ther 17(6):305–317, 1993

31. Wilson FD, Andrews JR, Blackburn TA, McCluskey G: Valgus extension overload in the pitching elbow. Am J Sports Med 11:83, 1983

13

Common Wrist Injuries

ROBERT S. RICHARDS
JAMES H. ROTH

EPIDEMIOLOGY

The wrist and hand are the most common sites of sporting injury to the upper limb, since the wrist has limited protection and the hand and wrist play a major role in sporting activities. Wrist and hand injuries account for 25 percent of athletic injuries, with the specific injury varying from sport to sport.[4] Football, basketball, and gymnastics have the highest rates of injury.[12]

Gymnasts have a high incidence of upper extremity injury, and 17 to 43 percent have chronic injuries.[30] Most gymnasts suffer acute injuries to the upper limb sometime during their career. Although shoulder and elbow problems are commonly recognized injuries, many gymnasts consider wrist pain a normal consequence of training.[5] Olympic gymnast Peter Kormann has been quoted as saying, "problems are only considered serious when the gymnast can no longer compete."[5] In an elite group of male gymnasts, 88 percent complained of wrist pain and 58 percent required chronic nonsteroidal anti-inflammatory drug (NSAID) medication to continue training.[30] The forces generated during pommel horse exercises are comparable to the load sustained at heel strike during running. The wrist is poorly adapted to a weight-bearing role, and the high incidence of wrist injuries is not surprising. In comparison with other sports, the high number of adolescent and preadolescent athletes in gymnastics creates unique injuries, especially to the growth plates.[10]

Different sporting activities are associated with different injury patterns. Scaphoid fractures are common in football and volleyball players. Hamate fractures are associated with racquet or stick sports such as baseball,

golf, hockey, tennis, and cricket. Growth plate injuries to the radius are common in young gymnasts. Rope avulsion injuries of the thumb occur in rodeo riders. Injuries due to single extreme stresses occur in contact sports such as wrestling, football, volleyball, and baseball. Repetitive stress injuries are more common in gymnasts, tennis, and racquetball players.

OSSEOUS INJURIES
Distal Radius Fractures

Fractures of the radius represent one of the most common fractures overall, accounting for approximately 10 percent of bony injuries and up to 75 percent of all fractures of the forearm.[3] Jupiter established the causal relationship between intra-articular displacement and subsequent degenerative arthritis. Reduction of articular surfaces must be anatomic, since a 2-mm step leads to subsequent degenerative arthritis.[24] Practical difficulties exist in obtaining an anatomic reduction in intra-articular fractures. Closed reduction does not allow accurate reduction, and open reduction is difficult in comminuted unstable fractures. Arthroscopy allows accurate reduction of the articular surface while preserving as much soft tissue stability as possible.

We now recognize that significant internal derangements of the carpus can occur in extra-articular fractures. Arthroscopy in these cases allows diagnosis and treatment of the associated scapholunate or lunotriquetral tears, ligament tears, triangular fibrocartilage complex (TFCC) injuries, or cartilage lesions. Nelaton in 1844 published the first description of TFCC injuries associated with distal radius fractures.[28] Subsequently, in 1940, Mayer demonstrated that dorsal or radial displacement of the distal fragment indicated damage to the disk. He stated that in most cases of distal radius fracture the force is sufficient to rupture the disk.[28] Using arthrography for diagnosis, estimates of the incidence of TFCC disruption in extra-articular distal radius fractures have ranged up to 45 percent.[34] Clinical symptoms with pain and laxity of the distal radioulnar joint have been reported to occur in 5 to 15 percent of fractures.[28] Arthroscopy has enabled us to delineate better the injuries associated with radius fractures. We perform arthroscopy of all intra-articular and many comminuted extra-articular fractures. A large number of associated injuries have been found. Most commonly, TFCC tears of the radial or central aspects were found (Fig. 13-1). Disruption of the ulnar insertion was uncommon. Unsuspected scapholunate ligament injuries were frequently found as well. We have treated TFCC tears with debridement rather than suture as the injuries have usually been central and radial. Small radial tears that open minimally with pronation and supination may be managed with immobilization.

Our ability to manage the TFCC and ligament injuries associated with these fractures is enhanced by arthroscopy, allowing better treatment of distal radial fractures.

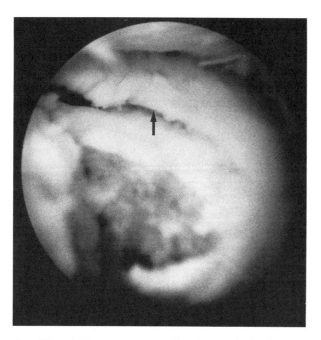

Fig. 13-1. Arthroscopic view of an intra-articular fracture with an associated TFCC avulsion (*arrow*).

Although reduction of these fractures is increasingly accurate with arthroscopy, wrist stiffness is a risk. We have used wrist continuous passive motion (CPM) in intra-articular radius fractures with excellent early return of motion. Use of wrist CPM has been effective in the rehabilitation of both acute injuries and established stiffness of the wrist.

Epiphyseal Injuries of the Radius and Ulna

Epiphyseal plate injuries have been reported in elite highly competitive gymnasts.[44] With increasing awareness, more reports of this injury are appearing in less advanced gymansts. It should be considered in the differential diagnosis of wrist pain in gymnasts at all levels.

Distal radial epiphyseal plate injury presents as dorsal wrist pain, aggravated by dorsiflexion. Radiographs show haziness and widening of the growth plate of the radius, generally on the radial aspect.[10] Early diagnosis is the key. Roy et al.[44] have shown that recovery was related to the severity of injury. Those patients without radiographic changes had resolution of pain and return to activities in 1 to 4 weeks. Those patients with radiographic changes had prolonged pain and may not return to activities for 6 months. Diagnosis of this injury prior to radiographic changes requires magnetic resonance imaging (MRI) scans, since bone scans do not distinguish between normal uptake in an open plate and growth plate injury. Treatment consists of immobilization and NSAID medication for the pain. Generally, the radiographic appearance of the epiphysis returns to normal over 6 to 8 weeks. Permanent morbidity with growth arrest in treated patients has not been commonly noted. However, concern does exist, since premature closure has been reported in one article, and gymnasts have been noted to have a higher incidence of positive ulnar variance, which may be related to chronic radial epiphyseal injury.[1] At this time treatment of asymptomatic radiographic changes is not indicated.

Scaphoid Fractures

The scaphoid is the carpal bone most commonly injured, accounting for two-thirds of all carpal fractures. The common occurrence of scaphoid fractures in young athletes makes a high incidence of suspicion essential. Approximately 1 percent of all college football players in the United States sustain a scaphoid fracture each year.[56] Scaphoid fractures can be difficult to diagnose acutely and are commonly missed. The natural history of untreated scaphoid fractures is for the pain to subside gradually, so the athlete may not seek treatment. Later, a second injury causes pain and a scaphoid fracture with delayed union or nonunion is diagnosed. Diagnosis can be difficult. If rapid diagnosis is needed, a negative bone scan after 3 to 5 days rules out injury.[35,48] If clinical suspicion exists, the best investigations to diagnose and evaluate fractures are conventional radiographs, tomograms, and computed tomography (CT). CT gives the best definition of cortex, trabecular bone, and fracture pattern among the available modalities.[45] The only difficulty is positioning the wrist for longitudinal axial scans in the injured patient with a limited range of motion (ROM). Longitudinal axial scans are important to allow assessment of angulation and displacement, both of which are associated with increased rates of nonunion. Recent work has shown that MRI is very sensitive in detecting scaphoid fractures; the disadvantage of MRI in the assessment of fractures is that the fracture line is visible on MRI long after radiographic and CT evidence of union exists.[21] Thus the decision regarding union of bone grafts and fractures should be made on CT or plain tomograms. This avoids prolonged unnecessary immobilization while waiting for MRI changes to occur. Occasionlly, one is asked to determine whether an apparent nonunion of the scaphoid is in reality a bipartite scaphoid. Although the existence of bipartite scaphoid has been questioned, it is now possible to differentiate the two on the basis of visualization of articular cartilage around the circumference of the segments on MRI.[17]

Undisplaced fractures of the scaphoid may be treated nonoperatively. Although long arm casts and casts incorporating the index and middle fingers have been suggested, our preferred treatment is a short arm thumb spica with the thumb interphalangeal joint free. Indications for open reduction include displacement greater than 1 mm or evidence of volar angulation of the distal fragment with early "humpback" deformity.[13,53]

Although the average time to union of scaphoid fractures treated nonoperatively is 12 weeks, a significant number take longer.[47] An advantage of open reduction with a compression screw is that return to sports may be quicker than with closed methods. Return to sports

after Herbert screw fixation may occur as soon as 1 month after surgery.[25] Insertion of either the cannulated or the standard Herbert screw is performed through a volar modified Russe approach for waist fractures. The cannulated Herbert screw may also be inserted arthroscopically (see Ch. 16). The jig may be inserted through an arthroscopy portal, avoiding the need for conventional volar arthrotomy and decreasing the potential morbidity. Fractures of the proximal one-fourth of the scaphoid require a modified technique. They are reduced and internally fixed through a dorsal approach, with the screw inserted from proximal to distal (Fig. 13-2).

Scaphoid nonunion remains a difficult problem. Early diagnosis and treatment generally results in scaphoid union rates of 90 to 95%. Factors leading to nonunion include delayed diagnosis, decreased vascularity in proximal pole fractures, presence of a dorsal intercalary segmental instability pattern, displacement of the fracture greater than 1 mm, and angulation of greater than 20 degrees between the proximal and distal fragments.[37,49] Treatment of scaphoid nonunion has involved both inlay grafts and corticocancellous wedge grafts. Although union rates using the Russe bone graft average 88 percent,[37] no correction of the angular deformity of the scaphoid is obtained. Use of Fernandez's wedge graft corrects the volar angular deformity but does require internal fixation.[18] No difference has been shown between compression screws and K-wires regarding the final union rate.[43] Electromagnetic stimulation (EBI) has been suggested as a treatment option, with high union rates of 80 to 90 percent.[37] Contraindications to EBI include synovial pseudarthrosis, a small proximal pole fragment, presence of a dorsal intercalated segmental instability (DISI) deformity or an angular deformity of the scaphoid. It is indicated in only a small number of patients and is not widely used.

Fractures of the Hook of the Hamate

Fractures of the hook of the hamate comprise 2 percent of carpal fractures.[25] They are most commonly associated with sports that require a club such as a baseball bat, hockey stick, golf club, or racquet to be gripped. The usual mechanism of injury is related to the type of grip used. Athletes who grip the equipment with the butt of the bat or stick in the palm are more likely to suffer this injury (Fig. 13-3).

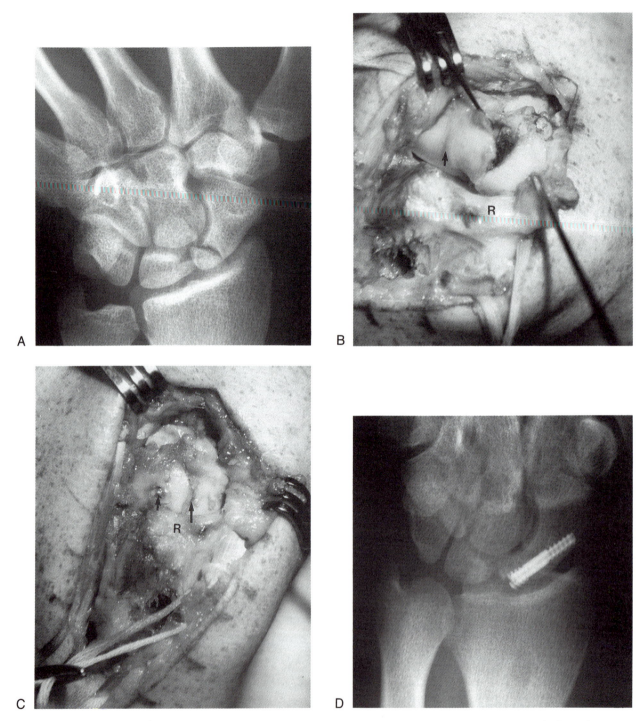

Fig. 13-2. (A) PA radiograph of a proximal pole scaphoid fracture. **(B)** Through a dorsal approach the radius (*R*), scapholunate ligament (*arrow*), and the fracture of the scaphoid are seen. **(C)** The radius (*R*) is seen. The fracture (*large arrow*) is reduced and internally fixed with a cannulated Herbert-Whipple screw (*small arrow*). **(D)** The postoperative radiograph.

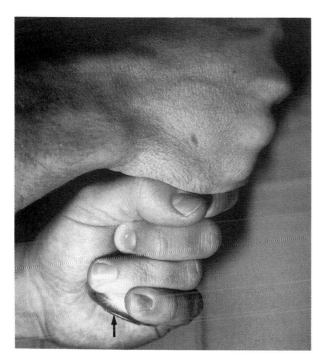

Fig. 13-3. Gripping the bat with the butt of the bat (*arrow*) held in the palm increases the risk of hook of hamate fracture.

The initial diagnosis is clinical. The patient presents with pain and weakness while gripping. At rest the hand is painless. Clinically the hook of the hamate is palpable along the hypothenar eminence distal and radial to the pisiform. Palpation here will elicit pain similar to the clinical discomfort. Ulnar nerve symptoms may or may not be present. Often diagnosis is delayed, since routine radiographs will not show a fracture and the patient may present for assessment after multiple normal radiographs. It is common for clinical suspicion not to exist until a bone scan (Fig. 13-4) is performed after multiple negative plain radio graphs. Carpal tunnel views or CT scan are needed to make the diagnosis (Fig. 13-5). If the diagnosis is made acutely, a trial of cast immobilization may result in union.[15] For symptomatic nonunion, excision of the hook of the hamate with repair of the transverse carpal ligament is indicated (Fig. 13-6). Excision of the hook of the hamate is also indicated in athletes wishing rapid return to competition, since the athlete will often return to competitive sports within 6 to 8 weeks after undergoing surgical excision.[9,25]

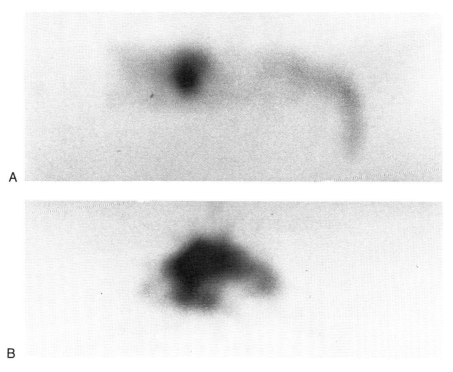

A

B

Fig. 13-4. Tomographic bone scans in the sagittal plane **(A)** and the axial plane **(B)** localize the uptake to the hamate.

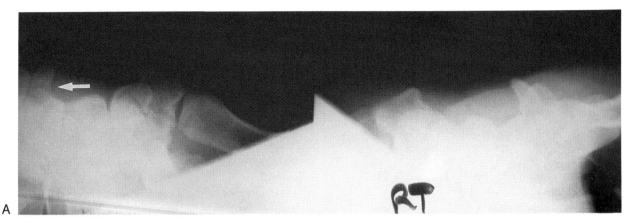

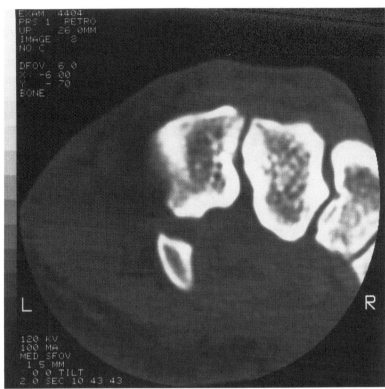

Fig. 13-5. **(A)** Carpal tunnel views of both wrists show the fracture of the hook of the hamate on the left (*arrow*). **(B)** CT shows the fracture clearly.

Triquetral Fractures

Triquetral fractures are common injuries, presenting as the third most common carpal bone fractured.[9] The mechanism of injury is again a fall on the outstretched hand, and the athlete presents with pain and swelling over the dorsal ulnar aspect of the wrist. Most com-

monly, they present as small avulsion fractures, with fractures through the body rarely seen. Fractures of the proximal pole of the triquetrum may be secondary to ulnar impaction.

Immobilization for a short period (4 weeks) with return to activity is recommended.[56] Not all triquetral fractures become pain-free, and this can be a long-

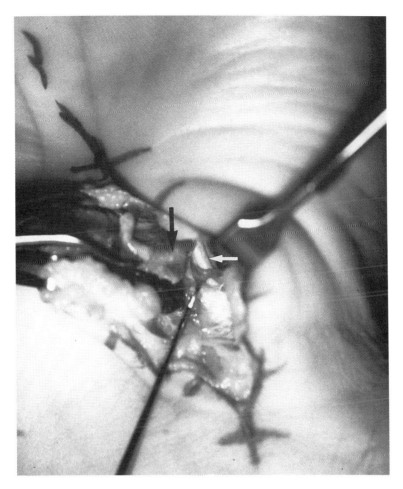

Fig. 13-6. An intraoperative view shows the excised hook of hamate (*black arrow*) with a flexor tendon (*white arrow*) visible in the wound. The skin hook retracts the edge of the flexor retinaculum.

term debilitating injury. The area of chondromalacia on the triquetrum can be a source of chronic pain. If conservative measures fail to improve the pain, arthroscopic debridement may be necessary.

Osteochondral Injuries

Osteochondral and cartilaginous injuries are becoming increasingly recognized as sources of wrist pain. Bilateral osteochondral flaps of the radius have been described as a cause of chronic wrist pain in weightlifters.[27] These injuries are not visible by radiographic diagnostic tests, leading to a lack of recognition in the past. Although osteochondral lesions have been identified on MRI in the knee, visualization in the wrist

has been poor due to the small size of the lesion.[11,23] Arthroscopic diagnosis remains the best method of visualizing these lesions. Diagnosis of any associated ligamentous injury is essential to treating these injuries.[25] If no other injuries exist, debridement has been an effective mode of treatment for this injury. If other ligamentous injuries exist, treatment of associated injuries must be undertaken; otherwise persistent pain from the underlying carpal instability will be present.[42]

Scaphoid Impaction Syndrome

Hyperextension of the wrist can result in impingement of the dorsal ridge of the scaphoid with the dorsal rim of the radius. This injury is difficult to diagnose, and its true incidence is unknown. It has been described in both gymnasts as well as weight lifters.[29] Clinically it presents with dorsal wrist pain. On examination, forced dorsiflexion reproduces the symptoms. Palpation of the dorsal ridge of the scaphoid produces localized tenderness. Although radiographic changes may show an osteophyte, they are often normal. The problem may exist as a capsulitis without radiographic changes. Often the diagnosis can only be made at arthrotomy. If definite radiographic changes exist, treatment consists of excision of the osteophytes and impinging bone. Good pain relief can be obtained in this instance. Nonoperative management is indicated in most cases to avoid the risk of morbidity associated with an exploratory arthrotomy in an athlete.

SOFT TISSUE INJURIES

Scapholunate Ligament Tears

Clinically, scapholunate ligament tears present like scaphoid fractures. Pain, swelling, and tenderness over the snuffbox may cause an initial suspicion of scaphoid fracture that is not confirmed on radiographs. These are often diagnosed as "clinical scaphoid" injuries but may be scapholunate ligament injuries. Early diagnosis of scapholunate injury has been difficult. Clinically, Watson and Hampton[51] have described a provocative test for ligament disruption, but dorsal pain over the scapholunate ligament has often been the only clinical sign. Early diagnosis and attempt at repair has been advocated, since the repair or reconstruction of chronic ligament tears is difficult.[8]

Acute ligament repair is most successful if performed less than 6 weeks after injury. The static subluxation seen on routine posteroanterior radiographs may not appear for months until the remaining ligamentous supports stretch. Provocative radiographic testing for scapholunate dissociation has included dynamic loading with the fist clenched[19] or distraction, as described by Johnson.[22] Again, these tests may be negative. Arthrography may be used to aid in the diagnosis. However, none of these tests allow definitive diagnosis of a complete versus partial tear. MRI imaging of intercarpal ligament tears has not proved as helpful as was hoped. Schweitzer[46] reports a sensitivity of only .25 percent with an accuracy of 64 percent in assessing the scapholunate ligament. Assessment of partial tears was poor, with a sensitivity of only 20 percent. Arthros-

copy remains the only method of identifying complete versus partial tears (Fig. 13-7). A decision to undergo diagnostic arthroscopy is based on persistent pain and tenderness after bony injury has been ruled out. Arthroscopy also allows accurate assessment and any associated pathology.

Treating scapholunate ligament injuries is a difficult problem. Open suture repair of the ligament is difficult. Often a dorsal reinforcement with a tendon graft or capsular flap must be performed.[26] Results are equivocal and the risk of stiffness after arthrotomy and prolonged immobilization is high. Because of this risk, arthroscopic reduction and pinning (Fig. 13-7B) have been suggested.[52] Arthroscopic reduction has the advantage of confirming the presence of an acute tear prior to further treatment. Two to four K-wires are placed across the reduced scapholunate interval (see Ch. 16). Satisfactory short-term results are noted, but prolonged immobilization is necessary, and healing of the ligament may not occur. No long-term results have been reported. Rehabilitation is prolonged after this injury. Immobilization is required for 6 to 8 weeks. ROM and gentle strengthening are started after cast removal. Pins are removed at 12 to 20 weeks. Maximal recovery may take 12 months.

Chronic scapholunate ligament tears may lead to the DISI pattern of carpal collapse. The long-term history is progressive arthritis leading to the scapholunate advanced collapse (SLAC) pattern of arthritis. Treatment of patients that present more than 6 weeks after injury is difficult. Primary ligament healing will probably not occur and other procedures are needed. Either ligament repair and capsulodesis[26] or scaphoid-trapezium-trapezoid fusion[52] are indicated in those patients with symptoms and no degenerative arthritis. Stabilization procedures in the asymptomatic patient with a scapholunate gap on radiographs is not indicated. In patients with advanced arthritic changes, pancarpal fusion may be required. Patients can return to sports after either limited wrist fusion or pancarpal fusion.

Lunotriquetral Tears

Arthroscopy has shown that lunotriquetral tears are more common than once thought.[55] Triquetrolunate instability may occur after a stage 3 perilunar instability in which the scapholunate ligament has been torn, but it is most often seen as an isolated injury.[31] It may be that a pattern of ligament injury exists in the reverse

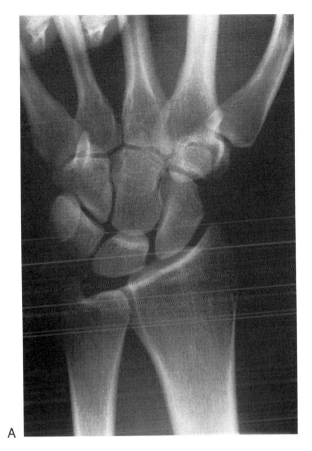 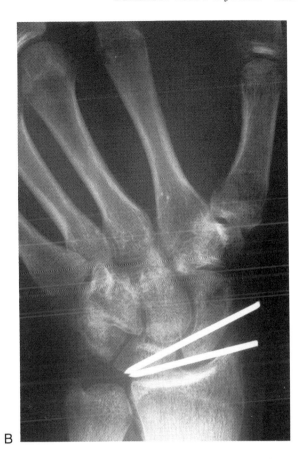

Fig. 13-7. (A) This patient presented 1 month after a hyperextension injury to his wrist with persistent dorsal tenderness. Plain radiographs were equivocal. **(B)** Arthroscopy revealed a complete scapholunate tear, which was treated with arthroscopic reduction and pinning.

order to a perilunate instability with the lunotriquetral ligament rupturing before the scapholunate.[41]

Clinically, the patient presents with ulnar wrist pain. The onset is often related to a specific trauma. The lunotriquetral ballottement test elicits pain and laxity at the lunotriquetral joint.[41] The differential diagnosis includes TFCC tears and midcarpal instability. Because of the multiple diagnostic possibilities, diagnosis has been difficult. Clinical assessment[41] and interruption of Gilula's arcs[19] have been used for evaluation. Radiographs may document a volar intercalated segmental instability (VISI) pattern with volar flexion of the lunate. Arthrography and arthroscopy have been used as the standards of diagnosis.

Assessment of lunotriquetral ligament tears with MRI is more difficult than scapholunate ligament injuries.

The reported sensitivity of MRI ranges from 23 to 50 percent.[46] MRI findings do not have the specificity or accuracy to allow clinical decisions to be made. Confirmation of MRI findings by arthroscopy must still take place. If the injury is diagnosed acutely, arthroscopic reduction and K-wire fixation are indicated. Postoperatively, the management and recovery is similar to scapholunate ligament injuries. Chronic ligament injuries are a difficult problem. Nonoperative management is indicated with anti-inflammatory medication and splints. Surgical reconstruction has been unpredictable. The results of ligament reconstruction and triquetrolunate arthrodesis alone are often poor.[14] If the patient is sufficiently symptomatic to accept the loss of motion, a four-corner fusion of the capitate, hamate, lunate, and triquetrum may be indicated.

Midcarpal Instability

Midcarpal instability can be intrinsic due to laxity at the triquetrohamate articulation or extrinsic secondary to fractures of the distal radius. Athletes most often have intrinsic midcarpal instability. In comparison with lunotriquetral injuries, a specific injury often cannot be elicited. The patient presents with pain and a "clunk," which appears during ulnar deviation of the wrist.[20] A volar sag is visible at rest that corrects during ulnar deviation (Fig. 13-8A and B). A neutral lateral radiograph may reveal a VISI pattern (Fig. 13-8A). Normally, the proximal row sits in volar flexion in radial deviation and with ulnar deviation a smooth transition to dorsiflexion occurs. With midcarpal instability, the proximal row reduces suddenly into a dorsiflexed position resulting in a catch-up "clunk." The pain and wrist clunk can be corrected by dorsally directed pressure on the

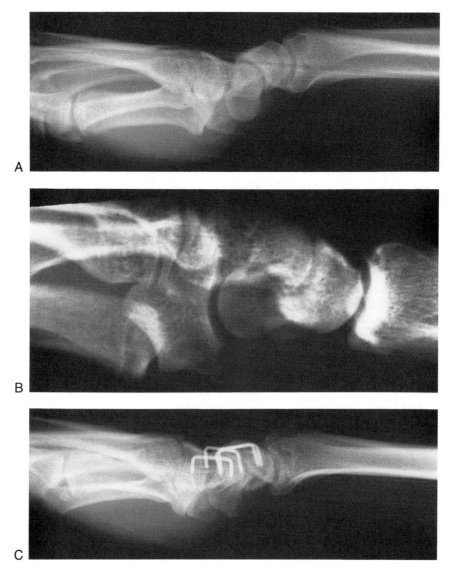

Fig. 13-8. **(A)** A lateral radiograph of a patient with midcarpal instability shows both the VISI deformity and volar sag. **(B)** A lateral radiograph in ulnar deviation shows correction of the VISI deformity. **(C)** A four-corner fusion corrects the VISI deformity and the volar sag.

pisiform, which corrects the proximal row palmar flexion deformity.[2] Similar laxity at the triquetrohamate articulation is often present on the contralateral side: an asymptomatic clunk can be elicited.

If the patient presents after an acute injury, casting in a long-arm cast in supination and radial deviation has been suggested.[20] This is a rare occurrence. In the chronic injury, treatment is initially nonoperative with supportive splints and anti-inflammatory medication. The splint provides dorsally directed pressure on the pisiform and eliminates the pain and clunk. The splint can be worn during sports.[2] If these measures fail, a four-corner fusion of the capitate, hamate, lunate, and triquetrum may be necessary (Fig. 13-8C).

Triangular Fibrocartilage Complex Injuries

TFCC injuries are a common cause of ulnar wrist pain. The TFCC consists of multiple structures blending to form a strong ulnar supporting complex that functions as the main stabilizer of the distal radioulnar joint and a major stabilizer of the ulnar carpus. The dorsal and palmar radioulnar ligaments provide stability to the distal radioulnar joint. The articular disc functions to transmit approximately 18 percent of an axial load at the wrist to the ulna.[39]

Causes of ulnar wrist pain include extensor carpi ulnaris subluxation or tendinitis, distal radioulnar joint subluxation with degenerative changes, ulnocarpal impingement, pisotriquetral arthritis, and TFCC perforations.[50]

Patients with TFCC tears present with ulnar pain. The pain can be aggravated by rotatory motion as well as ulnar deviation and compression. A click may or may not be present. The tears are often tender just distal to the ulnar styloid process. A single inciting incident can often be elicited. Diagnosis of TFCC tears can be made arthroscopically. Arthroscopy is superior to both arthrography and MRI (Fig. 13-9). Although MRI has the theoretical advantage of being noninvasive, diagnostic accuracy is poor, with both false positives

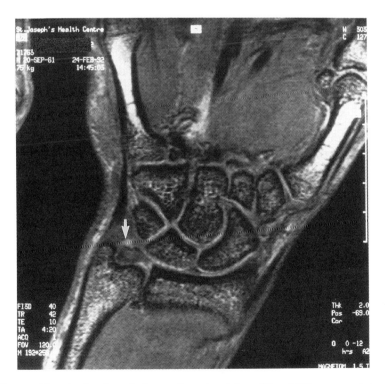

Fig. 13-9. This 30-year-old male developed ulnar wrist pain while golfing. MRI scan was interpreted as showing a possible TFCC tear (*arrow*). Arthroscopy revealed a normal TFCC. However, a lunotriquetral ligament tear not visualized by the MRI scan was present.

and negatives.[11,23] Diagnosis of TFCC tears on arthrography or MRI must take into account the increasing incidence of degenerative perforations with age. Clinical correlation is essential.

Palmer[39] and Blair et al.[7] have both described classification systems for TFCC lesions. Palmer classifies them into traumatic (I) and degenerative (II). Subclasses describe the presence of associated lunate and ulnar pathology as well as the location of the tear. Subclass 1A is a tear of the central portion of the TFCC; 1B is an avulsion of the TFCC from its attachment to the ulnar styloid; 1C is a peripheral tear adjacent to the lunate and triquetrum; and in 1D the attachments of the TFCC are avulsed from the radius. Blair classifies TFCC lesions into central, ulnar, or radial tears. The critical point in both classification systems involves separating the central or radial lesions from the ulnar peripheral lesions. The extrinsic blood supply to the articular disk is primarily from palmar, dorsal, and ulnar margins of the disk. The central and radial portions are avascular and have a limited capacity to heal. The proportion of the disc that is vascularized decreases from 33 percent in childhood to 25 percent in adults.[32]

Immobilization of acute TFCC injuries for 4 weeks in slight flexion and ulnar deviation is recommended. Commonly, TFCC injuries present as chronic perforations. The goal is to remove the redundant flaps of tissue without causing instability. Removing the redundant flaps may prevent the lunate from impinging on them with wrist motion and is the rationale for debridement.

Arthroscopic debridement of chronic perforations of the TFCC has been shown to be effective (see Ch. 16). Results of debridement have been good, with relief of pain in 73 percent of patients at 1 year. These results are similar to those reported from ulnar shortening, in which 28 of 36 patients (78 percent) had good pain relief.[16] Treatment depends on the location and size of the tear. Large central tears are resected. If the tear is peripheral and the edges are in apposition, then immobilization alone or supplemental suture of the tear are indicated. The objective of suture repair is to restore the normal tension and trampoline effect of the TFCC.

Arthroscopic treatment is associated with much less morbidity than open arthrotomy, and the magnification allows better visualization. The recovery of grip strength and motion is more rapid. Overall arthroscopy is now the modality of choice for diagnosis and treatment of lesions of the TFCC (see Ch. 16).

PREVENTION AND ORTHOTICS

Injuries of the upper limb related to a single force that exceeds the strength of the osseous and ligamentous structure of the wrist cannot be prevented by conditioning. The risk of injuries related to repetitive loading can be decreased by conditioning and orthoses.

The preventive aspects of sports medicine will vary from sport to sport. Learning the proper way to fall can decrease the stresses borne by the wrist and forearm. Falling properly involves learning to roll as one contacts the ground, absorbing the force on the shoulder and torso, and minimizing the force on the wrist. This skill is taught to gymnasts and judo participants and these groups have a low incidence of scaphoid fracture.[54] The same skills would decrease the incidence of scaphoid fracture in football players and volleyball players.

Gymnasts are the main group in which prevention has the greatest role to play. Dorsal wrist pain is related to conditioning and technique as well as the intensity of training and number of repetitions. A consistently identified factor in gymnasts with chronic wrist problems has been relative weakness of wrist and finger flexors.[54] Thus the limiting factor on wrist dorsiflexion is structural support from ligaments and the carpus rather than dynamic muscle action. Strengthening exercises allow dynamic control of wrist extension and decrease the loading and damage to dorsal tissues.

Modification of techniques is often useful. Changing the grip on the bat can decrease the risk of hook of hamate injuries.

Orthotics

Orthotic devices in sports can protect a previously injured part, prevent further injury, and allow participation of the injured player in sports with minimal interference with skill activities. The most common types of orthotic material are protective taping, low-temperature thermoplastics, and casting materials.

Most wrist orthotics are designed to prevent hyperextension. Protective taping procedures are well established.[40] If splints are designed for the wrist, the relationship of grip strength to wrist position should be considered.[36] Thus the wrist should be positioned in extension rather than neutral, and the athlete should be warned that positions less than 25 to 35 degrees of wrist extension will decrease grip strength.

Extension block splints allowing wrist flexion are useful in gymnasts who have dorsal wrist pain. After a period of immobilization, strengthening exercises for the wrist and finger flexors are instituted to allow the athlete to prevent wrist hyperextension dynamically. During this period resumption of activity is allowed with a dorsal blocking splint.

Soft playing splints are available to protect undisplaced scaphoid fractures during competition, with thumb spica casts used between games.[6] Functional bracing of the scaphoid has proved effective in maintenance of wrist flexion and extension.[25]

Returning to Competition

The timing of return to athletic activity can be difficult to determine. Often the pressure to compete is intense. Multiple factors are involved in the decision.[33] The timing will vary with the injury, the level of competition, the age of the athlete, and the specific sport. Return to competition should also wait until ROM and strength have recovered to the point that the athletes can protect themselves from further injury. Protective splinting and taping is essential at this stage.

CONCLUSIONS

Sport-related injuries of the wrist are common in many sporting activities. Accurate diagnosis of the underlying pathology is essential for treatment, since this group of patients has high expectations. Appropriate use of nonoperative and operative treatment methods are necessary to provide maximum return of function.

REFERENCES

1. Albanese SA, Palmer AK, Kerr DR et al: Wrist pain and distal growth plate closure of the radius in gymnasts. J Paediatr Orthop 9:23–28, 1989
2. Alexander CE, Lichtman DM: Triquetrolunate and midcarpal instability. p. 274. In Lichtman DM (ed): The Wrist and Its Disorders. WB Saunders, Philadelphia, 1988
3. Alffram PA, Bauer GC: Epidemiology of fractures of the forearm. A biomechanial investigation of bone strength. J Bone Joint Surg [Am] 44A:105–114, 1962
4. Amadio PC: Epidemiology of hand and wrist injuries in sports. Hand Clin 6:379–381, 1990
5. Aronen JG: Problems of the upper extremity in gymnasts. Clin Sports Med 4:61–71, 1985
6. Bergfield JA, Weiler GG, Andrish JJ et al: Soft playing splint for protection of significant hand and wrist injuries in sports. Am J Sports Med 10:293–296, 1982
7. Blair WF, Berger RA, El-Khoury GY: Arthromography of the wrist: an experimental and preliminary study. J Hand Surg 10A:350–359, 1985
8. Blatt G: Scapholunate instability. p. 251. In Lichtman DM (ed): The Wrist and Its Disorders. WB Saunders Philadelphia, 1988
9. Bryan RS, Dobyns JH: Fractures of the carpal bones other than lunate and navicular. Clin Orthop 149:107–111, 1980
10. Carek PJ, Fumich RM: Stress fracture of the distal radius. Physician Sportsmed 20:115–118, 1992
11. Cerofolini E, Luchetti R, Pederzini L et al: MR evaluation of triangular fibrocartilage complex tears in the wrist: comparison with arthrography and arthroscopy. J Comput Assist Tomogr 14:963–967, 1990
12. Chambers RB: Orthopaedic injuries in athletes (ages 6 and 17): comparison of injuries occurring in six sports. Am J Sports Med 7:195–197, 1979
13. Cooney WP, Dobyns JH, Linscheid RL: Fractures of the scaphoid: a rational approach to management. Clin Orthop 149:90–97, 1980
14. Culver JE: Instabilities of the wrist. Clin Sports Med 5:725–740, 1986
15. Culver JE: Sports related fractures of the hand and wrist. Clin Sports Med 9:85–109, 1990
16. Darrow JC, Linscheid RL, Dobyns JH et al: Distal ulnar recession for disorders of the distal radioulnar joint. J Hand Surg 10A:482–491, 1985
17. Doman AN, Marcus NW: Congenital bipartite scaphoid. J Hand Surg 15A:869–873, 1990
18. Fernandez DL: A technique for anterior wedge shaped grafts for scaphoid nonunions with carpal instability. J Hand Surg 9A:733–737, 1984
19. Gilula LA, Weeks PM: Post-traumatic ligamentous instabilities of the wrist. Radiology 129:641–651, 1978
20. Green DP: Midcarpal Instability. ASSH Instructional Course, Toronto, 1990
21. Imaeda T, Nakamura R, Miura T et al: Magnetic resonance imaging in scaphoid fractures. J Hand Surg [Br] 17B:20–27, 1992
22. Johnson J: Diagnosis of scapholunate dissociation with traction radiography. Presented at the Manus Canada Annual Meeting, Calgary, Alberta, Canada, June 1991

23. Kang HS, Kindynis P, Brahme SK et al: Triangular fibro-cartilage and intercarpal ligaments of the wrist: MR imaging. Cadaveric study with gross pathologic and histologic correlation. Radiology 181:401–404, 1991

24. Knirk JL, Jupiter JB: Intra-articular fractures of the distal end of the radius in young adults. J Bone Joint Surg 63A:647–659, 1986

25. Koman LA, Mooney JF, Poehling GG: Fractures and ligamentous injuries of the wrist. Hand Clin 6:477–491, 1990

26. Lavernia CJ, Cohen MS, Taleisnik J: Treatment of scapholunate dissociation by ligamentous repair and capsulodesis. J Hand Surg 17A:354–359, 1992

27. Levy HJ, Gardner RD, Lemak LJ: Bilateral osteochondral flaps of the wrists. Arthroscopy 7:118–119, 1991

28. Lidstrom A: Fractures of the distal end of the radius: a clinical and statistical study of end results. Acta Orthop Scand Suppl 41:7–118, 1959

29. Linscheid RL, Dobyns JH: Athletic injuries of the wrist. Clin Orthop 198:141–151, 1985

30. Mandelbaum BR, Bartolozzi AR, Davis CA et al: Wrist pain syndrome in the gymnast. Am J Sports Med 17:305–317, 1989

31. Mayfield JK, Johnson RP, Kilcoyne RK: Carpal dislocations: pathomechanics and progressive perilunar instability. J Hand Surg 5:226–241, 1980

32. Mikic Z: The blood supply of the human distal radioulnar joint and the microvasculature of its articular disk. Clin Orthop 275:19–28, 1992

33. Mirabello SC, Loeb PE, Andrews JR: The wrist: field evaluation and treatment. Clin Sports Med 11:1–25, 1992

34. Mohanti RC, Kar N: Study of triangular fibrocartilage of the wrist joint in Colles' fracture. Injury 11:321–324, 1980

35. Nielsen PT, Hedeboe J, Thommesen P: Bone scintigraphy in the evaluation of fracture of the carpal bone Acta Orthop Scand 54:303–306, 1983

36. O'Driscoll SW, Horii E, Richards RR et al: The relationship between wrist position, grasp size, and grip strength. J Hand Surg 17A:169–177, 1992

37. Osterman AL, Mikulics M: Scaphoid nonunion Hand Clin 14:437–455, 1988

38. Palmer AK: The distal radioulnar joint: anatomy, biomechanics, and triangular fibrocartilage complex abnormalities. Hand Clin 3:31–40, 1987

39. Palmer AK: Triangular fibrocartilage disorders: injury patterns and treatment. Arthroscopy 6:125–132, 1990

40. Press JM, Wiesner SL: Prevention: conditioning and orthotics. Hand Clin 6:383–392, 1990

41. Reagan DS, Linscheid RL, Dobyns DH: Lunotriquetral sprains. J Hand Surg 9:502–513, 1984

42. Roth JH, Poehling GG, Whipple T et al: Arthroscopic Surgery of the Wrist. Information Manual. Bowman-Gray School of Medicine, Winston-Salem, 1989

43. Roth JH, Reuter J: Comparison of cannulated scaphoid screw and nonthreaded pin fixation in volar bone grafting of primary scaphoid nonunions: a clinical review. Canadian Society for Surgery of the Hand Annual Meeting, Calgary, Alberta, June 2, 1991

44. Roy S, Caine D, Singer KM: Stress changes of the distal radial epiphysis in young gymnasts: a report of twenty-one cases and a review of the literature. Am J Sports Med 13:301–308, 1985

45. Sanders WE: Evaluation of the humpback scaphoid by computed tomography in the longitudinal axial plane of the scaphoid. J Hand Surg 13A:182–187, 1988

46. Schweitzer ME, Brahme SK, Hodler J et al: Chronic wrist pain: spin-echo and short tau inversion recovery MRI imaging and conventional and MRI arthrography. Radiology 182:205–211, 1992

47. Stewart MJ: Fractures of the carpal navicular (scaphoid): a report of 436 cases. J Bone Joint Surg [Am] 36A:998–1006, 1954

48. Stordahl A, Schjoth A, Woxholt G et al: Bone scanning of fractures of the scaphoid. J Hand Surg 9B:189–190, 1984

49. Szabo RM, Manske D: Displaced fractures of the scaphoid. Clin Orthop 230:30–38, 1988

50. Taleisnik J: Pain on the ulnar side of the wrist. Hand Clin 3:51–68, 1987

51. Watson HK, Hempton RF: Limited wrist arthrodesis part 1: the triscaphoid joint. J Hand Surg 5:320–327, 1980

52. Watson HK, Black DM: Instabilities of the wrist. Hand Clin 3:103–111, 1987

53. Weber ER: Biomechanical implications of scaphoid waist fractures Clin Orthop 149:83–89, 1980

54. Weiker GG: Hand and wrist problems in the gymnast. Clin Sports Med 11:189–202, 1992

55. Whipple TL: Wrist arthroscopy: clinical applications of wrist arthroscopy. p. 118. In Lichtman DM (ed): The Wrist and Its Disorders. WB Saunders Philadelphia, 1988

56. Zemel NP, Stark HH: Fractures and dislocations of the carpal bones. Clin Sports Med 5:709–723, 1986

14

Common Hand Fractures

M. MERLE
G. DAUTEL

INTRODUCTION

In the field of hand injuries, much attention has been given to fractures of metacarpal and phalangeal bones. Thanks to a good understanding of causal mechanisms, to numerous studies of deformities based on the biomechanical characteristics of the hand, and to development of techniques of osteosynthesis using miniaturized material, a variety of treatment methods currently exist that will ensure excellent restoration of hand anatomy in most cases and will also allow early mobilization. Most of the studies done in this field are in agreement on general principles, and they indicate which treatment (orthopaedic or surgical), would be best in each case.[5,6,20,49,64]

The therapeutic approach is entirely different in the case of top-notch athletes, either professional or amateur. The surgeon must deal with a patient who does not want to modify a schedule and stop activity for several weeks following a fracture of metacarpal or phalangeal bones. The coaches, sponsors, and relatives who make up the athlete's entourage insist that the surgeon select a method of treatment compatible with rapid or even immediate return to sports activity. Faced with this situation, the physician might be tempted to renounce standard treatment in order to satisfy the exceptional requests and needs of the patient. This can be a dangerous situation. It could lead to performance of an osteosynthesis with a high rate of complications—which would be a mistake—rather than application of an orthopaedic treatment that takes time but is safer. Relying on the alleged strength of the osteosynthesis, the athlete might apply great stress to the area, which may dismantle the repair and have adverse effects on function. Furthermore, even when surgical treatment yields a good functional result immediately after surgery, the results will not necessarily remain satisfactory in the long run.

The psychology of an athlete involved in competition leads to irrational behavior concerning the fracture. Athletes are so used to striving for performance and excellence that they feel the basic laws of biomechanics and bone consolidation do not apply to them. All too frequently, casts and splints that were meant to be kept in place for a period of several weeks are removed by the patient after only a few days because they hinder training. When these athletes retire from competition, they often present an interesting clinical and radiologic picture.

We recently examined a motorcycle champion who had suffered more than 29 articular, juxta-articular, and diaphyseal fractures of metacarpal and phalangeal bones in the course of his career. None of the digital chains was intact; they all had sequelae of fractures: malunions with bone angulation or rotation and post-traumatic arthritis involving the trapeziometacarpal, metacarpophalangeal, and interphalangeal articulations. Given this situation, one would expect the patient to be very dissatisfied. However, this was not the case; his hand was quite functional, each digital chain having a useful sector and range of motion (ROM). As for his pain, this retired champion would only say: "I can live with it; it's all in the head anyway," and he did not ask for pain-killing medication.

In these cases, the surgeon must be careful not to deviate from standard treatment and not to succumb to pressure by the athlete and the entourage. Nonobservance of anatomic and biomechanical principles, as well as the principles of bone healing, will only lead to failure. It is imperative to inform the patient and the entourage and to provide a detailed explanation of the risks involved in radical surgical treatment and in premature return to sports activity. The surgeon must foresee that excessive stress will be applied to the fracture site and must provide an especially strong protection, using nonelastic splints that will guard against direct blows to the region. With all these factors in mind, let us review the most frequent types of fracture of metacarpal and phalangeal bones observed in sports medicine.

CAUSAL MECHANISMS

Most hand fractures result from the practice of soccer, handball, basketball, and boxing.[2–57] Fractures of metacarpal bones are much more frequent than fractures of phalanges. Sprains are mostly observed at the level of metacarpophalangeal joints, followed by those of the proximal interphalangeal joints of long digits. On the whole, hand trauma represents 3 to 9 percent of all trauma caused by sports and is observed mainly in sports involving contact, speed, and energy.

ORGANIZATION OF THE HAND SKELETON AND MECHANISM OF DEFORMATION AFTER FRACTURE

Organization of the Hand Skeleton

The hand presents two arches: one is transverse, and corresponds to the metacarpophalangeal articulations; the other is longitudinal and is on the axis of the third ray. These two arches have a planar concavity and give the hand a cup-like shape, which aids in prehension. The second and third metacarpal bones are not mobile on the carpus, being strongly attached to its distal row. The first, fourth, and fifth metacarpal bones are mobile; in flexion, they augment hand concavity and thus improve prehension. Deformations or changes in orientation are not acceptable at the level of the nonmobile metacarpal bones; extreme care must be taken to restore the correct anatomic-configuration of these bones. Post-traumatic deformations of the fourth and fifth metacarpal bones have less adverse functional consequences given the mobility of the carpometacarpal joints.

Grasp strength is preserved if the metacarpal arch

is restored. Therefore, oblique and spiral fractures must be reduced in order to restore the length and axis of metacarpal bones. The digits are articulated on the metacarpophalangeal joints, which have an active range of flexion of 100 degrees; the ROMs of the proximal and distal interphalangeal joints are respectively 100 and 70 degrees. This range of function is obtained only if the lengths of metacarpal and phalangeal bones correspond to the numeric series of Fibonacci[0,1,1,2,3,5,8,13,21]. Thus the length of the proximal phalanx is equal to the sum of the lengths of the middle and distal phalanges. Treatment must restore the relative length of each component of the skeleton as best as possible.

Long digital chains, which are parallel when the fingers are extended, converge toward the tuberosity of the scaphoid bone when they are flexed. Function of the thumb is satisfactory as long as the trapeziometacarpal joint is normal and the first web space is not retracted; reduced mobility, and even complete stiffness, of the metacarpophalangeal and interphalangeal joints of the thumb are acceptable.

Mechanisms of Deformation

Metacarpal Fractures

The action of flexor tendons and interosseous muscles results in displacement in flexion of the distal bone fragment (Fig. 14-1). This displacement is more pronounced in fractures at the neck of the metacarpal bones, producing a protrusion of the metacarpophalangeal joint at the distal palmar crease. Interosseous muscles also cause axial rotation of the distal segment of the bone. The second and third metacarpal bones tend to rotate in pronation (ulnar rotation), whereas the fourth and fifth metacarpal bones tend to rotate in supination (radial rotation). These deformations might

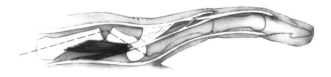

Fig. 14-1. The distal fragment of metacarpal bones is displaced in flexion by the simultaneous action of the flexor tendons and interosseous muscles. (From Merle and Dautel,[50] with permission.)

go unnoticed when the fingers are extended; they become visible only when the fingers are flexed, since the fractured ray is then superimposed on the adjacent one.

When reducing a fracture, the surgeon must take care to restore the convergence of the long fingers toward the tubercle of the scaphoid bone. Metacarpal bones that present spiral or long oblique fractures are shortened by the contraction of interosseous muscles. Restoring the length of metacarpal bones is indispensable to maintain the transverse arch of the hand.

Finally, it must be kept in mind that Bennett's fracture results in significant displacement due to the action of the abductor pollicis longus and thenar muscles. The first metacarpal bone is always displaced proximally and dorsally (Fig. 14-2). Similarly, fractures of the base of the fifth metacarpal bone are displaced by action of the extensor carpi ulnaris muscle.

Direct, axial trauma to the metacarpal bones of the index and long fingers produces fracture-dislocations at their bases. The palmar bone fragment remains attached to the carpal bones. The second and third metacarpal bones are readily displaced in a proximal and dorsal direction by the action of the extensor carpi radialis longus and brevis muscles, resulting in an S-shaped dorsal protrusion often masked by edema and hematoma.

Fractures of Phalanges

Diaphyseal Fractures of Proximal Phalanx

The interosseous muscles cause flexion of the proximal fragment, and the lateral strips of the extensor system cause extension of the distal fragment, resulting in a recurvatum of the first phalanx with dorsal concavity (Fig. 14-3A).

The lateral deviation of the distal fragment is readily visible clinically; it is due to the causal mechanism and to the orientation of the fracture. Axial rotation, although frequent, cannot be detected clinically or radiographically when the fingers are extended. It is imperative to verify the good convergence of the fingers in flexion after reduction of the fracture.

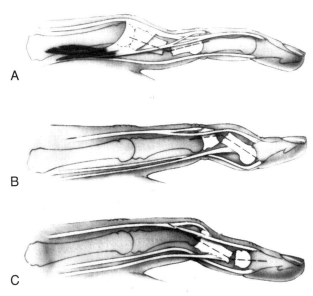

Fig. 14-3. **(A)** In cases of diaphyseal fracture of the first phalanx, the proximal fragment is flexed by the interosseous muscles, forming an angle with dorsal concavity. **(B)** Fracture of the middle phalanx: when the fracture is proximal to the insertion of the superficial flexor tendon, the distal fragment is displaced in flexion, forming an angle with palmar concavity. **(C)** Fracture of the middle phalanx: when the fracture is located distal to the insertion of the superficial flexor tendon, the resulting angle has a dorsal concavity. (From Merle and Dautel,[50] with permission.)

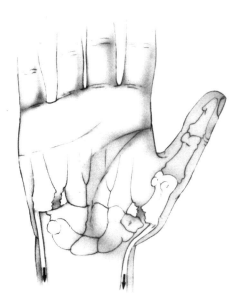

Fig. 14-2. In Bennett's fracture, the first metacarpal bone is displaced proximally and dorsally by the action of the abductor pollicis longus muscle. In cases of fracture at the base of the fifth metacarpal bone, a similar displacement is observed due to the action of the extensor carpi ulnaris muscle. (From Merle and Dautel,[50] with permission.)

Diaphyseal Fractures of Middle Phalanx

When the fracture is proximal to the insertion of the flexor sublimis digitorum tendon, the proximal fragment is displaced dorsally by the strip of the extensor tendon; the distal fragment is flexed by the action of the flexor sublimis digitorum muscle. The resultant deformation is an angulation with palmar concavity (Fig. 14-3B).

Conversely, a fracture distal to the insertion of the tendon of the flexor sublimis digitorum muscle causes the proximal fragment to flex; since the extensor system displaces the distal fragment dorsally, the deformation is an angulation with dorsal concavity (Fig. 14-3C).

CLINICAL AND RADIOLOGIC ASSESSMENT

Clinical Examination

Deformation of the hand skeleton after fracture is not always easy to analyze due to the edema or hematoma that can mask it. Recurvatum of the phalanges is readily visible. By contrast, oblique or spiral fractures often go unnoticed when fingers are extended. Gentle placing of the finger in flexion will then make its rotatory displacement apparent.

Flexion of the metacarpophalangeal joints increases the convexity of the metacarpal arch; in cases of fracture at the neck of a metacarpal bone, the head of the bone no longer protrudes. When the fragment is significantly displaced, it is easy to perceive this by palpating the palm of the hand at the distal palmar crease. Clinical examination ends with exploring the tendon system and the vascular and neural pedicles.

Radiologic Examination

Detecting a fracture on radiographs requires great care; frontal and sagittal radiographs of the hand are not sufficient. In the case of metacarpal bones, sagittal radiographs are also needed; the hand must be placed in pronation and supination at 30 degrees in order to visualize the second and fifth metacarpal bones. When lesions of the digits exist, frontal, sagittal, and oblique radiographs of each finger are necessary, so as to detect articular or juxta-articular lesions.

Brewerton's projection radiograph,[10] initially designed to evaluate erosion of metacarpal heads in cases of rheumatoid arthritis, is also very useful for assessing traumatic lesions of metacarpophalangeal joints[45] as well as fractures at the base of the fourth and fifth metacarpal bones.[42] The hand is placed with its dorsal aspect on the radiologic film and metacarpophalangeal joints flexed at 65 degrees; the x-ray tube is tilted 15 degrees toward the ulnar aspect of the hand.

TREATMENT

Treatment of fractures of the hand is well organized when patients, in order to have the best possible restoration of anatomy and function, are willing to accept a reliable method in spite of its drawbacks and inconvenience. On the contrary, the special case of athletes limits the choice of methods to orthopaedic ones because the stress that will be inflicted on the realigned skeleton during bone healing would threaten the best of osteosyntheses.

However, no method of treatment should be excluded; we will review the six categories according to Tubiana's classification[72]:

Immediate mobilization
Immobilization with splints
Orthopaedic reduction and early mobilization
Orthopaedic reduction and osteosynthesis by transcutaneous pins
Surgical reduction and minimal osteosynthesis, insufficient for early mobilization
Strong osteosynthesis followed by immediate mobilization

Immediate Mobilization

Weeks and Wray[74] and de la Caffinière and Mansat[15] reported that stiffness of the fingers resulted from a fracture of the hand in 25 percent of cases. Early, or even immediate, mobilization is the best way to prevent edema and joint stiffness and to preserve normal sliding of tendons.

In order to encourage the patient to move a broken finger while precluding excessive movement, it is advisable to attach the injured finger to the adjacent one

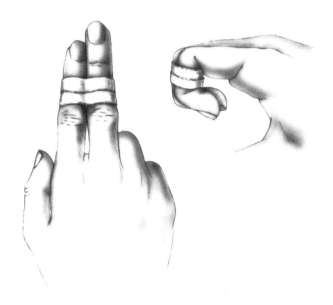

Fig. 14-4. Placing a digit with a stable fracture in syndactyly with the intact adjacent finger is the best possible dynamic splint, ensuring rapid functional recovery. (From Merle and Dautel,[50] with permission.)

with one or two adhesive bandages. This temporary syndactyly makes the best dynamic splint (Fig. 14-4). Three weeks are sufficient for the fracture site to harden; 6 weeks are needed before full stress can be applied. During athletic practice, additional protection is needed, and a thermoplastic gauntlet should be worn to ensure proper bone union.

Immobilization With Splints and on Bonvallet's Ball

Immobilization with splints is necessary for unstable fractures in which osteosynthesis is contraindicated. However, this method quite often results in malunion and articular stiffness, especially when metacarpophalangeal joints are not flexed to a minimum of 60 degrees and when the proximal interphalangeal joint is not maintained in extension. Too often, fingers continue to be placed on a tongue-depressor, an instrument that should be restricted to the field of otolaryngology. When immobilization is required, it is preferable to use thermoplastic splints, which can be adapted precisely to the patient's anatomy. Three weeks is a sufficient period to stabilize the fracture

site. After this time, active rehabilitation using dynamic splints will help to restore function. Three to 6 weeks are necessary to restore a useful ROM.

Bonvallet[9] suggested immobilizing the fingers on a plaster ball that is placed in the palm of the hand, while the wrist remains free. Use of this ball results in remolding and reorienting the digital chains. In the case of unstable fractures, immobilization for 3 weeks is appropriate. When the risk of secondary displacement is small, the syndactylized fingers should be mobilized once or twice a week in order to maintain joint ROM. Radiographs should be performed after mobilization to make sure that no secondary displacement exists. It is advisable to use a cylinder of thermoplastic material instead of a plaster ball, since this facilitates radiologic examination.

Orthopedic Reduction and Early Mobilization: The Functional Treatment

Thomine[68,69] was disappointed by results of standard orthopaedic treatment, noting that ROM was satisfactory in only 50 percent of cases. He suggested using a functional apparatus to treat diaphyseal fractures of the proximal phalanx. This apparatus is a thermoplastic gauntlet that stabilizes the wrist in extension (Fig. 14-5A), aligns the proximal interphalangeal joints of the digits in the frontal plane, and keeps the fourth and fifth carpometacarpal joints in flexion (Fig. 14-5B).

The metacarpophalangeal joints are flexed and the digits are placed in syndactyly distal to the proximal interphalangeal joint (Fig. 14-5C). In this so-called intrinsic plus position, little risk of secondary displacement with dorsal concavity exists in such cases of diaphyseal fracture of the proximal phalanx. Mobilization of proximal and distal interphalangeal joints is begun immediately; the device is left in place for 5 to 6 weeks. Clinical and radiologic follow-up must be meticulous in order to detect a possible secondary displacement.

This functional method could also be applied in cases of stable fractures of middle and distal phalanges: the distal interphalangeal joint must then be immobilized in extension with a trough-like dorsal splint kept in place by two adhesive bandages. In this way, the proximal interphalangeal joint can be mobilized without restriction.

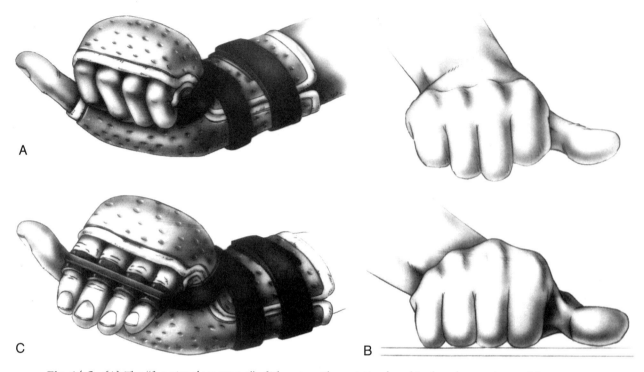

Fig. 14-5. (A) The "functional treatment" of Thomine. The wrist is placed in dorsal extension and the metacarpophalangeal joints at 90 degrees of flexion. The distal part of the palm is left out of the splint so that complete flexion of the digits is possible. **(B)** The proximal interphalangeal joints are aligned in the frontal plane by flexing of the fourth and fifth metacarpophalangeal joints. **(C)** The digital chains are placed in syndactylyl using rings held together by a small aluminum plate or thermoplastic material. The proximal interphalangeal joint and the digital pulp and nail remain free. (From Merle and Dautel,[50] with permission.)

Orthopedic Reduction and Osteosynthesis by Percutaneous Pins With Immobilization

Axial and X-Shaped Pin Assembly

Ever since Pratt[56] and von Saal[73] advised the use of Kirschner pins in hand surgery, many authors have used the method and refined the technique and indications. Kirschner pins are inserted percutaneously, which eliminates the need for surgical exposure of the fracture site; however, the technique must be meticulous, given the non-negligible risk of damage to vascular and neural pedicles. It is preferable to insert pins through the medial or lateral dorsal aspect of the finger, taking care not to damage or block the extensor system. Kirschner pins 10/10 and 12/10 mm in diameter are inserted with a powerful drill that rotates slowly so as to preclude heat damage to the cortical bone. Pins must not go through intact joints. It is advisable to insert the pins obliquely through the medial or lateral aspects of the heads of metacarpal bones and phalanges. A single pin is insufficient to stabilize the fracture site because it would act as an axis of rotation. A second pin must be used, inserted through the opposite side of the finger, resulting in an **X**-shaped assembly. Axial compression must be maintained at the fracture site during insertion of the second pin so as to prevent diastasis of the bone fragments. When positioning of the pins is difficult due to fracture instability, it is prudent to insert first an axial, temporary pin. This restores correct alignment. Once the two crossed pins are in place, the assembly is sufficiently secure and the axial pin can be removed. This assembly, called Eiffel Tower, was suggested by Tubiana[71]; it simplifies the surgical procedure and eliminates the risk of malunion (Fig. 14-6).

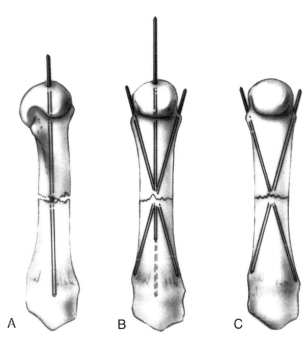

Fig. 14-6. Principle of treatment of a diaphyseal fracture by closed osteosynthesis with a Kirschner pin. **(A)** The Eiffel Tower assembly described by Tubiana starts with reduction and alignment of the skeleton by an axial pin. **(B)** Two oblique pins are inserted through the tubercles of the neck. **(C)** During these maneuvers, it is necessary to maintain compression at the fracture site to preclude diastasis. Finally, the axial pin is removed. (From Merle and Dautel,[50] with permission.)

Osteosynthesis of Metacarpal Bones by Grouped Pins

Kapandji[41] suggested treating nonarticular fractures of the first metacarpal bone with percutaneous pins. A double set of crossed, distal-to-proximal pins inserted through the medial and lateral aspects of the first meta carpal head ensures good stabilization of the fracture without surgical exposure and makes early mobilization possible (Fig. 14-7). The pins are removed under local anesthesia at 6 weeks.

Foucher et al.,[17] reviving the principle of Hacketal[30] and Ender, stabilize fractures of the fifth metacarpal head with grouped pins (Fig. 14-8). Pins are inserted through a cortical opening made on the posterior and medial aspect of the metacarpal bone after displacement of the head is reduced by the well-known Jahss maneuver[36] (Fig. 14-8A and B). This "bouquet" method

(Fig. 14-8C) can also be easily applied to the rare fractures of the second metacarpal head. On the other hand, it is difficult to apply to the third and fourth metacarpal bones given the narrowness of the metacarpal spaces.

Osteosynthesis of Metacarpal Bones by Transverse Pins

In 1973, Lamb et al.[44] published the results obtained with transverse pin osteosynthesis for unstable fractures of metacarpal bones. He thus popularized the little-known technique in 1943 described by Berkmann and Myles.[7] Furlong[25] used this method to immobilize unstable fractures of the neck of the fifth metacarpal bone.

James[37,38] also recommends this technique for treatment of unstable metacarpal fractures. Currently, this method is frequently used in cases of fracture-dislocation of metacarpal bones, and also when it is necessary to maintain the length of a metacarpal bone because of bone defect. (Fig. 14-9). Johnson[39] suggested using a single transverse pin to treat Bennett's fractures. With the same concept in mind, Iselin et al.[35] use two divergent pins for optimal stabilization of the first metacarpal bone and prevention of web space retraction.

Postoperative Care

Early mobilization is recommended after stabilization of the fracture by percutaneous pins. After a few days, as soon as edema has disappeared and the condition of the skin is satisfactory, dynamic splints are used to improve recovery of joint ROM. Depending on the type of fracture, the pins can be removed at any time between the beginning of the fourth week and the end of the sixth week. Most of these methods are not compatible with a return to sports activity without additional protection such as splints and protective shells.

Open Reduction and Minimal Osteosynthesis, Insufficient for Early Mobilization

Complex open lesions of the hand caused by crush trauma are usually observed in motorcyclists; in these cases osteosynthesis with early mobilization cannot be considered, because primary repair of tendons is not feasible and skin coverage can only be obtained at a later time. It is then appropriate to realign the digital

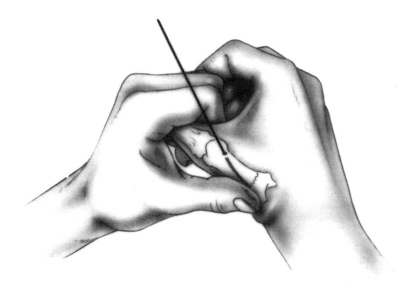

Fig. 14-7. Principle of reduction and stabilization of closed fracture of the proximal part of the first metacarpal bone with percutaneous pins using the method of Kapandji. The first, round-tipped pin is inserted until it reaches the site of fracture. After reduction and compression, it is pushed in until it reaches the base of the first metacarpal bone. The second, lateral pin is inserted using the same technique. (From Merle and Dautel,[50] with permission.)

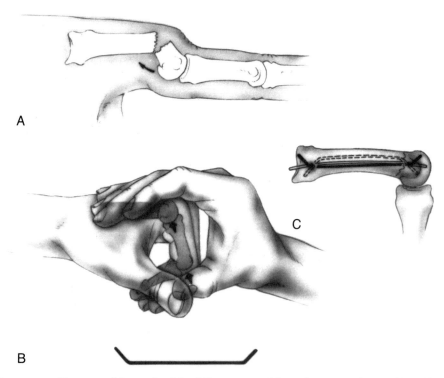

Fig. 14-8. Treatment of fracture of the neck of the fifth metacarpal bone by grouped pins. (**A** & **B**). The fracture is reduced by the maneuver of Jahss. The finger is flexed at 90 degrees and force is applied along the axis of the proximal phalanx. (**C**) Three round-tipped, preshaped pins are inserted through a short corticotomy made at the dorsal and medial aspect of the proximal part of the metacarpal bone. Pushing these pins into the distal fragment in three different planes ensures stabilization of the fracture. (From Merle and Dautel,[50] with permission.)

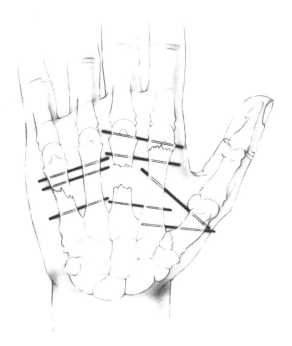

Fig. 14-9. Immobilization of metacarpal bones by transverse pins. Bennett's fracture is treated with diverging pins placed in the first and second metacarpal bones. Bone defect of the third metacarpal bone is perpetuated by transverse pins anchored in the second metacarpal bone. Unstable fractures of the fifth metacarpal bone and fractures of the neck of the second metacarpal bone can be treated using the same technique. (From Merle and Dautel,[50] with permission.)

chains with pins and to place transverse and axial pins as needed depending on the type of fractures and dislocations. In cases of carpometacarpal dislocations, the choice of treatment is similar: it is especially important to restore the correct anatomic configuration of the fourth and fifth carpometacarpal joints, since they are mobile.

Strong Osteosynthesis With Immediate Mobilization

A period of enthusiasm accompanied introduction of AO material. Subsequently, many surgeons complained that the material was too bulky, especially the screws and plates: when they were affixed to the dorsal aspects of metacarpal and phalangeal bones, they tended to damage the extensor tendon system. Heim

and Pfeiffer,[32] who promoted the method, reported in 1974 that operative procedures were sometimes very difficult and that treatment of fractures of phalanges with this material yielded unsatisfactory long-term results. This explains why many surgeons went back to using Kirschner pins inserted with a back-and-forth motion through the fracture site or to using the various procedures described in the chapter on percutaneous osteosynthesis. Lister[46] reports favorable results with a combination of cerclage and pins in fracture treatment, and in replantations and arthrodeses. Cerclage provides the necessary compression, and the pin ensures proper orientation (Fig. 14-10).

We were not satisfied with the results of pin fixation in fractures—nor was Foucher[20]—because the assembly is not sufficiently stable to permit early mobilization. Moreover, pins placed in the vicinity of joints interfere with movements of capsular elements and ligaments; also, the risk of lesion to vascular and neural pedicles is not negligible. Finally, the rate of septic complications, nonunion, and malunion is relatively high (25.3 percent).[18]

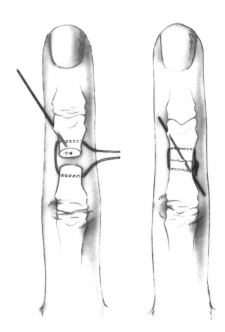

Fig. 14-10. Transverse fractures can be stabilized by a combination of cerclage and an oblique pin. Cerclage, parallel to the site of fracture, precludes rotation and displacement of the bone fragments in the frontal plane, while the pin precludes their displacement in the sagittal plane. (From Merle and Dautel,[50] with permission.)

However, use of Kirschner pins should not be rejected completely; they can be useful in treatment of articular and juxta-articular fractures of proximal and distal interphalangeal joints with a small bone fragment, and also in fractures of the phalanges. In open fractures of the distal phalanx by dorsal section of the distal phalanx, ungual synthesis can be used in place of an axial pin: a needle going through the nail and ungual bed coapts the two bone fragments. A metallic thread placed around the needle provides the needed compression to the assembly.

Biomechanical studies showed that stress applied to the digital chain during movements in extension and flexion remains minimal. Based on these data, the Ostéo Company developed miniaturized apposition material (Fig. 14-11) and equipment for intramedullary osteosynthesis, which is the preferred approach for complex fractures and replantations.

Intramedullary Methods: The Intramedullary Pin and Its Variations

In intramedullary methods, solidity of the assembly is supplied by a triangular, grooved pin that comes in three sizes and by a small amount of cement, which precludes rotation. When use of cement is judged inappropriate, Foucher[20] advocates use of a "locked" pin; the body of this triangular, grooved pin is pierced obliquely at 45 degrees; a 8/10-mm Kirschner pin is inserted into this hole with a back-and-forth motion through the site of fracture.

Bioabsorbable substances of great mechanical strength have recently become available: intramedullary pins made of polylactic acid were developed by Johnson and Johnson Orthopaedic, based on the principle of the locked pin. A 5/10-mm Kirschner pin, also made of bioabsorbable material, ensures stability of

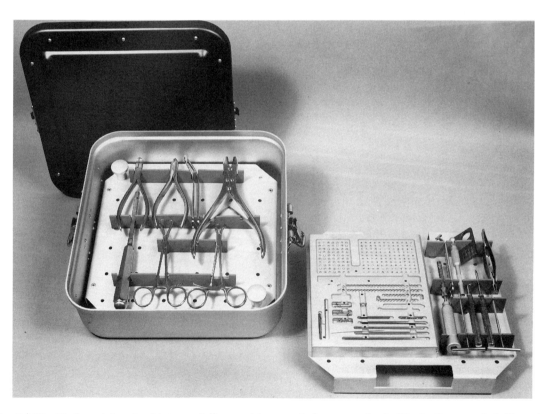

Fig. 14-11. Kit for miniaturized intramedullary and juxtacortical osteosynthesis (Ostéo Company). Self-tapping cortical screws (1.5 mm in diameter), cancellous bone screws (2.2 mm in diameter), and minibolts (1 mm in diameter) are useful to synthesize small fragments. (From Merle and Dautel,[50] with permission.)

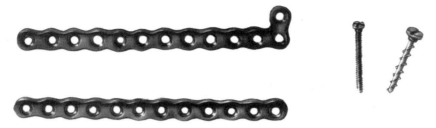

Fig. 14-12. Plain or L-shaped plates can be cut to the desired length and bent to the desired shape; they accommodate both cortical screws (1.5 mm in diameter) and cancellous bone screws (2.2 mm in diameter). (From Merle and Dautel,[50] with permission.)

the osteosynthesis. The material is hydrolyzed within 14 months without causing a foreign body reaction. Bioabsorbable miniscrews will soon become available to complete this equipment.

Use of these techniques remains the exception in sports traumatology; they apply only to cases of comminuted open fractures or to final arthrodeses of the metacarpophalangeal joint of the thumb and of the distal interphalangeal joints.

Juxtacortical Material

Juxtacortical equipment is composed of 0.8-mm-thick plates that can be molded and cut to the desired dimensions (Fig. 14-12). These plates can be affixed to the sides of metacarpal bones and the first two phalanges without hindering tendon movements. They are used mainly in treatment of unstable closed fractures, malunions, and nonunions. These plates can accommodate either self-tapping cortical screws, 1.5 mm in diameter, which can also be used to stabilize oblique or spiral fractures (or small fragments), or self-tapping cancellous screws, 2.2 mm in diameter, which provide very strong anchorage in metacarpal bases and heads. In this last case, it is preferable to use a reverse L-shaped miniature plate, which accomodates two screws, to stabilize proximal or distal fragments. A 1.1-mm drill is used for the 1.5-mm screws.

Miniaturized plates for osteosynthesis ensure satisfactory stability of the fracture site but are not compatible with mobilization or work involving stress. In athletes, it is imperative to protect the repair by attaching the osteosynthesized finger to the adjacent finger. This constitutes the best possible dynamic splint and provides excellent protection for the operated finger. As far as the thumb is concerned, a thermoplastic splint is indispensable.

In cases of unstable articular fracture with a small bone fragment, we use minibolts, 1 mm in diameter, which can be implanted either sideways or transversally (Fig. 14-13). The risk of palmar tilt of a condylar fragment can be prevented by adding a 6/10 minipin.

When the articular bone fragment is too small to accommodate this material, it is preferable to use Jenning's "barbed wire." The barb of the hook keeps the fragment in proper position without piercing it. A prerequisite of this technique is a skin area in good condition; the skin must be able to tolerate the rubber washer and the lead weight that immobilize the bone repair for a period of 3 weeks (Fig. 14-14).

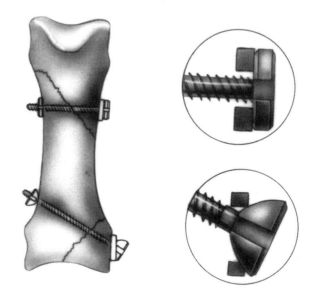

Fig. 14-13. Minibolts (1 mm in diameter) are used to stabilize articular fragments. In obliquely oriented assemblies, hemispherical minibolts are used together with a washer. Flat minibolts are used only in transverse assemblies. (From Merle and Dautel,[50] with permission.)

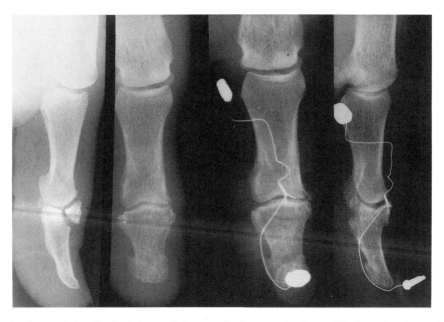

Fig. 14-14. The base of the distal phalanx of the thumb that was broken off is kept in place with Jenning's barbed wire.

External Fixation

In 1974, Crockett[14] suggested using an external prop to immobilize arthrodeses of the fingers. Kirschner pins are held together by acrylic cement. Scott and Mulligan,[61] and later Vilain and his team[58] refined the indications of external fixation in treatment of complex trauma of the hand and in osteoarthritis. In 1973, Allieu[1] adapted the principle of Hoffman's external fixation to the hand, and recommended a "simple frame" assembly combined with frontal transfixing pins. This type of repair is appropriate in cases of complex trauma of the column of the thumb. When external fixation is used on digits, it is advisable to use dorsal oblique pins held together by small coupling bars to preserve joint ROM.

Miniaturized Hoffmann's external fixation makes it possible to obtain osteosyntheses of digits compatible with early mobilization. However, using this type of apparatus can be difficult when the pins must be anchored in small juxta-articular fragments. In such cases, it is necessary to include adjacent bones in the assembly and to bridge intact articulations. This is done only in cases of complex trauma of the column of the thumb.

Surgical Exposure and Technical Problems of Osteosynthesis

Intramedullary and juxtacortical osteosynthesis require mastering the techniques of skin cover in order to protect the fracture site and the implanted material. Surgical exposure (Fig. 14-15) must be planned with great precision in order to minimize skin devascularization and removal of periosteum. In cases of closed diaphyseal fractures of phalanges, we prefer exposure through a seagull-shaped skin incision, which causes little damage, preserves gliding space of tendons, and allows early mobilization since no pain exists. Diaphyseal fractures of metacarpal bones are usually exposed by longitudinal incisions oriented along intermetacarpal spaces.

At the level of metacarpophalangeal joints, we advise using an S-shaped skin incision oriented along the intermetacarpal depression and extended as far as the medial or lateral dorsal aspect of the phalanx. In cases of articular fracture, we advise an S-shaped dorsal skin incision to expose the proximal interphalangeal joint. This provides excellent access to the articulation and facilitates reduction and placement of minibolts, miniscrews, and pins.

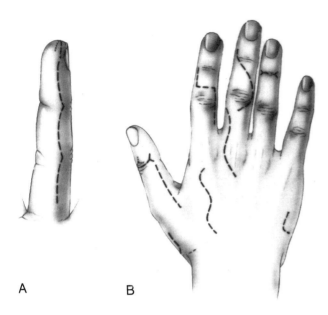

A   B

Fig. 14-15. (A) Seagull-shaped incision to expose diaphyseal fractures of the phalanges. **(B)** Z-shaped or S-shaped incisions to expose the dorsal aspect of the digital chains. Transverse incision to expose the interphalangeal joint of the thumb. A Gedda-Möberg incision to expose the base of the thumb, and J-shaped incision to expose the base of the fifth metacarpal bone. (From Merle and Dautel,[50] with permission.)

Some proximal fractures of the distal phalanx can be osteosynthesized with a 22-mm-long, flat-head, axial cancellous-bone screw. Appropriate exposure for this procedure is obtained by a "shark's jaw" incision at the junction of nail bed and finger pulp. Articular fractures of the interphalangeal joint of the thumb can be exposed through a transverse incision along the dorsal interphalangeal crease, extended on each side by a V/Y-shaped incision in order to expose the medial and lateral aspects. Finally, direct exposure of Bennett's fractures with a large fragment is achieved by a J-shaped incision on the medial or lateral dorsal aspect of the first metacarpal bone and extended transversally toward the palmar aspect of the trapeziometacarpal joint, as suggested by Gedda and Möberg.[26,54]

The goal of these methods of osteosynthesis is early mobilization. Mobilization should be done under the direct supervision of rehabilitation specialists familiar with hand pathology and with the principle of "all at once" treatment. Close monitoring of edema and skin condition, as well as detection of associated lesions, makes it possible to modulate active and passive rehabilitation. Once edema has subsided, it becomes possible to use dynamic splints with pressure points localized at sufficient distance from the site of fracture. Whenever a significant risk of secondary displacement exists, athletes should refrain from sports practice for 3 weeks (i.e., the period during which hardening of the ossification site takes place). After 6 weeks, most fractures have healed, and the era can be submitted to the full stress of sports activity.

INDICATIONS FOR TREATMENT

The choice of treatment to stabilize the fracture of an athlete is very difficult, one must take into consideration the kind of sport involved and the need for early return to activity before bone healing, the risk of dismantling the repair must be assessed, and in the event of a mishap, a secondary treatment that could salvage the patient's condition must be foreseen. Whenever possible, orthopaedic treatment is preferable. Osteosynthesis should be used only in cases of unstable articular or juxta-articular fractures; it must be kept in mind that miniaturized material for osteosynthesis is not strong enough to withstand the stresses inflicted during sports activity and must be reinforced by addition of a splint. It must be emphasized that indications can only be outlined and that in the specific field of sports trauma no absolute rules exist.

Functional Orthopaedic Treatment

The best treatment for stable fractures is the functional orthopaedic approach. Results are consistently satisfactory when the patient can be closely observed so as to detect any secondary displacement that could occur during the first 3 weeks. Whenever possible, placing the fingers in syndactyly speeds up functional recovery, because the adjacent finger is the best possible dynamic splint.

Bonvallet's ball has the advantage of reshaping the transverse and longitudinal arches of the hand and fingers; it also maintains convergence of long digits toward the tubercle of the scaphoid bone.

The functional method suggested by Thomine[69] in the treatment of fractures of the proximal phalanx is logical but requires close observation of the lesion. In his series of 14 fractures, the author did not observe any malunion with rotational displacement but did note three cases of bone shortening, one ulnar deviation, three recurvations, and one flexion deformity.

Percutaneous Pins

In cases of extremely unstable closed fractures, it is appropriate to obtain stabilization after reduction by percutaneous pins. The goal of this type of osteosynthesis is to preclude secondary displacement, which always has an adverse consequence on function; also this method aims to obtain mobilization as early as possible. Therefore strict immobilization is rarely indicated, since it frequently results in stiffness.

In a review of 415 fractures of phalanges, Strickland et al.[64,65] observe that 75 to 80 percent of total active motion was recovered when immobilization was not longer than 4 weeks; when immobilization lasted longer, functional recovery was only 66 percent because of stiffness of metacarpophalangeal and proximal and distal interphalangeal joints.

Open Osteosynthesis

Open osteosynthesis is used mainly in cases of open fractures that are very unstable or cannot be properly reduced, and in cases of articular and juxta-articular fractures. It is also justifiable in cases of closed diaphyseal fractures that cannot be properly reduced and immobilized by orthopaedic treatment (Fig. 14-16).

Comminuted Fractures

Comminuted fractures are usually osteosynthetized by intramedullary pins. Repair must be strong in order to preserve joint motion and preclude tendon adhesion at the fracture site. In these crush fractures, in which numerous associated lesions are seen, the material of osteosynthesis should be embedded whenever cutaneous cover can be obtained.

Screws for Unstable, Very Oblique, or Spiral Fractures

We do not use pins in open fractures because such repairs are often difficult to do and are insufficiently strong. Quite frequently, reduction is improper, and pins interfere with juxta-articular structures, hamper tendon gliding, and damage vascular and neural pedi-

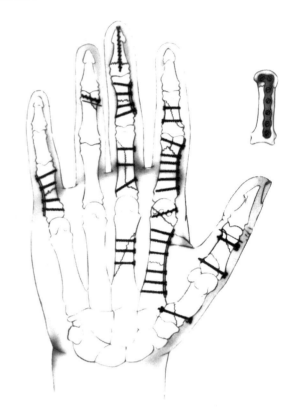

Fig. 14-16. Indications for use of juxtacortical material. Articular fragments of the column of the thumb are stabilized by minibolts. Unstable metacarpal and phalangeal fractures of the second ray are treated with a lateral or medial plate. An **L**-shaped plate is useful in the treatment of bicondylar fractures. Long oblique fractures can be treated with three cortical screws. (From Merle and Dautel,[50] with permission.)

cles. Foucher and Merle[18] reported their experience with 664 open fractures of the digits. It is difficult to establish precise comparisons among methods because osteosyntheses by cemented intramedullary pin, locked pin, or Kirschner pins were not applied to the same types of lesions. Nonetheless, their results indicate complications in:

12.2 percent of cemented osteosyntheses
15.6 percent of locked pins
25.3 percent of Kirschner pins

These rates include acute and chronic infection, nonunion, malunion, and amputations. In 310 osteosyntheses of metacarpal bones, Frère et al.[23] noted complications in only 6.5 percent of the cases. ROMs were

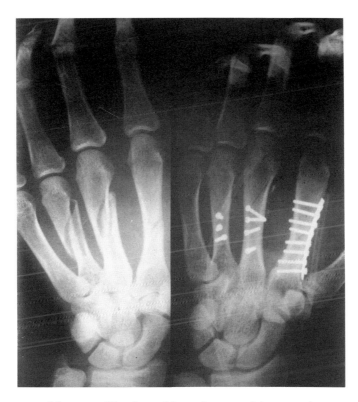

Fig. 14-17. Triple metacarpal fractures. The short oblique fracture of the second metacarpal bone is stabilized with a lateral plate. The other two long oblique fractures are osteosynthesized with cortical bone screws (1 mm in diameter). (From Merle and Dautel,[50] with permission.)

normal in 97 percent. These findings indicate that pins have a high rate of complications. When a fracture must be osteosynthesized, it is preferable to apply a rigorous method that ensures anatomic restoration and strength.

Actually, satisfactory restoration of anatomic bone configuration does not necessarily suffice to obtain a useful functional result, especially when tendon lesions are associated. Strickland et al.[65] have shown that the percentage of total active motion was 52 percent when a comminuted fracture was associated with tendon lesions, whereas it was 68% in similar fractures with no associated tendon lesions. In a series of 49 fractures of the proximal phalanx, we noted 80 percent excellent results when the fractures were not associated with lesions of other elements, whereas only 35 percent of the results were rated excellent when lesions of the extensor tendon system were associated. However, the unsatisfactory results of these fractures at Cauchoix and Dupard stages II and III can be corrected subsequently by osteosynthesis.

In most cases, restoration of normal anatomic configuration of the hand skeleton ensures that a tenolysis or a tenoarthrolysis performed a few months later will have a satisfactory result; this cannot be obtained after orthopaedic treatment.

Articular and Juxta-Articular Fractures

In most cases, articular and juxta-articular fractures require osteosynthesis because the fragments are displaced and often reduction cannot be obtained orthopaedically. It is essential to restore perfect anatomy of articular surfaces in order to recover function and prevent arthritis which would cause pain and reduce ROM (Figs. 14-18, 14-19).

The osteosynthesis must be performed with great care, using minibolts or miniscrews; disinsertion of capsular and ligamentous elements must be kept to a strict minimum in order to limit risk of necrosis of bone fragments.

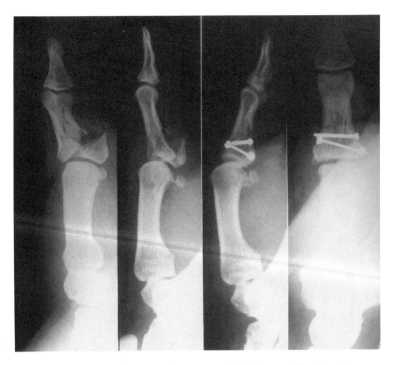

Fig. 14-18. Articular multifragmented fracture of the proximal phalanx of the thumb, osteosynthesized with a minibolt and a cortical bone screw. (From Merle and Dautel,[50] with permission.)

Slight imperfections in the alignment of metacarpophalangeal joints are tolerable; by contrast, even minor imperfections are unacceptable at the proximal interphalangeal joints. In a series of 38 cases of fractures of the proximal interphalangeal joints, we noted that results were rated excellent or satisfactory in 76.47 percent of cases in which anatomic reduction was perfect, whereas only 22.23 percent reached this level when reduction was imperfect.

Fractures of one condyle have a satisfactory outcome, whereas fractures of both condyles always result in articular stiffness. This is due to the difficulty of this type of osteosynthesis and to the high proportion of condylar necrosis. Impacted fractures are usually best treated by orthopaedic methods. However, anatomic reduction of the articular surfaces is impossible due to the causal mechanism; even when the fibrocartilage functions well over an extended period of time, secondary arthritis with pain and reduced ROM is frequently observed. We disagree with the optimistic opinion expressed by Trojan,[70] who reported excellent results after this type of impacted fracture.

Fractures of the Thumb

In athletes, lesions bear on the metacarpophalangeal joint and on the first metacarpal bone. Avulsion of a bone fragment attached to the medial ligament must be treated by fixation with barbed wire, pin, or cerclage. Bennett's fractures are more severe. If only one voluminous fragment exists, fixation is obtained with a minibolt or miniscrew. On the other hand, when the single fragment is small or when several are present, we advise using pins according to the technique of Iselin[35] or Wiggins.

Nonarticular fractures of the first metacarpal bone can be treated orthopaedically in most cases. Even when reduction is not anatomically perfect, the normal ROM of the trapeziometacarpal joint can compensate for some angular or rotational imperfection.

However, nonarticular fractures of the base of the first metacarpal bone can be treated by distal-to-proximal pin according to the technique of Kapandji.[41] In previous work, we indicated that external fixation is the only treatment appropriate for the complex open

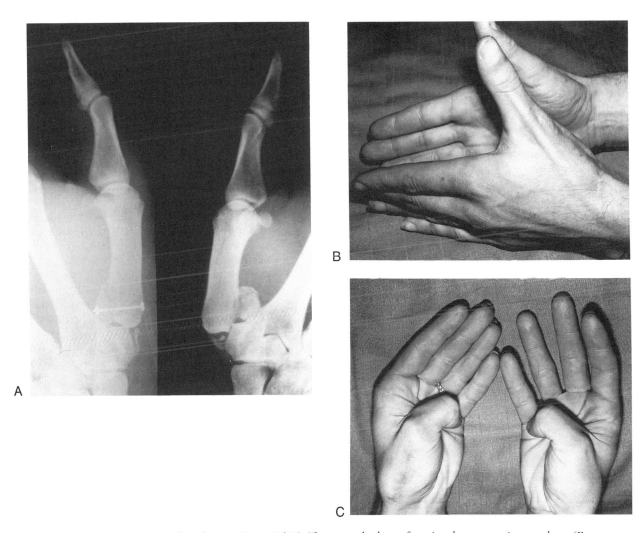

Fig. 14-19. (A–C): Same hand as in Figure 14-18. Three weeks later, functional recovery is complete. (From Merle and Dautel,[50] with permission.)

lesions of the column of the thumb that are sometimes seen in motorcycle accidents.

CONCLUSIONS

Appropriate treatment of sports-related fractures of metacarpal and phalangeal bones implies that the athlete understand fully what the surgeon aims to achieve. The athlete should be aware that the requirements of competition must be set aside for a while and that a constraining orthopaedic treatment must be applied in most cases. It is often necessary to protect the frac-

ture site for 3 weeks, the period of time needed for the repair to harden. Returning too early to sports activity will result in secondary displacements, which may have adverse consequences on function and necessitate additional procedures that may prove especially difficult. In general, the preferred treatment for athletes is orthopaedic; however, articular, juxta-articular, long oblique, and spiral fractures should be osteosynthesized. Even though miniaturized osteosynthesis material is compatible with early mobilization, it cannot ensure an immediate return to sports activity without the additional protection of the fracture site given by a splint.

REFERENCES

1. Allieu Y: L'utilisation du tuteur externe en chirurgie de la main. Acta Orthop Belg 39:98–1001, 1973
2. Amadio PC: Epidemiology of hand and wrist injuries in sports. Hand Clin 6:379–381, 1990
3. Amend P, Dap F, Girot J et al: L'ostéosynthèse des fractures articulaires des doigts longs. Réunion de Printemps du GEM, Marseille, 1986.
4. Barton NJ: Fractures of the phalange of the hand. Hand 9:1–10, 1977
5. Barton NJ: Fractures of the shafts of the phalanges of the hand. Hand 11:119–133, 1979
6. Barton NJ: Fracture of the Hand and Wrist. Churchill Livingstone, Edinburgh, 1988
7. Berkmann EF, Myles GJ: Internal fixation of metacarpal fractures exclusive of the thumb. J Bone Joint Surg 25:816–821, 1943
8. Blalock HS, Pearce H, Kleinert H et al: An instrument designed to help reduce and percutaneously pin fractured phalanges. J Bone Joint Surg 57A:792–796, 1975
9. Bonvallet JM: Immobilisation des fractures digitales sur boule plâtrée. In: Traumatismes Ostéoarticulaires de la Main. Monographie du GEM. Expansion Scientifique Française, Paris, 1971
10. Brewerton DA: A tangential radiographic projection for demonstrating involvement of metacarpal heads in rhumatoid arthritis. Br J Radiol 40:233, 1967
11. Castaing J, Lapierre F: Anatomie pathologique et étude des résultats des fractures des métacarpiens et des phalanges. Ann Orthop Ouest 4:61–64, 1972
12. Clifford RH: Intramedullary wire fixation of hand fractures. Plast Reconstr Surg 11:366–371, 1953
13. Constantinesco A, Foucher G, Merle M et al: Système non traumatique de mesure du comportement élastique des tendons. Application à la chirurgie réparatrice des traumatismes de la main. J Techn Biomed 1977
14. Crockett DJ: Rigid fixation of bones of the hand using K-wires bonded with acrylic resin. Hand 6:106–107, 1974
15. de la Caffinière JY, Mansat M: Raideur post-traumatique des doigts longs. Rev Chir Orthop 67:515–571, 1981
16. Evrard H, Nokerman B: L'enclouage centro-médullaire dans les fractures des métacarpiens. Acta Orthop Belg 39:1035–1044, 1973
17. Foucher G: L'ostéosynthèse des fractures des phalanges et des métacarpiens. p. 213. In: Cahiers d'Enseignement de la S.O.F.C.O.T. Expansion Scientifique Française, Paris, 1988
18. Foucher G, Merle M: Complications des fractures ouvertes des doigts. Comparaison des méthodes de traitement. A propos de 664 cas. Réunion de Printemps du GEM, Marseille, 1986
19. Foucher G, Chemorin C, Sibilly A: Nouveau procédé d'ostéosynthèse original dans les fractures du tiers distal du cinquième métacarpien. Nouv Presse Med 5:1139–1140, 1976
20. Foucher G, Merle M, Michon J: Intérêt de l'ostéosynthèse dans la stabilisation des fractures du squelette métacarpophalangien. Ann Chir 31:1065–1069, 1977
21. Foucher G, Merle M, Michon J: Ostéosynthèse miniaturisée en chirurgie de la main. p. 407. In Tubiana R (ed): Traité de Chirurgie de la Main. Vol. 2. Masson, Paris, 1984
22. Foucher G, Merle M, Van Genechten F, Denuit P: La synthèse unguéale. Ann Chir Main 3:168–169, 1984
23. Frère G, Hoel G, Moutet F, Ravet D: Les fractures du col du cinquième métacarpien. An Chir Main 1:221–226, 1982
24. Frère G, Massart P, Hoel G: Trois cent dix ostéosynthèses de métacarpiens. Ann Chir 35:771–777, 1981
25. Furlong R: Injuries of the Hand. JA Churchill, 1957
26. Gedda KO, Möberg E: Open reduction and osteosynthesis of the so-called Bennett's fracture in the carpometacarpal joint of the thumb. Acta Orthop Scand 22:249–257, 1953
27. Goudot B, Voche P, Bour C, Merle M: Ostéosynthèse par mini plaque en "L" des fractures métaphysaires et métaphysoépiphysaires des métacarpiens et des phalanges. Rev Chir Orthop 77:130–134, 1991
28. Green DP, Anderson JM: Closed reduction and percutaneous pin fixation of fractured phalanges. J Bone Joint Surg [Am] 55A:1651–1654, 1973
29. Grundberg AB: Intramedullary fixation for fractures of the hand. J Hand Surg 6:568–573, 1981
30. Hackethal K: Die Bundelnegelung. Springer-Verlag, Berlin, 1961
31. Hankin FM, Peel SM: Sport related fracture and dislocation in the hand. Hand Clin 6:429–453, 1990
32. Heim U, Pfeiffer KM: Small Fragment Set Manual: Technique Recommended by the A.S.I.F. Group. Springer-Verlag, New York, 1974
33. Ikuta Y, Tsuge K: Micro-bolts and micro-screws for fixation of small bones in the hand. Hand 6:261–265, 1974
34. Irigaray A: New fixing screw for completely amputated finger. J Hand Surg 5:381, 1980
35. Iselin M, Blangueron S, Benoit D: Fracture de la base du premier métacarpien. Mem Acad Chir 82:771–774, 1956
36. Jahss SA: Fractures of the metacarpals. A new method of reduction and immobilisation. J Bone Joint Surg [Am] 20A:178–186, 1938
37. James JIP: Fracture of the proximal and middle phalanges of the fingers. Acta Orthop Scand 32:401–402, 1962
38. James JIP: Fractures of the phalanges and metacarpals. Proc Br Soc Surg Hand 379–381, 1966
39. Johnson EC: Fractures of the base of the thumb: a new method of fixation. JAMA 126:27, 1944

40. Joshi BB: Percutaneous internal fixation of fractures of the proximal phalanges. Hand 8:86–92, 1976

41. Kapandji IA: Ostéosynthèse à foyer fermé des fractures proximales non articulaires du premier métcarpien: double brochage croisé ascendant. Ann Chir Main 2:179–185, 1983

42. Kaye JJ, Lister GD: An other use for the Brewerton view. J Hand Surg 3:603, 1978

43. Kilbourne BC, Paul EG: The use of small bone screws in the treatment of metacarpal metatarsal and phalangeal fractures. J Bone Joint Surg [Am] 40A:375–383, 1958

44. Lamb DW, Abernethy PA, Raine PAM: Unstable fractures of the metacarpals: a method of treatment by transverse wire fixation to intact metacarpals. Hand 5:43–48, 1973

45. Lane CS: Detecting occult fractures of the metacarpal head: the Brewerton view. J Hand Surg 2:131–133, 1977

46. Lister G: Intraosseous wiring of the digital skeleton. J Hand Surg 3:427–435, 1978

47. Mannerfelt L, Malmste M: Arthrodesis of the wrist in rheumatoid arthritis. A technique without external fixation. Scand J Plast Reconstr Surg 5:124–130, 1971

48. Marin-Braun F, Vaienti L, Dap F et al: Les ostéosynthèses de la colonne du pouce. A propos d'une série de 228 cas. Réunion de Printemps du GEM, Marseille, 1986

49. Merle M, Foucher G: Internal fixation for complex hand injuries. Tech Orthop 2:14–17, 1986

50. Merle M, Dautel G: La Main Traumatique. Masson, Paris, 1992

51. Merle M, Foucher G, Mole D, Michon J: Résultats fonctionnels des fractures ostéosynthésées de la première phalange des doigts longs. Ann Chir 35:765–770, 1981

52. Merle M, Foucher G, Isselin J et al: La stabilisation en urgence des traumatismes complexes ouverts du poignet. Ann Chir 35:275–280, 1981

53. Michon J, Merle M, Foucher G: Traumatismes complexes de la main, traitement tout en un temps avec mobilisation précoce. Chirurgie 103:956–964, 1977

54. Moberg E: Dringliche Handchirurgie. Georg Thieme Verlag, Stuttgart, 1972

55. Nemethi CE: Phalangeal fractures treated by open reduction and Kirschner wire fixation. Ind Med Surg 23:148–150, 1954

56. Pratt DR: Internal splint for closed and open treatment of injuries of the extensor tendon at the distal joint of the finger. J Bone Joint Surg [Am] 34A:785–788, 1952

57. Rettig AC, Ryan R, Stone JA: Epidemiology of hand injuries in sports. p. 37. In Strickland JW, Rettig AC (eds): Hand Injuries in Athletes. WB Saunders, Philadelphia, 1992

58. Richard JC, Latouche X, Lemerle JP et al: La place du fixateur externe dans le traitement en urgence des traumatismes graves ouverts de la main. Ann Chir 34:679–701, 1980

59. Robertson RC, Cawley JJ, Faris AM: Treatment of fracture dislocation of the interphalangeal joint of the hand. J Bone Joint Surg [Am] 28A:68–70, 1946

60. Robins RHC: Injuries and Infections of the Hand. Edward Arnold, London, 1961

61. Scott MM, Mullingan PJ: Stabilising severe phalangeal fractures. Hand 12:44–49, 1980

62. Simonetta C: The use of AO plates in the hand. Hand 2:43–45, 1970

63. Steel WM: The AO small fragment set in hand fractures. Hand 10:246–253, 1978

64. Strickland JW, Rettig AC: Hand injuries in athletes. WB Saunders, Philadelphia, 1992

65. Strickland JW, Steichen JB, Kleinmann WB, Flynn N: Factors influencing digital performance after phalangeal fracture. p. 126. In: Difficult Problems in Hand Surgery. Vol. 15. CV Mosby, St Louis, 1982

66. Tamai S: Digital replantation: analysis of 163 replantations in an 11 year-period. Clin Past Surg 5:195–209, 1978

67. Thevenin R, Iselin F, Pradet G. Ostéosynthèse des phalanges par vis souples centro-médullaires. Nouv Presse Med 1:2771–2774, 1972

68. Thomine JM: Fractures récentes des phalanges des métacarpiens et leur traitement. p. 609. In Tubiana R (ed): Traité de Chirurgie de la Main. Vol. 2. Masson, Paris, 1984

69. Thomine JM, Gibon Y, Bendjeddou MS, Biga N: L'appareillage fonctionnel dans le traitement des fractures diaphysaires des phalanges proximales des quatre derniers doigts. Ann Chir Main 2:298–306, 1983

70. Trojan E: Fracture dislocation of the bases of the proximal and middle phalanges of the fingers. Hand 4:60–61, 1972

71. Tubiana R: A propos du traitement chirurgical des fractures des métacarpiens et des phalanges. Ann Chir 35:757–758, 1981

72. Tubiana R: La mobilisation précoce des fractures des métacarpiens et des phalanges. Ann Chir Main 2:293–297, 1983

73. Von Saal FH: Intramedullary fixation in fractures of the hand and fingers. J Bone Joint Surg [Am] 35A:5–16, 1953

74. Weeks PM, Wray RC: Management of Acute Hand Injuries: A Biological Approach. 2nd Ed. CV Mosby, St Louis, 1973

75. Wright TA: Early mobilization in fractures of the metacarpals and phalanges. Can J Surg 11:491–498, 1968

15

Soft Tissue Injuries and Tendinitis

G. FOUCHER

INTRODUCTION

As an avocational activity, sport has grown considerably in the last few years. Simultaneously and consequently, professional sport has also attracted more people, increasing the level of performance, concurrence, and money involved. It is surprising to note that an activity supposed to promote health is responsible for so many injuries. Prevalence of injury, according to the few data available, is around 50 percent, which means that one in every two athletes will suffer some type of injury. It is logical that the hand would be especially exposed when it is used to grasp or hit balls or opponents. Some traumas are common in all sports and others are specific to activities like water skiing or rodeo (soft tissue avulsion) or trap shooting (gun shot lesion). This discussion separates the more frequent injuries into those secondary to a single trauma and those resulting from multiple and repetitive trauma, generally termed *overuse lesions*. Better knowledge on the part of coaches, physicians, and surgeons is the only way to avoid delay in presentation, and over- or undertreatment (with a possible career disaster), as well as to promote prevention through special training and protection by garments, padding, or taping.

ACUTE SOFT TISSUE INJURIES

Tendons and ligaments are the soft tissues most commonly injured.

Extensor Tendon Lesions

Rupture or attrition of the extensor tendon at the distal interphalangeal (DIP) level is frequent, not only in baseball (baseball finger) but in all ball activities. The "drop" of the distal phalanx is variable. A radiograph is necessary to rule out the infrequent chip avulsion, which has the same treatment and prognosis; an articular fracture and a proximal interphalangeal (PIP) lesion resembling chip avulsion are seen in the classic jammed finger.

Splinting remains the best treatment, and we favor a dorsal, custom-made splint (Elliott type), which frees the pulp; the Stack's splint is most frequently used, however. For recent injuries 6 weeks is enough, while cases of delayed presentation (even of 1 month) require 8 weeks followed by night splinting for a few more weeks. It is not a "simple" treatment, and any flexion during cleansing or extension loss in the splint is followed by a residual extension lack. In lax athletes, a swan neck deformity can occur, which is not only unattractive but exposes the PIP to further injury. Surgery is not generally necessary, but, for example, a Fowler tenotomy of the medial band is an acceptable alternative in a supple swan neck to a permanent check-rein taping.

Frequently seen in combat sports, injury of the medial band at the PIP level is more serious and initially more hidden. Any painful PIP enlargement suggests this lesion. If left undiagnosed or untreated, it will proceed to a full-blown boutonnière deformity, the head of the first phalanx engaging in the extensor slit with PIP flexion and the lateral band migrating volar to the axis of the joint, producing DIP hyperextension; while the deformity is reducible at the beginning, ultimately it becomes fixed, rendering treatment difficult and unpredictable. Different diagnostic tests have been described: lack of the last 15 or 20 degrees of extension at the PIP level, lack of strength when extension is opposed, or lack of passive flexion at the DIP level (in PIP extension). A radiograph may show a chip avulsion, thus ruling out any other fracture. At the initial stage, an orthosis that fixes the PIP joint in extension and leaves the DIP joint free is the best treatment. After 4 weeks, a "dynamic" splint of the Capener type is worn constantly for an additional 3 weeks, followed by night splinting if necessary. Depending on the rules of the sport, activity can be authorized using the "tube." Treatment of a neglected boutonnière is outside the scope of this chapter, but it is sufficient to say that such treatment is long and frequently unpredictable.

Rupture of an extensor tendon occurs infrequently after an episode of tendinitis, usually of the extensor pollicis longus.

Rupture at the extensor hood level is more frequent. Two types have been described: noncontact rupture, involving a total or partial tear of the sagittal band, usually the radial one; or contact extensor split injury. The exact mechanism of the former is not fully understood; it occurs in power grip or in forced flexion of the metacarpophalangeal (MP) joint while the wrist is in flexion and ulnar deviation.[5] The radial sagittal band of the middle finger is most commonly affected,[25] with luxation of the extensor tendon (difficult to see initially due to edema). Active extension of the MP joint is lost, but passive extension is possible and is actively maintained by the patient. When this injury is seen immediately, 3 weeks of immobilization with full extension of the MP joint (PIP being free) is sufficient. When neglected, the injury requires surgical repair, usually by a strip of extensor or a junctura tendinum. Partial tears are rarely seen initially but can cause long-standing pain with some limitation of function at the MP joint. Koniuch et al.[27] have demonstrated the necessity of surgical repair. The second type is more frequent in our experience, mainly because we take care of a boxing team. With insufficient protection, longitudinal rupture of the MP capsule can occur. Presentation is a local painful swelling with a sensation of depression in the center. It must be differentiated from bursitis, which is quite frequently chronic at the third ray level. Posner et al.[50] recently stressed the surgical indications. Our experience is less aggressive, and we have seen cases secondarily with very moderate trouble. In case of persistent pain, surgery is indicated, with repair and 4 weeks of immobilization. Return to punching is not advised before 3 to 5 months (advice rarely accepted).

Flexor Tendon Lesions

Rutpure of the pulley in climbing calls for protection, using external support; the appropriate treatment has been debated. Even seen early, orthopaedic treatment seems insufficient, and surgical repair is preferable.

The most frequent lesion is the "jersey finger": distal flexor tendon avulsion occurs when a player grasps the opponent by the clothes in rugby and in American football. Many authors have attempted to determine why the ring finger is usually involved. Lack of independence (flexor, lumbrical, and extensor), weaker distal insertion, and prominence during grip have all been implicated.[7,33,40]

Among the three types described type II is more frequent: retraction of the distal extremity around the PIP leaves the long vinculum intact.[33] The two other types are less frequent: palmar retraction (type I), or limited retraction due to a bony fragment (type III). Clinically, the lack of DIP flexion, the pain along the finger (or in the palm), and the weakness do not constitute a major disability, which explains the frequent delay in presentation. When these injuries are seen in the acute stage, agreement is general that reinsertion provides satisfactory results; later treatment is a matter of debate. Some patients need no treatment, and others, who have palmar pain and weakness, can benefit from distal arthrodesis; we favor proximal resection associated with side anastomosis of the two flexor tendons. Loss of independence is balanced by improvement in strength. Finally, because of the long treatment period and possible loss of PIP flexion, the most controversial solution remains grafting of the profundus through the intact superficialis. However, Curtis has demonstrated that excellent results can be obtained.[41]

Ligament Injury of the Fingers

Ligament injuries are frequently associated with bone avulsion or more complex fracture-luxations. A frequent problem is immediate so-called reduction by a friend or a coach on the playing field. This cannot be advised, since it often makes assessment difficult later on. A radiograph ray before (and after) manipulation is strongly advised to complete the clinical assessment and to rule out associated bone lesions. Some lesions, such as the DIP are extremely rare; volar plate lesions described by Bowers.[3] Others, such as carpometacarpal luxations of the first and fifth ray, are treated like fractures. We focus here on the lesions more frequently found at the PIP and MP levels.

Proximal Interphalangeal Joint

The PIP joint is exposed to trauma in either extension, flexion, or lateral stress. Disruption of ligaments with or without joint dislocation is frequent in all sport activities; a preponderance is seen in combat and ball sports.

Flexion Injury

Volar PIP joint luxation is accompanied by avulsion of the central slip of the extensor; after reduction, immobilization in extension is required for 4 weeks followed by dynamic splinting and protection during activity for an additional month.

Extension Injury

For chip avulsion injuries of the volar plate, a figure-of-eight splint is worn for 3 weeks, followed by protection during any sport activity. Dorsal luxation occurs more frequently, can be opened anteriorly, and is accompanied by volar plate avulsion or rupture. Distal avulsion is more common than proximal or rupture through the substance. Reduction must be gentle, avoiding strong traction and soft tissue interposition, stability through the range of motion is assessed. Immobilization is controversial, and stiffness rather than instability has been observed. We favor immobilization in 15 degrees of flexion for 1 week followed by extension restriction using a figure-of-eight splint, leaving the flexion arc free for an additional 3 weeks. Protection by buddy taping is advised for 2 months. A lack of full extension with local swelling and cold intolerance is commonly observed after such an injury. Night splinting is useful in extension. Even though recurrent dorsal dislocation is extremely rare,[46] two complications should be mentioned[42–44]: the "pseudoboutonnière deformity with marked PIP flexion deformity can be accompanied radiologically by calcification of the proximal check-rein ligaments. Swan neck deformity can also develop and in our experience is more frequent in rupture through the substance of the volar plate; this rupture does not heal due to circulation of synovial fluid, and we have observed that very late repair, even years later, can be performed.

Lateral Stress Injury

Complete collateral ligament ruptures has been controversial. Our experience using both surgery and conservative treatment has led us to favor the latter. Collateral ligament injuries have been studied biomechanically by Kliefhaber et al.[26] and Schernberg[53] and clinically graded into four stages, ranging from tenderness to instability, by Green and Rowland.[18] For partial lesions of the collateral ligament, buddy taping for 1 month is sufficient for continuous use in sport activity (2 months). For total rupture, 1 week of immobilization is followed by a laterally reinforced figure-of-eight splint in 20 degrees of flexion for 3 weeks and buddy taping for an additional 4 weeks. Prevention by the same type of buddy taping or special gloves is recommended in some sports such as football (linemen), hockey, or judo.

Metacarpophalangeal Joint

The thumb is the most frequent ray involved. Special anatomic considerations explain the frequent indication for surgery. In dorsal luxation, traction can interpose the sesamoid bones, requiring surgical intervention; gentle reduction without traction avoids this pitfall. In collateral ligament ruptures, which are exceedingly frequent in skiing but also in other activities like hockey, football, or boxing (and in still other activities using a stick or racquet), several points need to be emphasized. Radiographs must be performed before any stress, to avoid displacing an otherwise undisplaced bone fragment. Second, clinical assessment must be thorough, because combined lesions are frequent (dorsal and lateral lesions or lateral and palmar ruptures). For assessment of the ulnar collateral ligament, we have been pleased with the Lundborg sign, which consists of palpating the Stener lesion instead of performing a stress view. In a series of 20 cases, he demonstrated that migration of the collateral ligament over the expansion of the adductor pollicis can be predicted.[1] In such cases an operation is mandatory within the first week; we use a pullout of Jenning's barbed wire for bone reinsertion without transfixion of the MP by a K-wire. Three weeks of immobilization in a thumb spica is followed by protection for an additional month during any sport activity.

Other MPJ joints are less vulnerable, but border digits can be involved with collateral ligament rupture. Conservative treatment with immobilization in slight flexion is needed for 4 weeks followed by buddy taping. Finally, a rare lesion mentioned in the literature is the attenuation or rupture of the deep transverse metacarpal ligament, which can occur while punching a ball or an opponent. Volar subluxation of the ray is associated with swelling and abnormal mobility in anteroposterior translation. Cast immobilization is recommended by the authors for 4 to 6 weeks with the joint at 80 degrees of flexion. Dislocations are less frequent than at the PIP level but are more commonly associated with soft tissue interposition, which calls for surgical exposure. Volar plate interposition in the vicinity of the neurovascular bundle has been extensively described in the literature opposing the dorsal and volar approach. Protective splinting should be used for 4 weeks followed by protection.

Neurovascular Injuries

Neurovascular injuries are quite rare but need a brief mention. Any type of nerve compression can occur after a discrete trauma, but chronic entrapment is more frequent, without special presenting signs. Some injuries are typical to special sports like cycling (Guyon's ulnar nerve compression, known as *handlebar palsy* among cyclists). Smail demonstrated from his own clinical experience that one-third of the body weight is borne by the bar. We noted the same finding in two top-level motorcyclists involved in the Paris-Dakar race. One of them did not recover spontaneously, and an electromyogram (EMG) performed 6 months later demonstrated denervation. Neurolysis was performed with excellent results; the patient returned 1 year later because of a recurrence after the same race! Fortunately spontaneous recovery finally occurred. Padded gloves and bars are helpful.

In bowler's thumb, external pressure leads to fibrosis around the ulnar digital thumb collateral nerve. Protection and prevention are efficacious, and neurolysis is rarely necessary. Vascular trauma is more frequently repetitive than isolated.[31]

OVERUSE INJURIES OF THE HAND AND WRIST

In contrast to injuries resulting from a single macrotrauma (the force exceeding the failure threshold of a given tissue), overuse injuries result from repetitive microtrauma. According to Herring and Nilson,[21] 30 to 50 percent of all sport-related injuries are due to overuse. Each tissue can be affected, tendinitis being the major overuse injury of the tendon; other common injuries include bursitis, stress fracture, chondromalacia, apophysitis, muscle soreness and compartment syndrome, fasciitis and nerve friction-compression.[58] Risk factors can be related to training errors (technical mistakes, abrupt changes in intensity, duration or frequency, defective equipment) or to the athlete (musculoskeletal imbalance, anatomic malalignment, associated disease). Among these overuse injuries, tendinitis has a definite prevalence. The name of the condition has been disputed, for neither the tendon itself nor the compressive compartment present any inflammatory signs (Ippolito).[23a] Any tendon in the hand can be involved, but some locations are more frequent, and it seems that small-diameter tendons with an angulated track are more prone to the disease. However, in our experience, trigger finger and De Quervain's disease, for example, do not have the same prevalence as in non-sport-related tendinitis.

Clinical symptoms are dominated by pain with variable functional impairment and loss of strength. This pain is spontaneous, usually localized, and triggered by movements. It can be reproduced by direct palpation or by opposed active movements and passive elongation of the tendon. Any doubt vanishes after a local infiltration of xylocaine (generally with corticoids), enabling us to rule out an associated disease and providing us with the first step of treatment. Indeed, conservative treatment needs a trial period and is generally effective if associated with rest (sometimes with a splint). A splint alone, transverse deep massage, electrotherapy, acupuncture, anti-inflammatory drugs, and local infiltration of corticoids have all been used successfully; the choice depends on the severity of the disease and the time off the athlete can accept. A precise, progressive, and correct program of retraining is mandatory until the previous level of performance is reached (the rule of 10 percent increase is a good one and the phrase "no pain no gain" must be retired).

Dorsal Tendinitis

Classically, frequency of tendinitis decreases from the first to the sixth compartment.

De Quervain's Disease

Tenovaginitis of the first dorsal compartment of the extensor was first reported in 1895 by a Swiss surgeon, Fritz De Quervain, assistant professor of Kocher. However, two previous descriptions can be found as early as 1892 by Tillaux (*aï crepitant*) and 1893 by Gray (*maladie des lavandières*), both in anatomic books. One-third of the patients report a previous local trauma, and the sports most frequently involved are racket sports and weight lifting.[32] Clinically, passive elongation of the abductor pollicis longus (APL) and extensor pollicis brevis (EPB) is obtained by ulnar inclination of the wrist and MP flexion, a maneuver described by Eichoff and later by Finkelstein.[11] This sign is not specific and can be positive in intersection syndrome and Wartenberg radial neuritis.[60] The association with this neuritis is interesting; we have found it in 18 percent of our De Quervain cases.[14] Pronation of the forearm triggers dysesthesia in the radial cutaneous territory.[39] Besides the ligual problem, which can arise in cases of infiltration or surgery, simple liberation of the first compartment can worsen the neurologic pathology by tethering the nerve distally. If surgery on the first compartment is anticipated, a splint is usually worn for 3 weeks and the Tinel sign checked again; in the absence of progression, a neurolysis of the radial cutaneous branch, 9.5 cm proximal to the styloid process where it crosses the brachioradialis tendon, is performed at the same stage as the De Quervain treatment.

Medical treatment, first by infiltration and, if this is not effective, by repetition combined with a splint is usually successful. Engel[10a] used tenography and was able to predict efficiency: in cases of the opacification stopping, medical treatment was positive in only 30 percent. Many series stressed the complications (found in 3 to 10 percent) of surgery[30,35,64]: incomplete liberation, neuroma of the radial nerve, tendon adhesions, keloids, and luxation of the APL (more frequently ante-

rior than posterior). All of these complications are easily avoided by a rigorous technique. Anatomic studies have demonstrated several relevant points. The cutaneous branch of the radial nerve crosses the area either without (36 percent) or with division (50 percent with two branches and 14 percent with three).[32] The APL frequently presents many strips (2 to 5) in 56 to 89 percent of cases.[17,24,28,32,48,56,59,64] The EPB is either double (4 percent for Stein[56]) or absent (6 percent for Leao[32]). It is of major surgical relevance that Schenck,[52] in a series of 300 cadaverous hands, found that 40 percent presented a separate compartment for APL and EPB. Similar findings occurred in two-thirds of the patients in the clinical series. Therefore observation of two tendons after the opening of one compartment is not a guarantee, and a second compartment needs to be checked systematically. The distal fascia does not warrant liberation and is one of the retaining factors to avoid luxation. Another method we have described to avoid postoperative splinting in athletes is to fix the retinaculum roof to the skin anteriorly with a resorbable stitch.[13]

Intersection Syndrome

Intersection syndrome, which occurs at the intersection between the APL and EPB muscle bellies and radial extensors is frequent among rowers, skiers, and weightlifters. Friction produces either a bursitis[62] or an inflammatory peritendinitis.[23] The pain elicited is more proximal than in De Quervain's disease, and crepitation is frequent. Conservative treatment was effective in 89 percent of our cases, usually a splint in 20 degrees of extension of the wrist. In surgical cases we consistently found a bursitis, which was excised. Other authors recommend division of the second dorsal compartment and synovectomy.[19]

Tendinitis of the Extensor Pollicis Longus

We have not observed extensor pollicis longus tendinitis in sports (except in undisplaced fracture of the distal radius), but only in musicians or in occupational diseases. Historically it was called *drummer palsy* by Dums due to the repetitive thumb motion that produced tendinitis and ultimate rupture.[20] It is a rare contraindication to local corticoid injection, due to the risk of rupture. In an elegant injection study Lundborg[1] demonstrated the paucity of the vascularization around the Lister tubercle, and Froimson[15] recommended incising the compartment to reroute the tendon superficially.

Extensor Indicis Proprius Syndrome and Extensor Manus Brevis

In 1969, Ritter and Inglis[51] defined the extensor indicis proprius (EIP) syndrome in two athletes in a classic paper. Pain and swelling of the fourth compartment were noticed. Both needed an operation, and muscle belly was found in the compartment. Pain could be reproduced through resisted active extension of the index in maximal flexion of the wrist.[55] Muscle fibers begin to create a compartment syndrome more than a tendinitis following hypertrophy. Indeed, in an anatomic study, muscular fibers were found underneath the fourth compartment in 75 percent of the 263 specimens.[8] We observed two cases with the same type of symptoms with an extensor indicis manus brevis, a rare supplementary muscle, classically nonengaging under the dorsal retinaculum. In both cases, swelling was visible and contracted with extension of the index; in one case it was associated with a dorsal ganglion.

Extensor Proprius Digiti Quinti Tendinitis

We observed no clinical cases of tendinitis of the fifth compartment, but extensor proprius digiti quinti tendinitis can be presented with either lower muscular fibers engaging the compartment[2] or with true tendinitis.[22] In his anatomic study, Schenck found two tendinous slips in 84 percent and more than two in 9 percent.

Tenovitis of the Extensor Carpi Ulnaris

Anatomically, the sixth compartment is different from the others and presents an independent fibroosseous tunnel on the dorsum of the lower end of the ulna. In athletes, true tenosynovitis is rare, unlike the general elderly population. A more frequent mechanism is tendinitis secondary to friction after a traumatic rupture of the ulnar septum of the compartment. This rupture happens mainly after a sudden movement of the wrist in ulnar inclination, flexion, and hyperpronation. Racquet sports were responsible for three of our five cases. Snapping of the tendon is not always easy to perceive,

and because of the usual delay in presentation conservative treatment through immobilization in supination and radial inclination is rarely possible. Reconstruction can be performed either with a free graft[10] or with a sling of retinaculum.[6]

Palmar Tendinitis

Digital Flexor Tendinitis

Trigger finger, even if it sometimes occurs after an isolated trauma or a fall, is quite rare in athletes compared with the general population. No clinical aspect calls for different treatment in this special population. In our series a simple infiltration was effective in 84% of cases.

Inflammation with visible swelling and tenderness at the distal forearm level is not exceptional. Acute carpal tunnel syndrome can be associated. Any repetitive activity in extension-flexion of the wrist and finger can be responsible, but the prevalence in our series is among weight lifters. Medical treatment is usually effective, and synovectomy is rarely necessary. However, in surgically treated cases, it is mandatory to reconstruct the carpal ligament in athletes according to our data comparing strength after a simple open incision, reconstruction, and endoscopic release. The last "tendinitis" that can be observed in this area is secondary to a frequent anatomic observation by Linburg and Comstock[34] of an anastomosis between the flexor pollicis longus and flexor profundus of the index. A prevalence of 31 percent in clinical studies and 25 percent in cadavers was noted by this author, but Lombardi et al.[37] found that only 57 percent of the patients presenting a distal index flexion when the thumb was actively flexed across the palm still had this connection at surgery; the others had only dense synovitis. Despite this relative frequency, no athletes we have seen have been disturbed by this "anomaly" in their activity. Perhaps "pulling," an exclusively Nordic sport activity, can trigger this type of pathology.

Flexor Carpi Radialis Tendinitis

Flexor carpi radialis tendinitis may develop after repetitive flexion of the wrist or direct trauma on the tendon. It is quite rare in sportsmen compared with the usual tendinitis of the 60-year-old woman who presents with associated scaphotrapezial arthritis. In our series of 24 cases of such tendinitis, none was triggered by a sports activity. Anyway, pain and tenderness are located close to the scaphoid tubercle, and a true ganglion or bursitis can be observed. Conservative treatment was effective in 30 percent of our cases. In the case of surgery we favor a transcanal carpal approach, perhaps together with the transverse incision mentioned by Stern[57] or the radial approach described by Steichen to avoid opening the carpal canal, with the risk of decreased strength.

Flexor Carpi Ulnaris Tendinitis

Simple tendinitis can occur, but athletes in their forties can also develop an acute syndrome with calcinosis circumscripta, including crystal deposit arthritis. In such cases, the patient presents as an emergency with intractable pain, skin redness, and total wrist incapacity. A radiograph with wrist flexion and semipronation demonstrates a cloudy calcification. Simple splinting is enough to alleviate the pain of this self-limited disease. Chronic tendinitis is much less incapacitating and must be distinguished from post-traumatic fractures or instability of the pisiform and fractures of the hook of the hamate. Conservative treatment is usually sufficient. In cases of recurrence or persistence, Palmieri[47] has demonstrated the efficiency of pisiform excision without any loss of strength.

CONCLUSIONS

Due to their frequency, soft tissue injuries through simple trauma or overuse need to be brought to the attention of both the medical and nonmedical people who take care of athletes. Most of them can be prevented by simple measures such as garment protection or preventive splint or taping. Mistakes in diagnosis and treatment can have devastating effects on the income and career of professionals. Iatrogenic injuries are to be avoided, and conservative treatment has to be tried despite frequent pressure from the patient, who is eager to get back early and is attracted by an unrealistic confidence in surgery. Most patients will complain of returning late to work because of compensation injuries, but returning to an activity too early can be highly detrimental in some cases, and progressive retraining is of the greatest importance.

REFERENCES

1. Abrahamsson SO, Sollerman C, Lundborg G et al: Diagnosis of displaced ulnar collateral ligament of the metacarpophalangeal joint of the thumb. J Hand Surg 15a:457–460, 1990
2. Ambrose J, Goldstone R: Anomalous extensor digiti minimi proprius causing tunnel syndrome in the dorsal compartment. J Bone Joint Surg 57:706–707, 1975
3. Bowers WH: The proximal interphalangeal volar plate II: a clinical study of hyperextension injury. J Hand Surg 6:77–81, 1981
4. Bowers WH, Wolf JW, Nehil JL et al: The proximal interphalangeal joint volar plate I: an anatomical and biomechanical study. J Hand Surg 5:79–88, 1980
5. Bunnell S: Surgery of the Hand. 3rd Ed. JB Lippincott, Philadelphia, 1964
6. Burkhart SS, Wood MB, Linscheid RL: Posttraumatic recurrent subluxation of the extensor carpi ulnaris tendon. J Hand Surg 7:1–3, 1982
7. Bynum DK Jr, Gilbert JA: Avulsion of the flexor digitorum profundus: anatomic and biomechanical considerations. J Hand Surg 13A:222–227, 1988
8. Cauldwell EW, Anson BJ, Wright RR: The extensor indicis proprius muscle. A study of 263 consecutive specimens, abstracted. Q Bull Northwestern Univ Med School 17:267, 1943
9. Drury BJ: Traumatic tendovaginitis of the fifth dorsal compartment of the wrist. Arch Surg 80:554–556, 1960
10. Eckhardt WA, Palmer AK: Recurrent dislocation of extensor carpi ulnaris tendon. J Hand Surg 6:629–631, 1981
10a. Engel J, Luboshitz S, Israeli A, Ganel A: Tenography in De Quervain's disease. Hand 13:142–146, 1981
11. Finkelstein H: Stenosing tendovaginitis at the radial styloid process. J Bone Joint Surg [Am] 12A:509, 1930
12. Fitton JM, Shea FW, Goldie W: Lesions of the flexor carpi radialis tendon and sheath causing pain in the wrist. J Bone Joint Surg [Br] 50B:359–363, 1968
13. Foucher G: Les tendinites de la main et du poignet du sportif. p. 60. In: Livre du Congrès d'Euromédecine, Montpellier, 1991
14. Foucher G, Greant P, Sammut D, Buch N: Nevrites et névromes des branches sensitives du nerf radial. A propos de quarante-quatre cas. Ann Chir Main 10:108–112, 1991
15. Froimson AI: Tenosynovitis and tennis elbow. p. 2126. In Green DP (ed): Operative Hand Surgery. 2nd Ed. Churchill Livingstone, New York, 1988
16. Gazarian A, Foucher G: La tendinite du grand palmaire. A propos de 24 cas. Ann Chir Main 11:14–18, 1992
17. Giles KW: Anatomical variations affecting the surgery of De Quervain's disease. J Bone Joint Surg [Br] 42B:352, 1960

18. Green DP, Rowland SA: Fractures and dislocations in the hand. p. 313. In Rockwood CA, Green DP (eds): Fractures in Adults. JB Lippincott, Philadelphia, 1984

19. Grundberg AB, Reagan DS: Pathologic anatomy of the forearm: intersection syndrome. J Hand Surg 10A:299–302, 1985

20. Hajj AA, Wood MB: Stenosing tenosynovitis of the extensor carpi ulnaris. J Hand Surg 11A:519–520, 1986

21. Herring SA, Nilson KL: Introduction to overuse injuries. Clin Sports Med 6:225–239, 1987

22. Hooper G, McMaster MJ: Stenosing tenovaginitis affecting the tendon of extensor digiti minimi at the wrist. Hand 11:299–301, 1979

23. Howard NJ: Peritendinitis crepitans. J Bone Joint Surg 19:447–459, 1976

23a. Ippolito E, Postacchini F, Scola E et al: De Quervain's disease. Int Orthop 9:41–47, 1985

24. Keon-Cohen B: De Quervain's disease. J Bone Joint Surg 33:96–99, 1951

25. Kettelkamp DB, Flatt AE, Moulds R: Traumatic dislocation of the long finger extensor tendon. A clinical, anatomical and biomechanical study. J Bone Joint Surg 53:229–240, 1971

26. Kiefhaber TR, Stern PJ, Grood ES: Lateral stability of the proximal interphalangeal joint. J Hand Surg 11A:661–669, 1986

27. Koniuch MP, Peimer CA, Van Gorder T et al: Closed crush injury of the metacarpophalangeal joint. J Hand Surg 12A:750–757, 1987

28. Lacey T, Goldstein LA, Tobin CE: Anatomical and clinical study of the variations in the insertions of the abductor pollicis longus tendon, associated with stenosing tendovaginitis. J Bone Joint Surg 33:347–350, 1951

29. Lapidus PW, Fenton R: Stenosing tenovaginitis at the wrist and fingers: report of 423 cases in 369 patients with 354 operations. Arch Surg 64:475, 1952

30. Lapidus PW, Guidotti FP: Stenosing tenovaginitis of the wrist and fingers. Clin Orthop 83:87–90, 1972

31. Laporte G, Dunat L: La Main des Pelotaris. Un "modèle" de pathologie traumatique. Ann Chir 29:499–507, 1975

32. Leao L: De Quervain's disease. J Bone Joint Surg [Am] 40A:1063–1070, 1958

33. Leddy JP, Packer JW: Avulsion of the profundus tendon insertion in athletes. J Hand Surg 2:66–69, 1977

34. Linburg RM, Comstock BE: Anomalous tendon slips from the flexor pollicis longus to the flexor digitorum profundus. J Hand Surg 4:79–83, 1979

35. Lipscomb PR: Chronic nonspecific tenosynovitis and peritendinitis. Surg Clin North Am 24:780, 1944

36. Lipscomb PR: Stenosing tenosynovitis at the radial styloid process (de Quervain's disease). Am J Surg 134:110–115, 1951

37. Lombardi RM, Wood MB, Linscheid RL: Symptomatic restrictive thumb-index flexor tenosynovitis: incidence of musculotendinous anomalies and results of treatment. J Hand Surg 13A:337–340, 1988

38. Loomis LK: Variations of stenosing tenosynovitis at the radial styloid process. J Bone Joint Surg [Am] 33A:340, 1951

39. Mackinnon SE, Dellon AL: The overlap pattern of the lateral antebrachial cutaneous nerve and the superficial radial nerve. J Hand Surg 10A:522–526, 1985

40. Manske PR, Lesker PA: Avulsion of the ring finger flexor digitorum profundus tendon: an experimental study. Hand 10:52–55, 1978

41. McClinton MA, Curtis RM, Wilgis EFS: One hundred tendon grafts for isolated flexor digitorum profundus injuries. J Hand Surg 7:224–229, 1982

42. McCue F, Honner R, Johnson MC, Gieck JH: Athletic injuries of the proximal interphalangeal joint requiring surgical treatment. J Bone Joint Surg [Am] 52A:937–956, 1970

43. McCue FC, Honner R, Gieck JH: A pseudo-boutonnière deformity. Hand 7:166–170, 1975

44. McCue FC, Andrew WF: Athletic injuries of the proximal interphalangeal joint, "coach's finger." Contemp Orthop 3:516–524, 1981

45. Moberg E, Stener B: Injuries to the ligaments of the thumb and fingers. Acta Chir Scand 106:166–186, 1953

46. Palmer AK, Linscheid RL: Chronic recurrent dislocation of the proximal interphalangeal joint of the finger. J Hand Surg 3:95–97, 1978

47. Palmieri TJ: Pisiform area pain treatment by pisiform excision. J Hand Surg 7:477–480, 1982

48. Parsons FG, Robinson A: Eighth report of the Committee of Collective Investigation of the Anatomical Society of Great Britain and Ireland, for the Year 1897–98. J Anat Physiol 33:189–203, 1899

49. Patel MR, Desai SS, Bassini-Lipson L: Conservative management of chronic mallet finger. J Hand Surg 11A:570–573, 1986

50. Posner MA, Ambrose L: Boxer's knuckle—dorsal capsular rupture of the metacarpophalangeal joint of a finger. J Hand Surg 14A:229–236, 1989

51. Ritter MA, Inglis AE: The extensor indicis proprius syndrome. J Bone Joint Surg [Am] 51A:1645, 1969

52. Schenk RR: Variations of the extensor tendons of the fingers. Surgical significance. J Bone Joint Surg [Am] 46A:103–110, 1964

53. Schernberg F, Elzein F, Gillier P, Gerard Y: Les Luxations des articulations interphalangiennes proximales des doigts longs. Ann Chir Main 1:18–28, 1982

54. Spinner M, Kaplan E: Extensor carpi ulnaris: its relationship to the stability of the distal radioulnar joint. Clin Orthop 68:124–129, 1970

55. Spinner M, Olshansky K: The extensor indicis proprius syndrome: a clinical test. Plast Reconstr Surg 51:134–138, 1973

56. Stein AH: Variations of the tendons of insertion of the abductor pollicis longus and the extensor pollicis brevis. Anat Rec 110:49–55, 1951

57. Stern PJ: Tendinitis, overuse syndromes and tendon injuries. Hand Clin 6:467–475, 1990

58. Trepman E, Micheli LJ: Overuse injuries in sports. Semin Orthop 3:217–222, 1988

59. Wagenseil F: Untersuchungen über die Muskulatur der Chinesen. Z Morphol Anthropol 36:39–150, 1937

60. Wartenberg R: Cheiralgia parestetica (isolierte Neuritis des Ramus superficialis nerve radialis). Z Ger Neurol Psychiatr 141:145–155, 1932

61. Weeks PM: A cause of wrist pain: nonspecific tenosynovitis involving the flexor carpi radialis. Plast Reconstr Surg 62:263–266, 1978

62. Wood MB, Linscheid RL: Abductor pollicis longus bursitis. Clin Orthop 93:293–296, 1973

63. Wood MB, Dobyns JH: Sports-related extraarticular wrist syndromes. Clin Orthop 202:93–102, 1986

64. Woods THE: De Quervain's disease: a plea for early operation. A report on 40 cases. Br J Surg 51:358–359, 1964

16

Arthroscopy of the Wrist

ROBERT S. RICHARDS
JAMES H. ROTH

INTRODUCTION

During the 1980s arthroscopy gained wide acceptance in the management of sports-related injuries. Concerns about visualization in the face of hemarthrosis and the effectiveness of arthroscopy in the acutely injured joint have diminished as experience has been gained. Arthroscopy of the wrist has become widespread and is proving to be a valuable tool in the athlete. The early diagnosis and treatment of many lesions is now possible with high accuracy and a lower morbidity than arthrotomy.

TECHNIQUE

Portals

In wrist arthroscopy, multiple dorsal portals are used (Fig. 16-1). The radiocarpal portals are numbered by their relation to the extensor tendons.[2,30] The 1–2 portal is situated between the first and second extensor compartments. To avoid radial artery injury, it is located in the extreme dorsum of the snuff box just radial to the extensor pollicis longus tendon.[30] The 1–2 portal might be used during reduction and K-wire fixation of radial styloid fractures or when inserting K-wires for pinning of the scapholunate interval.

The 3–4 and 6–R portals are the two main working portals for radiocarpal arthroscopy. The 3–4 portal lies between the extensor pollicis longus and the extensor digitorum communis tendons. This portal is established 1 cm distal to Lister's tubercle between the tendons of the third and fourth compartments. The 6–R portal is located distal to the ulnar head and radial to the extensor carpi ulnaris (ECU) tendon. This portal

is established at the proximal pole of the triquetrum. It is best established under direct vision after advancing the arthroscope ulnarly and transilluminating the ulnar side of the wrist. Transillumination allows the superficial veins to be avoided. The 6–U portal is distal to the ulnar styloid on the ulnar side of the ECU tendon. The 6–U portal has been recommended for use as an inflow or outflow portal but generally is unnecessary.

The midcarpal portals are named differently. The midcarpal radial portal (MCR) is located along the radial side of the third metacarpal 1 cm distal to the 3–4 portal. A depression between the proximal and distal carpal rows can be palpated. The midcarpal ulnar (MCU) portal is established along the midline of the fourth metacarpal roughly at the same level as the MCR portal. This is best located under direct vision after establishing the MCR portal. A gap between the proximal and distal carpal row can be palpated along the midline of the fourth metacarpal and the needle inserted.

The final dorsal portal is used for arthroscopy of the distal radioulnar joint. This is located along the radial head of the ulna.[30] This portal is located by palpation of the radial edge of the ulnar head. Supinate the wrist to relax the capsule and facilitate entry. Insert the arthroscope sheath proximal to the triangular fibrocartilage complex (TFCC).

Technique of Radiocarpal and Midcarpal Arthroscopy

General or regional anesthesia is essential both in the acutely injured joint and in chronic conditions. Regional anesthesia can be axillary block or intravenous regional (Bier) block.[22] In contrast to experience with knee arthroscopy, local anesthesia is insufficient for

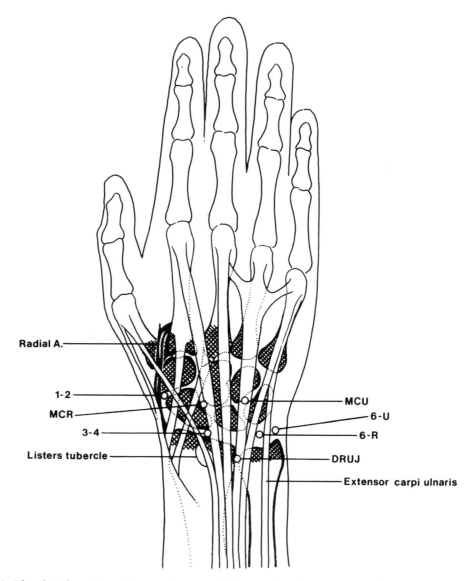

Fig. 16-1. The dorsal wrist portals are diagrammed. Numbering of the radiocarpal portals is based on their relationship to the extensor compartments of the wrist. Midcarpal portals are identified by their position in relationship to the capitate.

wrist arthroscopy. The wrist joint is small, with a volume of only 5 to 8 ml, and the intercarpal spaces are difficult to enter. Merely distending the joint does not give sufficient exposure to perform wrist arthroscopy. The greater relaxation and distraction allowed by regional or general anesthesia is essential for success.

Arthroscopic examination of the wrist should include both the midcarpal and radiocarpal joints. Radiocarpal arthroscopy alone does not permit complete diagnosis and is not sufficient for many of the operative procedures on the carpus. A systematic approach allows complete examination of both radiocarpal and midcarpal joints in a very short time. Midcarpal arthroscopy adds little additional morbidity or operative time.

After induction of anesthesia, the patient is positioned supine on the operating table with the shoulder abducted, allowing the arm to hang free. All procedures are performed with an above-elbow tourniquet elevated to 250 mmHg. The arm is prepped with tincture of iodine and the fingers are then placed in sterile traps prior to application of the drapes. For most cases of diagnostic arthroscopy, distraction is obtained by placing the index and long fingers in the finger traps. Occasionally more ulnar distraction is needed and the traps may be placed on the ulnar fingers. The risk of skin damage can be decreased by placing more fingers in the traps.

The finger traps may be suspended from intravenous poles, overhead hooks, or static arms attached to the table. Distraction towers on the hand table may also be used. Our personal preference is for an articulated arm system attached to the operating room table, which allows easy positioning of the arm prior to final drape application. Previously, a ceiling-mounted sky hook was used, but this limits the flexibility of positioning and makes adjustment of table height awkward. Final positioning of the arm and operating table is performed before drape application to prevent the drapes from pivoting and pulling on the arm. Use of a suspension apparatus rather than a distraction tower allows easier rotation of the wrist. Countertraction of 7 lb is applied to a wide sling placed over the tourniquet on the arm. A chair with arm rests is desirable to allow the surgeon to work while sitting with the elbows supported. Working with the arms and elbows extended is fatiguing.

Arthroscopy remains an equipment-dependent procedure. Ideal arthroscope diameters are in the 2.5- to 2.7-mm range and may be used for radiocarpal, midcarpal, and distal radioulnar joint arthroscopy. The 1.7-mm arthroscope is no longer recommended due to a limited field of view. The 4.0-mm diameter arthroscope is too large and increases the risk of articular damage. Shorter arthroscopes with a lever arm of 100 mm are preferred. The limited depth of the wrist joint makes it awkward to control a longer arthroscope. An oblique viewing angle of 30 degrees allows a wider arc of visualization. A complete set of small joint equipment should include probes, suction punches, graspers, and a small powered shaver system. The power shaver should include both 2.0- and 3.5-mm full radius shavers as well as joint burrs. The large shaver system has too large a handle and too long a lever arm for easy manipulation in the wrist. A probe of approximately 1.5 to 2.0 mm in diameter and approximately 100 mm in length is ideal. Shorter, finer probes are produced, but they are awkward to use and bend easily.

The wrist is now examined and the landmarks palpated. The 3–4 portal is established first. An 18- to 21-gauge needle is inserted 1 cm distal to Lister's tubercle. Angling the needle 10 degrees volarly aids insertion of the needle and decreases the risk of articular damage. The joint is then distended with 5 to 7 ml of lactated Ringer's solution. To maintain orientation the surgeon should avoid moving the thumb from Lister's tubercle. A 15 blade is used to make a longitudinal stab incision at the 3–4 portal site; this stab is carried down through the joint capsule. A longitudinal incision minimizes the risk to soft tissue structures. Avoid using a hemostat to spread the soft tissues in order to decrease the extravasation of irrigation fluid into the soft tissues. The blunt trocar is used for insertion, since a sharp trocar increases the risk of articular damage. After introduction of the arthroscope into the 3–4 portal, the next portal to be established is the 6–R portal. The arthroscope is advanced ulnarly from the 3–4 portal and the ulnar side of the wrist is transilluminated. It is useful to note the amount of transillumination. A wide area of transillumination indicates that one is in the radiocarpal joint. A more limited area of transillumination indicates that the arthroscope is probably in the midcarpal joint. The 6–R portal is established distal to the ulnar head and radial to the ECU tendon. The triquetrum is palpated and an 18-gauge needle inserted at the proximal edge of the triquetrum. Transillumination allows the veins to be avoided. Once the needle is visualized, a stab incision is made and the capsule incised. The return of saline indicates entry into the joint. An adequate capsular incision provides sufficient outflow without the use of accessory portals. Inflow is gravity fed through the arthroscope sheath. This provides more effective cleansing of the operative site than a separate inflow. Unlike other joints, infusion pumps have not been necessary, since wrist distraction avoids the need for high-pressure distension.[16]

A hook probe is now inserted into the 6–R portal and the camera oriented properly. A consistent examination routine speeds the arthroscopy. First start radially with the arthroscope in the 3–4 portal. The radial styloid is visualized, and then the radioscaphocapitate, radiolunatotriquetral, and radioscapholunate (RSL) ligaments. An important anatomic landmark is the synovial fold, which is associated with the RSL. Retraction of this fold exposes the RSL (Fig. 16-2). The scaphoid and lunate fossae should then be examined. Finally, the scapholunate interosseous liga-

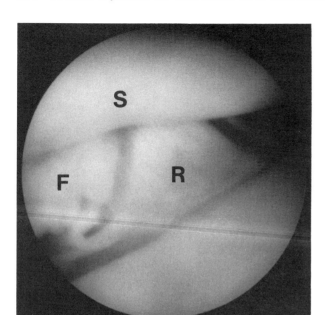

Fig. 16-2. The fold of synovium (*F*) overlying the radio-scapholunate ligament (*R*) is retracted allowing it and the scapholunate ligament (*S*) to be visualized.

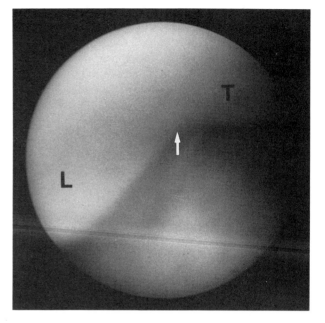

Fig. 16-3. Through the 6–R portal the lunate (*L*), triquetrum (*T*), and lunotriquetral ligament (*arrow*) between them are seen.

ment and articular surfaces of the scaphoid and lunate are examined.

The arthroscope is now inserted into the 6–R portal and the hook into the 3–4 portal. Use of the probe is essential to permit a complete arthroscopy, since much of the information to be obtained is tactile as well as visual. Visualize the triquetrum, lunotriquetral ligament, and lunate first (Fig. 16-3). Now visualize the TFCC and the ulnocarpal ligaments (Fig. 16-4). Finally, the pisotriquetral joint can be visualized. Probe all surfaces with the hook probe. Incomplete tears of the interosseous ligaments may not be diagnosed on visual examination alone. An intact TFCC will have a firm surface much like a trampoline. TFCC tears will cause loss of this normal tension.

Diagnostic arthroscopy must also include the mid-carpal joints. Midcarpal arthroscopy using a 3-mm-diameter scope can be accomplished quite readily. Establish the MCR portal 1 cm distal to the 3–4 portal along the radial border of the third metacarpal. This portal overlies the scaphocapitate joint. Again, slight volar angulation of both needle and the arthroscope aids in entering the joint space. Now establish the MCU portal. The depression between the proximal and distal carpal

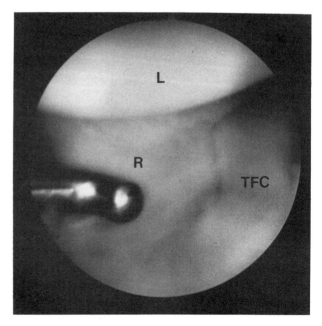

Fig. 16-4. The lunate (*L*), radius (*R*), and TFCC (*TFC*) are seen through the 6–R portal.

rows can be palpated along the midline of the fourth metacarpal. Insert a needle into the joint to allow direct visual confirmation of the portal position and establish the portal with a 15 blade. The scaphotrapeziotrapezoid joint, the scapholunate interval, the capitate, and the lunate are visualized. Carefully examine the lunate facets and the articulation for arthrosis with the proximal pole of the hamate, as suggested by Viegas.[25] Fractures of the scaphoid, as well as separation at the scapholunate joint, are more easily seen and reduced through the midcarpal joint than the radiocarpal joint.

Most arthroscopies are performed on an outpatient basis. Bupivacaine (Marcaine) is injected intra-articularly prior to application of the dressing. The patients are placed in a bulky below-elbow sterile dressing for 7 days. The portal sites are not sutured to allow egress of the fluid into the dressing. After the dressing is removed the patient is started on a course of active range of motion (ROM).

Complications

Complications after any arthroscopic procedure are rare, and the wrist is no exception. A major national survey in the United States has revealed an overall complication rate of 0.56 percent.[24] Most of the 545,000 patients reported, however, had knee arthroscopy. In the wrist the major potential complications include the following: infections, neuromas, tendon ruptures or damage, reflex sympathetic dystrophy, skin slough, finger joint injury or stiffness from the finger traps, skin slough in the fingers from the finger trap pressure, skin slough over the dorsum of the wrist, nerve injury from the tourniquet, and compartment syndromes. Adequate precautions during arthroscopy will prevent most of the above complications.[28] None of these complications have been noted in our patients. However, wrist arthroscopy is not to be taken lightly. Cartilage injury from instruments and increased pain and stiffness have been seen. Fluid extravasation either in the subcutaneous space or the deep compartments has not been a clinical problem. To minimize the risk of compartment syndrome, we avoid arthroscopy of acute fractures in the first 72 hours after injury. Avoidance of irrigation pumps and minimal use of irrigation are further safeguards. Ringer's lactate is the most physiologic of the irrigation fluids and minimizes the risk from extravasation.

TRIANGULAR FIBROCARTILAGE COMPLEX INJURIES

Assessment of TFCC injuries can be difficult. Arthroscopy has been shown to be superior to arthrography in the assessment of TFCC perforations.[20,23] Assessment of three-compartment arthrography revealed only two-thirds of all complete TFCC tears; 11 of 16 scapholunate and 18 of 21 lunotriquetral perforations were identified preoperatively by arthrography.[11] Also, the false-positive rate varied from 10 to 20 percent. Magnetic resonance imaging (MRI) has similar limitations.[3,20] A second weakness of MRI and arthrography is an inability to detect the cartilage erosions associated with TFCC tears. Cerofolini et al.[3] noted that in none of their 10 cases was MRI able to visualize cartilaginous lesions later seen at arthroscopy.

The anatomy[13,19] and blood supply of the TFCC[14] have been well documented. The important structures from the arthroscopist's viewpoint are the dorsal and volar radioulnar ligaments surrounding the central triangular disk. These ligaments become taut during rotation to maintain stability of the distal radioulnar joint. These ligaments must be preserved during arthroscopic resections of the TFCC to maintain stability of the joint. The extrinsic blood supply to the articular disk supplies primarily the palmar, dorsal, and ulnar margins of the disk. The central and radial portions remain avascular. The proportion of the disc that is vascularized decreases from 33 percent in childhood to 25 percent in adults.[14]

Palmer[18] and Blair et al.[1] have both described classification systems for TFCC lesions. Palmer classifies them into traumatic (I) and degenerative (II). Subclasses describe the presence of associated lunate and ulnar pathology as well as the location of the tear (see Ch 13). Blair classifies TFCC lesions into central, ulnar, or radial tears. The critical point in both classification systems involves separating the central or radial lesions from the ulnar peripheral lesions. Neither arthrography nor MRI provide sufficient anatomic detail to make this decision. Arthroscopy is essential for proper classification.

Treatment depends on the location and size of the tear. Agreement exists that lesions of the central avascular disc or its radial attachment will not heal and that repair is futile. Peripheral lesions have the potential to heal, and either suture repair or immobilization of acute peripheral TFCC injuries for 4 weeks has been recommended. Large central tears are resected. If the tear is peripheral and the edges are in apposition, then immobilization alone or supplemental suture of the tear is indicated. The objective of suture repair is to restore the normal tension and trampoline effect of the TFCC.

Currently our treatment of central (class 1A) and radial (class 1D) tears (Fig. 16-5) is debridement of the damaged portion of the TFCC. Acute or chronic tears are treated in a similar fashion. Acute TFCC tears are commonly seen in association with distal radius fractures. Often a history of trauma can be elicited in those patients with long-standing pain and chronic perforations. Chronic perforations are often seen in association with positive or neutral ulnar variance. The goal is to remove the redundant flaps of tissue without causing instability (Fig. 16-6). Removing the redundant flaps may prevent the lunate from impinging on them with wrist motion, causing pain.

Arthroscopic debridement of chronic perforations of the TFCC has been shown to be effective. If the dorsal and volar radioulnar ligaments are left intact, no biomechanical instability has been seen. Results of debridement have been good, with relief of pain in 73 percent of patients at 1 year.[17] These results are similar

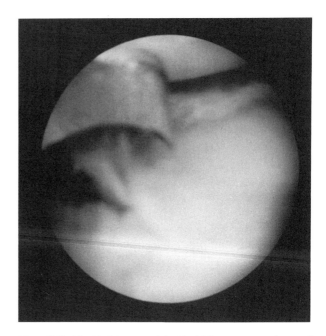

Fig. 16-6. The TFCC tear is debrided. The poor vascularity of the TFCC here makes suture repair unlikely to be successful.

to those reported from ulnar shortening, in which 28 of 36 (78 percent) patients had good pain relief.[5] Arthroscopic resection gives good decompression of the ulnar side of the joint without the risks and immobilization involved in osteotomy. Additional decompression in ulnar-positive patients can be achieved by the use of the Wafer procedure.[18] In this technique the distal 2 mm of the ulnar head is removed using a burr after the tear has been resected. The burr is introduced through the 6–R portal. The forearm must be put through a range of pronation and supination to ensure that the ulnar head has been completely and evenly resected. The ulnar head is removed underneath the horizontal portion of the TFCC, leaving the origin and insertion intact. Again, good early results are reported.

Arthroscopic treatment is associated with much less morbidity than open arthrotomy, and the magnification allows better visualization. The recovery of grip strength and motion is more rapid. Treatment of TFCC lesions has included suture repair, debridement, or excision of the TFCC, as well as ulnar head resection and ulnar-shortening osteotomy. All but ulnar shortening can now be performed arthroscopically, enhancing its potential to treat these lesions. Overall, arthroscopy is now the modality of choice for diagnosis and initial treatment of lesions of the TFCC.

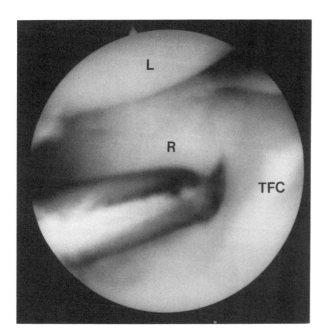

Fig. 16-5. A radial TFCC tear is seen here with the probe through the tear. The lunate (*L*) and radius (*R*) are seen.

SCAPHOLUNATE TEARS

Arthroscopy is an important tool in the diagnosis and treatment of ligamentous injuries of the wrist. Scapholunate injuries are more easily treated in the acute rather than the chronic stage (see Ch. 13). However, only arthroscopy allows definitive early diagnosis. Clinical examination and provocative radiographic testing remain unreliable.[6,7,26] Arthrography has been used but cannot distinguish partial from complete tears. MRI has poor sensitivity and specificity. Arthroscopy remains the best method of distinguishing complete tears from partial tears. Arthroscopy also allows assessment of the edges of the tear and of any associated pathology.

Treating scapholunate ligament injuries is a difficult problem. Open suture repair of the ligament is difficult since it is a small, tight interosseous ligament. Often a dorsal reinforcement with a tendon graft or capsular flap must be performed. Results are equivocal, and the risk of stiffness after arthrotomy and prolonged immobilization is high. Because of this risk, early arthroscopic reduction and pinning has been suggested.[22] Midcarpal arthroscopy gives a better view of the joint surfaces, since the scapholunate ligament does not obscure the joint on the midcarpal aspect. Placement of K-wires in the scaphoid and lunate allow correction of the dorsiflexed lunate and palmarflexed scaphoid. Reduction is accomplished with the arthroscope in the midcarpal portals. This allows accurate reduction of the scapholunate interosseous interval. K-wire fixation can then be performed (Fig. 16-7A and B). Generally, two to four K-wires are used. Early short-term results are encouraging (Fig. 16-7C), but the ligament may not heal.[29] K-wire breakage is also a possible complication.

Generally, treatment of acute scapholunate ligament injuries has been recommended only within the first 6 weeks. However, waiting to treat the athlete in the off season can be undertaken. Whipple[29] reports that arthroscopic reduction and pinning has been successful in inducing arthrofibrosis up to 3 months after the injury if the scapholunate gap is less then 3 mm.

LUNOTRIQUETRAL TEARS

Clinically, the patient presents with pain along the ulnar aspect of the wrist. The onset is often related to a specific trauma. The lunotriquetral ballottement test elicits pain and laxity at the lunotriquetral joint.[21] The differential diagnosis includes TFCC tears and midcarpal instability (see Ch. 13).

Arthroscopy is the standard of diagnosis, since assessment of lunotriquetral ligament tears with MRI is more difficult than scapholunate ligament injuries. This is due to the size and the oblique orientation of the ligament to the plane of the coronal images. Arthroscopic reduction of lunotriquetral ligament tears should also be performed with the arthroscope in the midcarpal joint. The lunotriquetral articulation is difficult to define exactly from the radial joint because the lunotriquetral ligament covers the articulation.

The triquetrum is pinned to the lunate using multiple K-wires. Results similar to scapholunate pinning are reported with formation of an arthrofibrosis and correction of the lunotriquetral instability.

OSTEOCHONDRAL INJURIES

Arthroscopy has revealed that chondral lesions are commonly seen in patients with chronic pain. Bilateral osteochondral flaps of the radius have been described as a cause of chronic wrist pain in weightlifters. These injuries are not visible by radiographic diagnostic tests, including MRI, leading to a lack of recognition in the past.[3,8] Arthroscopic diagnosis remains the best method of visualizing these lesions. Diagnosis of any associated ligamentous injury is essential to treating these injuries.[10] If no other injuries exist, debridement has been an effective mode of treatment for this injury. If other ligamentous injuries exist, then treatment of associated injuries must be undertaken or else persistent pain from the underlying carpal instability will be present.

SCAPHOID FRACTURES

Obtaining and maintaining reduction of displaced scaphoid fractures is difficult using closed methods, so open reduction and internal fixation is often necessary. The primary disadvantage of the volar approach is that division and repair of the strong volar ligaments is necessary. Postoperatively, volar scarring may limit wrist dorsiflexion. A dorsal approach may compromise the blood supply to the scaphoid. Arthroscopic reduction and internal fixation of scaphoid fractures avoids these problems.[27] Fixation has been accomplished us-

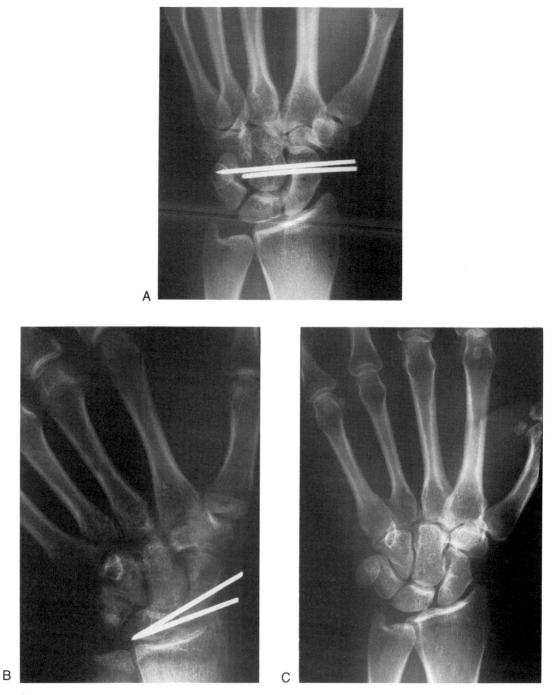

Fig. 16-7. **(A)** This 28-year-old woman sustained a complete scapholunate ligament tear while playing volleyball. Arthroscopic reduction of her scapholunate ligament tear and stabilization with K-wires allowed healing. We no longer place pins across the midcarpal joints. **(B)** Our preferred pin placement is across the scapholunate interosseous interval alone. Two to four K-wires are used. **(C)** Follow-up radiographs at 2½ years after injury reveal maintenance of a normal scapholunate interval. Wrist range of motion averages 80% of the contralateral wrist, and she has returned to work as a physiotherapist.

ing both the original Herbert screw as well as the Herbert-Whipple cannulated screw system. Reduction of the scaphoid fracture should be performed with the arthroscope in the midcarpal joint, since this allows the most accurate visualization of the fracture. Two wires are then placed down the long axis of the scaphoid. After drilling over one guidewire, the cannulated screw is inserted while the second guide wire prevents rotational displacement. The second wire is then removed. Arthroscopic reduction and fixation remains a promising treatment option in anyone with a displaced scaphoid fracture and may be indicated in selected athletes with undisplaced scaphoid fractures.

RADIUS FRACTURES

Jupiter established the causal relationship between intra-articular displacement and subsequent degenerative arthritis. Reduction of articular surfaces must be anatomic, since a 2-mm step leads to subsequent de-

generative arthritis.[9] Practical difficulties exist in obtaining an anatomic reduction in intra-articular fractures. Closed reduction does not allow accurate visualization, and open reduction is difficult in comminuted unstable fractures. Arthroscopy combines accurate reduction of the articular surface with preservation of maximal soft tissue stability. Magnification aids in obtaining the desired anatomic reduction. Although technically demanding, excellent visualization is obtained by washing the joint and debriding adherent clots using a powered abrader. The use of suction also minimizes the extravasation of fluid.

Arthroscopy of fractures after fluoroscopic closed reduction and percutaneous pinning has often revealed significant intra-articular steps greater than 1 mm. We have achieved better reduction of these fractures with manipulation of the fractures under arthroscopic visualization. Depressed die punch fractures may be elevated using the angled probe, and any small osteochondral fragments that may block anatomic reduction can be removed (Fig. 16-8A). Assessment of

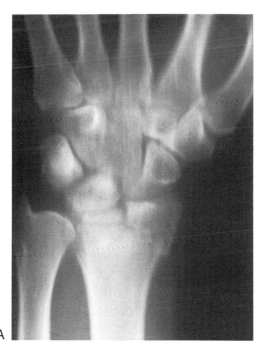
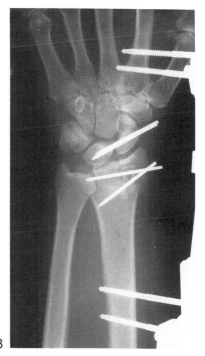

A   B

Fig. 16-8. (A) This patient presented with an intra-articular distal radius fracture. Tomography reveals the depressed lunate fossa and intra-articular step. Arthroscopic reduction and bone grafting were necessary to restore the intra-articular surface. **(B)** Arthroscopy also revealed a complete scapholunate ligament tear not evident on the original radiographs, as well as a TFCC tear. The TFCC tear was debrided and the scapholunate ligament tear treated with arthroscopic reduction and K-wire fixation.

stability after reduction and the need for bone graft to support the articular surface is also facilitated (Fig. 16-8B). Arthroscopy allows diagnosis and simultaneous treatment of associated ligamentous and TFCC injuries. Associated scapholunate ligament tears are managed by arthroscopic reduction and K-wire fixation, as previously described.

In addition to using arthroscopy in intra-articular fractures, arthroscopy may be indicated in extra-articular fractures. The association between extra-articular radius fractures and wrist ligamentous injury has been recognized for some time. Nelaton in 1844 published the first description of TFCC injuries associated with distal radius fractures.[12] Subsequently, in 1940, Mayer demonstrated that in most cases of distal radius fracture the force is sufficient to rupture the TFCC.[12] Using arthrography for diagnosis, estimates of the incidence of TFCC disruption in extra-articular distal radius fractures have ranged up to 45 percent.[15] Clinical symptoms with pain and laxity of the distal radioulnar joint have been reported to occur in 5 to 15 percent of fractures.[4,12]

Arthroscopy has enabled us to delineate better the injuries associated with radius fractures. We perform arthroscopy of all intra-articular and some of the comminuted extra-articular fractures. A large number of associated injuries have been found. TFCC tears of the radial or central aspects are usually present. Disruption of the ulnar insertion is uncommon. Unsuspected scapholunate ligament injuries are frequently found as well. We have treated TFCC tears with debridement rather than suture as the injuries have usually been central and radial. Small radial tears that open minimally with pronation and supination may be managed with immobilization.

Our ability to manage the TFCC and ligament injuries associated with these fractures is enhanced by arthroscopy, allowing better treatment of distal radius fractures.

CONCLUSIONS

Wrist arthroscopy is useful in the evaluation and treatment of many different forms of intra-articular pathology. The treatment of ligamentous disruptions, triangular fibrocartilage tears, fractures of the distal radius, and scaphoid injuries has been enhanced by increasingly sophisticated arthroscopic surgery.

REFERENCES

1. Blair WF, Berger RA, El-Khoury GY: Arthrotomography of the wrist: an experimental and preliminary study. J Hand Surg 10A:350–359, 1985
2. Botte MJ, Cooney WP, Linscheid RL: Arthroscopy of the wrist: anatomy and technique. J Hand Surg 14A:313–316, 1989
3. Cerofolini E, Luchetti R, Pederzini L et al: MRI evaluation of triangular fibrocartilage complex tears in the wrist: comparison with arthrography and arthroscopy. J Comput Assist Tomogr 14:963–967, 1990
4. Cooney WP, Dobyns JH, Linscheid RL: Complications of Colles' fractures. J Bone Joint Surg [Am] 62A:613–619, 1980
5. Darrow JC, Linscheid RL, Dobyns JH et al: Distal ulnar recession for disorders of the distal radioulnar joint. J Hand Surg 10A:482–491, 1985
6. Gilula LA, Weeks PM: Post-traumatic ligamentous instability of the wrist. Radiology 129:641–651, 1978
7. Johnson J: Diagnosis of scapholunate dissociation with traction radiography. Canadian Society for Surgery of the Hand Annual Meeting, Calgary, Alberta, June 2, 1991.
8. Kang HS, Kindynis P, Brahme SK et al: Triangular fibrocartilage and intercarpal ligaments of the wrist: MRI imaging. Cadaveric study with gross pathologic and histologic correlation. Radiology 181:401–404, 1991
9. Knirk JL, Jupiter JB: Intra-articular fractures of the distal end of the radius in young adults. J Bone Joint Surg [Am] 63A:647–659, 1986
10. Koman LA, Mooney JF, Poehling GG: Fractures and ligamentous injuries of the wrist. Hand Clin 6:477–491, 1990
11. Levinsohn EM, Rosen DI, Palmer AK: Wrist arthrography: value of the three-compartment injection method. Radiology 179:231–239, 1991
12. Lidstrom A: Fractures of the distal end of the radius: a clinical and statistical study of end results. Acta Orthop Scand Suppl 41:7–118, 1959
13. Linscheid RL: Biomechanics of the distal radioulnar joint. Clin Orthop 275:46–55, 1992
14. Mikic Z: The blood supply of the human distal radioulnar joint and the microvasculature of its articular disk. Clin Orthop 275:19–28, 1992
15. Mohanti RC, Kar N: Study of triangular fibrocartilage of the wrist joint in Colles' fracture. Injury 11:321–324, 1980
16. Oretorp N, Elmersson S: Arthroscopy and irrigation control. Arthroscopy 2:46–50, 1986
17. Osterman AL: Arthroscopic debridement of triangular complex tears. Arthroscopy 6:120–124, 1990
18. Palmer AK: Triangular fibrocartilage disorders: injury patterns and treatment. Arthroscopy 6:125–132, 1990
19. Palmer AK, Werner FW: The triangular fibrocartilage complex of the wrist—anatomy and function. J Hand Surg 6:153–162, 1981

20. Pederzini L, Luchetti R, Soragni O et al: Evaluation of the triangular fibrocartilage complex tears by arthroscopy, arthrography, and magnetic resonance imaging. Arthroscopy 8:191–197, 1992

21. Reagan DS, Linscheid RL, Dobyns DH: Lunotriquetral sprains. J Hand Surg 9:502–513, 1984

22. Roth JH: Wrist arthroscopy. Radiocarpal arthroscopy: technique and selected cases. p. 108. In Lichtman DM (ed): The Wrist and Its Disorders. WB Saunders, Philadelphia, 1988

23. Roth JH, Haddad RG. Radiocarpal arthroscopy and arthrography in the diagnosis of ulnar wrist pain. Arthroscopy 2:234–243, 1986

24. Small NC: Complications in arthroscopy: the knee and other joints. Arthroscopy 2:253–258, 1986

25. Viegas SF: The lunatohamate articulation of the midcarpal joint. Arthroscopy 6:5–10, 1990

26. Watson HK, Hempton RF: Limited wrist arthrodesis part 1: the triscaphoid joint. J Hand Surg 5:320–327, 1980

27. Whipple TL: Wrist arthroscopy: clinical applications of wrist arthroscopy. p. 118. In Lichtman DM (ed): The Wrist and Its Disorders. WB Saunders, Philadelphia, 1988

28. Whipple TL: Precautions for arthroscopy of the wrist. Arthroscopy 6:3–4, 1990

29. Whipple TL: The role of arthroscopy in the treatment of wrist injuries in the athlete. Clin Sports Med 11:227–238, 1992

30. Whipple TL, Marotta JJ, Powell JH: Techniques of wrist arthroscopy. Arthroscopy 2:244–252, 1986

17

Brachial Plexus Injuries

NATHANIEL L. TINDEL
ELLIOTT B. HERSHMAN
JOHN A. BERGFELD

INTRODUCTION

Athletic injuries to the upper extremity in contact sports are common. Even though the brachial plexus and its branches are particularly vulnerable, they are often overlooked as sources of pain and weakness. Such injuries should be considered in the differential diagnosis of any upper extremity trauma. These injuries can be quite severe, and a delay in diagnosis may affect an athlete's ability to use the upper extremity, let alone return to sport. Any part of the plexus may be injured, from avulsion of the spinal roots to stretching of peripheral nerves. All physicians treating athletes should have a thorough understanding of the anatomy, mechanism, presentation, diagnosis, prognosis, and treatment of brachial plexus injuries.

ANATOMY

The brachial plexus is a network of nerves formed by the union of the ventral rami of nerves C5 to C8 and T1 (Fig. 17-1). Above the clavicle, these rami lie in the posterior triangle of the neck and run between the scalenus anterior and scalenus medius muscles. Below the clavicle, the brachial plexus lies in the axilla. Anatomically, the plexus is divided from proximal to distal into five rami, three trunks, and six divisions (supraclavicular); three cords passing beneath the clavicle); and five terminal nerves (infraclavicular).

The terminology and anatomy of rami and roots can be confusing.[54] Each spinal nerve is formed by the union of one ventral and one dorsal root, each of which is attached to the spinal cord. Each ventral root leaves the cord containing efferent (motor) fibers, whereas each dorsal root enters the cord containing afferent (sensory) fibers. The cell bodies of the axons of the ventral roots are in the ventral gray horn of the spinal cord. The cell bodies of axons of the dorsal roots are found in the spinal ganglia (dorsal root ganglia), which lie in the intervertebral foramen. Upon exiting the intervertebral foramen, each spinal nerve then divides into a ventral and dorsal ramus. The dorsal rami supply the skin and muscles of the back. The ventral rami supply the skin and muscle and joints of the neck, trunk, and extremities. Only ventral rami unite to form networks of nerves, or plexi. Dorsal rami do not form plexi and therefore exist only as unisegmental peripheral nerves.[3]

The ventral rami of C5 and C6, C7, and C8 and T1 unite to form the superior, middle, and inferior trunks, respectively. The brachial plexus may be considered prefixed if a contribution from the fourth cervical spinal nerve is present or postfixed if a contribution from the second thoracic spinal nerve is present.[22] Anatomically, the inferior trunk lies on the first rib, posterior to the subclavian artery.[54] Each of these trunks then divides into anterior and posterior divisions. The three posterior divisions unite to form the posterior cord (the cords are named in relationship to the axillary artery), which supplies the extensor muscles of the limb. The anterior divisions of the superior and middle trunks unite to form the lateral cord, and the anterior division of the inferior trunk continues as the medial cord.

269

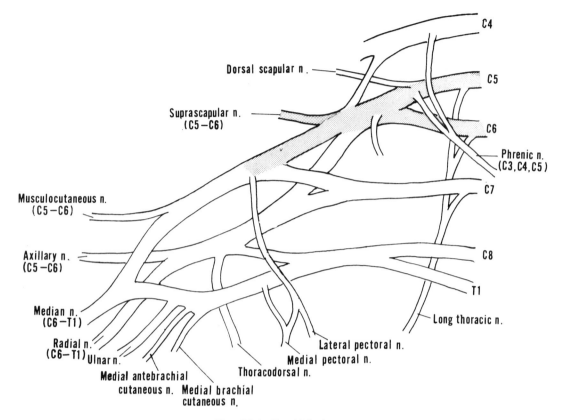

Fig. 17-1. Brachial plexus.

Each cord of the brachial plexus divides into two major and several minor terminal nerves.[3,54] The lateral cord has three branches: (1) the lateral root of the median nerve (not to be confused with the dorsal and ventral roots above); (2) the lateral pectoral nerve, which supplies the pectoralis major; and then continues as (3) the musculocutaneous nerve. The medial cord has five branches: (1) the medial root of the median nerve; (2) the medial pectoral nerve, supplying the pectoralis major and minor; (3) the medial brachial cutaneous nerve; (4) the antebrachial cutaneous nerve; and then continues as (5) the ulnar nerve. The posterior cord also has five branches: (1) the lower subscapularis nerve; and (2) the upper subscapularis nerve (both supply the subscapularis muscles, with the latter supplying the teres major); (3) the thoracodorsal nerve, supplying the latissimus dorsi muscle; and the posterior cord terminates by dividing into the (4) axillary; and (5) radial nerves. The axillary nerve moves to the posterior aspect of the humerus by passing through the quadrangular space along with the posterior circumflex humeral vessels. The axillary nerve supplies the teres minor and deltoid muscles as well as a small, variable patch of skin overlying the inferior aspect of the deltoid muscle. The radial nerve leaves the axilla and passes between the long and medial heads of the triceps muscle to enter the radial groove of the humerus.[54]

The brachial plexus has four supraclavicular branches to the upper limb. Two nerves arise from the rami and two from the trunks. The long thoracic nerve arises from C5 to C7 and innervates the serratus anterior muscle. The dorsal scapular nerve arises predominantly from C5, with minor contributions from C4, and innervates the rhomboids and levator scapulae muscles. Two nerves arise from the upper trunk (C5 and C6). The nerve to the subclavius muscle supplies the subclavius. The suprascapular nerve, which passes laterally across the posterior triangle of the neck, superior to the plexus and through the suprascapular notch, innervates the supraspinatus and infraspinatus muscles.

The autonomic nervous system takes on importance when the clinician attempts to localize lesions in the brachial plexus.[20] The parasympathetic portion arises from cells in the brain stem (cranial nerves III, VII, IX, and X) and sacral region of the spinal cord (sacral nerves 2, 3, and 4). The parasympathetic nervous system has little to do with localizing brachial plexus injuries. The sympathetic portion, however, which arises from cells in the thoracic and upper lumbar regions of the spinal cord (T1 to L3), can certainly be affected. To reach parts of the body superior and inferior to the T1 and L3 levels, respectively, the preganglionic fibers arise from the spinal cord but only traverse ventral roots T1 to L3 to exit the corresponding spinal nerve by a white ramus communicans. The white ramus communicans connects the spinal nerve with the sympathetic cervical chain. Once within the chain, the preganglionic fiber then ascends into the neck via the cervical extension of the chain to its appropriate level. At this point, it synapses with a postganglionic fiber within the ganglion. Postganglionic fibers arise from the synapse within the ganglion and join the spinal nerve at each spinal level via a gray ramus communicans. Thus, as a rule, all spinal nerves have gray rami communicantes (postganglionic fibers), but only thoracic and upper lumbar nerves have white rami (preganglionic fibers). Functionally, the importance of this arrangement is seen when the inferior aspect of the brachial plexus is injured, specifically the T1 nerve root: the sympathetic nerve supply to the head on the ipsilateral side is interrupted. The injury results in a clinical syndrome known as Horner syndrome, which consists of the following symptoms:

1. Pupillary constriction due to paralysis of the dilator pupillae muscle
2. Ptosis due to paralysis of the smooth muscle in the levator palpebrae muscle
3. Vasodilation and loss of sweating on the ipsilateral face and neck due to lack of sympathetic nerve supply to the blood vessels and sweat glands.

It is important to diagnose the Horner syndrome, which localizes the site of the brachial plexus injury and thus allows more complete prognosis and treatment.

MECHANISM OF INJURY

Several modes of injury to the brachial plexus have been recognized. Mechanisms fall into one of two main categories: direct compression and traction injury. Compression type injuries occur when structures about the shoulder and neck cause direct pressure to the brachial plexus. Cervical ribs in young athletes have been reported to compress the lower trunks of the brachial plexus.[64] Likewise, the suprascapular nerve has been shown to be compressed where it passes either through the coracoid notch or into the infraspinous fossa in volleyball players[28] (Fig. 17-2). Fractures of the clavicle are common injuries and often occur in athletic competition, but they rarely cause plexus injury acutely.[40] The plexus can become compressed, however, by hyperabundant callus formation.[52,53] Generally, favorable results are obtained with excision of the offending fracture callus.[52]

A more common mechanism of injury to the brachial plexus is traction. In the athlete, forcible separation of the head and shoulder can stretch the interposing soft tissue structures. Stretching of the head and shoulder with the arm at the side most often stresses the upper roots of the plexus, sparing the lower roots.[4] With increasing elevation or abduction of the arm, more

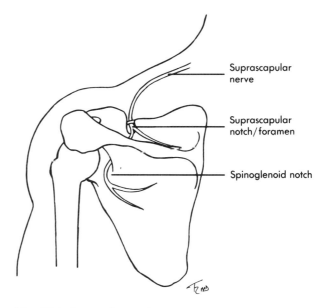

Fig. 17-2. Potential sites of suprascapular nerve entrapment. (From Pianka and Hershman,[59] with permission).

tension is placed on the lower roots.[79] The relative position of the shoulder and head is also known to increase the differential tension among the nerve roots. Cadaveric studies show that tension is exerted on all roots of the plexus when the abducted arm is forced behind the trunk and the head is thrust toward the opposite side.[14] Forced lateral-flexion injuries of the neck (called stingers, burners, or nerve pinch by athletes and trainers), notably seen in football injuries, have been associated with stretching of both the lower[17] and upper[19] cervical nerve roots.

Substantial stretching of a nerve is possible before rupture occurs. Denny-Brown et al.[23] created neurapraxic states in animal nerves by varying amounts of tension. They showed that the effects of stretching a peripheral nerve beyond the physiologic elastic limit correspond to the degree of injury found. Initially, with stretch of a nerve, the epineural vasculature is damaged, with patches of ischemic changes and loss of segments of myelin sheath of the nerve. Further stretch leads to rupture of the perineurium and herniation of the nerve fibers. Recovery of the nerve varies in proportion to the extent of stretch.

CLASSIFICATIONS

Many classifications of the brachial plexus injuries exist. The two main ones attempt to provide a correlation between the degree of nerve injury and the clinical symptomatology. In 1943 Seddon[73] proposed a three-grade system for injury to peripheral nerves. He categorized them from least severe to worst, as follows: (1) neurapraxia, (2) axonotmesis, and (3) neurotmesis. Sunderland[77] later expanded this grouping to a five-grade system, with degrees of increasingly severe nerve injury.

Neurapraxia, the least severe injury (Sunderland's first degree), is a transient episode of motor paralysis or sensory weakness, or both. It involves a local conduction block in the nerve with segmental demyelination. No axonal abnormality is present. Neurapraxia carries a good prognosis, and recovery is usually rapid and complete.

Axonotmesis is the second category. Injury occurs to both the axon and the myelin sheath, and wallerian degeneration occurs distal to the level of injury. However, the nerve is not physically transected. The conti-

nuity of the Schwann tube remains intact to act as a pathway for the regenerating axon and myelin sheath.[77] Predicted recovery time is based on the distance of the end organs from the site of injury. Recovery may be incomplete.

Seddon's third, and most severe, category of injury is neurotmesis (corresponding to Sunderland's third, fourth, and fifth degrees of injury). In Sunderland's third-degree injury, nerve fibers and their Schwann tubes are severed within intact nerve fascicles. Recovery is variable but never complete. In a fourth-degree injury, the perineurium surrounding each fascicle is damaged as well. The fifth degree of injury involves either transection of the nerve or extensive scarring with a loss of continuity that prevents nerve regeneration across the area of injury. No recovery is expected from this last type of injury.

Based on Seddon's classification, Clancy et al.[19] proposed a three-grade clinical system of closed, traction brachial plexus injuries. Grade I corresponds to Seddon's neurapraxia. This results in a temporary loss of motor and sensory function that may last for minutes or hours. Complete recovery is expected within a few weeks. This injury is referred to as a *burner* or *stinger* by athletes because of the burning pain experienced when making a block or tackle. Electromyograms (EMGs) performed 2 to 3 weeks after the injury are normal with a grade I injury. By contrast, grade II injuries fail to regain full motor or sensory recovery (or both) as quickly, and EMGs reveal changes consistent with axonotmesis.

Robertson et al.[67] reported on 10 football players who sustained grade II brachial plexus injuries. Each had clinical and electrodiagnostic evidence of injury to the upper trunk of the brachial plexus following an injury to the shoulder region. Six of the 10 recalled having experienced several previous episodes. In 9 of the 10, weakness followed the burning paresthesias 1 to 7 days after the injury. All the athletes demonstrated gradual regain of strength. In seven players, the examination returned to normal in 1 to 6 weeks. In three players, mild-to-minimal weakness persisted for up to 9 months. Their experience suggests that this syndrome is due to stretching of the brachial plexus.

Grade III injuries in Clancy's classification have the worst prognosis. They are analogous to neurotmesis and carry a dismal chance of recovery. Fortunately, these are rare.

DIAGNOSIS

The prognosis after injuries of the brachial plexus depends on the location, type, and severity of the injury. On the one hand, avulsion of a nerve root as it exists from the spinal cord is not likely to undergo spontaneous recovery, nor is surgical repair likely to be successful. On the other hand, traction or compression of a peripheral nerve has a far better prognosis. The problem then becomes one of determining at which level the plexus has been injured. Therefore an accurate and complete assessment of the level and extent of the injury is essential.

A careful history should be taken first, including the mechanism of injury, particularly the position of the limb and head at the time of impact as well as the type and amount of force used to create the injury. A detailed description of symptoms, including paralysis, numbness, and burning sensations, with their locations and duration should be elicited. Any symptom related to the cervical spine, including a stiff neck, pain with motion of the neck, or tenderness of the bony structures of the neck, requires a careful evaluation of the cervical spine.

It is of utmost importance to distinguish between a spinal cord and a nerve root injury. Both can produce pain, numbness, and weakness about the shoulder. In the acutely ruptured disc, for example, a player will hold the head tilted toward the side of the root affected. Pain in the interscapular region is often present. Pain is made worse by extending the neck while tilting it toward the affected side.[68] Lhermitte's sign, indicative of spinal cord compression, can be elicited if the patient complains of an electric shock through the body on flexion of the neck. One must always "assume every neck injury is a broken neck until proven otherwise."[3]

Inspection begins by watching the athlete walk off the field. Symmetry of motion is important to note. An Erb's palsy (also called Duchenne-Erb palsy), in which the arm is internally rotated and adducted (the classic "waiter's tip" position of the limb) is readily noticed.[39] This upper trunk lesion, which involves C5 and C6, produces paralysis of the abductors and lateral rotators of the arm, the elbow flexors and supinators, the rhomboids, and the clavicular head of the pectoralis major.[46] Deltoid atrophy, which is too often overlooked, can be seen when the deltoid no longer fills out the lateral contours of the shoulder. Atrophy can also be noted

in the infraspinatus and supraspinatus fossa when the spinati are involved (Fig. 17-3). The trapezius muscle should also be palpated. Paralysis of the trapezius can be disabling and leads to drooping of the shoulder, winging of the scapula, and weakness of forward elevation and abduction.[7,8] The scapula should be closely evaluated for winging, which may be related to a long thoracic nerve lesion.

Middle trunk lesions are essentially those of C7 and involve the extensors of the elbow, wrist, and fingers. Lower trunk lesions (Dejerine-Klumpe) have a pattern of C8 and T1 damage. This results in a combined median and ulnar palsy with sparing of the pronator teres and flexor carpi radialis muscles as well as sensory loss along the ulnar aspect of the hand and forearm and the medial aspect of the arm. In summary, lesions of the upper trunk affect the shoulder and arm, those of the middle trunk affect the extensors of the elbow and hand, and those of the lower trunk affect the hand and forearm.[22]

A sensory examination must be carried out. Isolated C5 lesions do not necessarily produce sensory loss. C6 involvement leads to loss of sensation over the lateral aspect of the upper extremity. C7 innervates the middle finger and C8 and T1 the ulnar forearm and midial upper arm, respectively. Athletes' reflexes are often hyporeflexic or even absent, so little is gained by a reflex examination unless response is asymetric. The supraclavicular fossa should be palpated and percussed for the presence of swelling or a positive Tinel sign.

After a spinal cord injury has been ruled out, the next important question is whether the injury is preganglionic or postganglionic: postganglionic lesions tend to be more treatable and thus lead to a better prognosis. The two types may be differentiated in several ways, although not always easily, and many injuries involve combinations of both anatomic areas.

In preganglionic injuries, the spinal roots are avulsed from the cord. The motor axons are disconnected from their cell bodies, the anterior horn cells, and undergo degeneration. The sensory axons, having lost their central connection from the cord, still remain attached to the dorsal root ganglions (which contain their cell bodies) and do not degenerate. In addition, the posterior primary divisions of the root, which supplies the posterior muscles and skin, are also denervated. In upper plexus lesions, C5 contributions to the phrenic nerve (predominantly a C4 innervated nerve) can leave

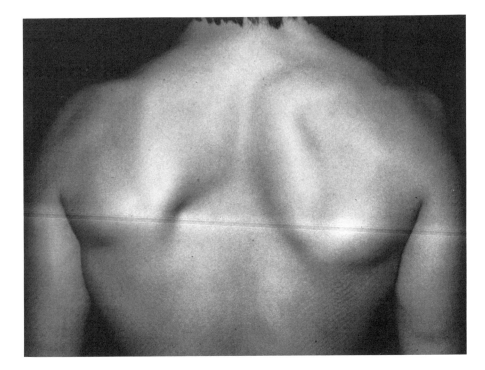

Fig. 17-3. Infraspinatus atrophy. (From Pianka and Hershman,[59] with permission).

the ipsilateral hemidiaphragm paralyzed. Dorsal scapular and long thoracic nerves arise from the upper plexus spinal nerve roots just after their exit from their foramen. Thus, in upper plexus injuries, paralysis of the rhomboids or serratus anterior also implies nerve root or preganglionic damage. If, however, the above muscles are preserved, with paralysis of the lateral rotators of the humerus, the lesion is located at Erb's point, where the fifth and sixth cervical roots join to form the upper trunk.[46] In the lower plexus, the presence of Horner syndrome suggests a preganglionic lesion of the T1 nerve root.

Adjunctive Testing

In 1954, Bonney[11] described the classic triple response to 1 percent histamine acid phosphate solution as a means of distinguishing preganglionic from postganglionic lesions. The response depends on the integrity of the sensory axons to a particular dermatomal area. In a preganglionic lesion, the sensory axons are preserved, as they remain in continuity with their cell bodies in the dorsal root ganglion. Thus the normal reaction is preserved. This is the tripled response noted by the appearance of local vasodilation, formation of a wheal, and then further vasodilation (flare). This would be considered a positive response to the test and is a poor prognostic sign. In a postganglionic lesion, the sensory axons degenerate and the reaction to histamine is altered. In these lesions, local vasodilation and whealing are not followed by the formation of a flare. The absence of a flare is considered a negative response to the test, implies that the lesion is postganglionic, and therefore carries a better prognosis.

Electrodiagnostic Testing

EMG can add useful information for both prognosis and diagnosis. The EMG is a two-part procedure composed of (1) the needle electrode examination, and (2) nerve conduction studies.[85] Motor conduction, muscle activity, and sensory conduction can all be used to localize lesions.

The needle electrode examination is performed by inserting a needle electrode into a muscle and assessing the electrical activity within the muscle at rest and during voluntary movement. This examination has the advantage of high sensitivity to motor axon loss. Since each motor axon innervates several hundred individual muscle fibers, the loss of a single axon is readily apparent. In the voluntary part of the examination, denervation of the muscle is represented by fibrillation potentials long before weakness can be detected by physical examination.[85] Fibrillation potential is the spontaneous activity seen when a muscle is at rest after it has been denervated. Unfortunately, these action potentials do not appear until 21 days after nerve injury.[85] Needle electrode examination can also discern preganglionic from postganglionic lesions. Bufalini and Pescatori[15] demonstrated the use of posterior cervical needle electrode examination in distinguishing intraforaminal from extraforaminal brachial plexus injuries. Since the deep posterior cervical muscles are innervated by the posterior branches of spinal nerves, which branch off immediately after the root emerges from the intervertebral foramen, denervation implies an intraforaminal, or preganglionic lesion.

The second part of the needle electrode examination is the evaluation of voluntary muscle activity with the motor unit potential. The action potential is seen when the athlete contracts the muscle. This allows the examiner to distinguish between an axonal lesion and an upper motor neuron lesion. Axon lesions result in decreased numbers of impulses, but the rate of transmission remains rapid, while upper motor neuron lesions and poor effort also result in decreased numbers, but transmit at slower rates.[85]

The nerve conduction study is the second part of the EMG examination. Unlike the needle electrode examination, which only assesses motor function, the nerve conduction study can assess both motor and sensory nerve function. By stimulating a nerve proximally with one electrode, the surface response distally to muscle or skin is recorded with a second electrode. The important point to remember is that conduction velocity is only affected by some demyelinating diseases and that it is the amplitude of the responses that is informative of an axonal lesion in the nerve distal to the cell body. This is extremely valuable in assesing preganglionic lesions. In this type of injury, the sensory nerve action potential amplitude is not affected because the axon is still in continuity with its cell body in the dorsal root ganglion. In contrast, the muscle action potential amplitude is diminished because the axon has lost its continuity with the cell body in the

anterior horn of the spinal cord.[85] The advantages of the nerve conduction study are that it does not require patient cooperation, it assesses both motor and sensory function, and it is far less uncomfortable for the patient.[85]

Somatosensory evoked potentials have also proved to be of significant value in the evaluation of brachial-plexus lesions. Landi et al.[44] showed that preoperatively they aid in predicting outcome in certain lesions and that intraoperatively they serve as useful guides to the most appropriate surgical procedures.[44] Date et al.[21] have analyzed dermatomal somatosensory evoked potentials and found them to be a useful adjunct to other studies for localizing the site of a brachial plexus lesion.

Radiography

Plain radiographs of the cervical spine and shoulder are always obtained when evaluating individuals with brachial plexus trauma. Shoulder dislocation and clavicular fracture are easily noticed. However, a fractured cervical transverse process or first rib may be missed. These latter injuries may be the only direct evidence of a brachial plexus injury. As the deep cervical fascia invests both the nerve root and the transverse process, the root can easily be avulsed with these injuries.[46] Cervical scoliosis can be associated with multiple root avulsions.[65]

Marshall and De Silva[51] reported good visualization of the cervical nerve roots with computed tomography (CT) myelography. Contrast-enhanced CT can provide good visualization of the cervical nerve roots. They noted that the important fifth and sixth cervical roots, which are least visualized with conventional myelography, are shown well by CT scans.[51] However, they pointed out that the the increasing obliquity of the lower cervical roots makes them more difficult to assess.[51]

Myelography

In 1947, Murphey et al.[55] accidently demonstrated the association of traumatic meningocele with spinal root avulsion on cervical myelogram while looking for a herniated disc.[66] For quite some time, the finding of pseudomeningocele on myelogram has been considered pathognomonic of spinal root avulsion. It has been shown, however, that a false-negative result may appear when the meningeal tear undergoes repair by scar tissue, and the meningocele defect may disappear.[78] In addition, Heon[34] demonstrated that meningeal tears can exist without rupture of the root. Yeoman[89] later demonstrated that a periarachnoid scar may give the false-positive apperance of a filling defect in the meningeal sac.[89] He also showed a lack of concordance with findings from myelography and the axon reflex test.

Magnetic Resonance Imaging

Interest has recently developed in imaging of the brachial plexus with magnetic resonance imaging (MRI). The multiplanar capability of MRI (Fig. 17-4) can follow the course of the nerves more easily than other imaging techniques such as CT scan.[74] MRI can be used in traumatic injury to the plexus to evaluate neuroma formation, the presence of meningoceles, or extrinsic compression due to fracture callus or hematoma.[33,69,74] Neoplasms compressing or infiltrating the plexus can be identified with MRI.[16,62,83] Brachial neuritis with nerve enlargement on MRI has also been reported.[74] MRI is also useful in intraspinal cases of upper extremity symptoms when evaluating patients with confusing clinical signs.

BRACHIAL PLEXUS INJURIES

Fractures

Acute fractures can be associated with brachial plexus trauma,[64,65,66] and sometimes injury to the brachial vessels is also present.[27,52,53] These neurovascular injuries often occur with high-enery trauma to the clavicle and shoulder girdle. The clavicle fracture may be highly comminuted, consistent with a high-energy impact. Evidence of vascular compromise following clavicle injury requires arteriographic evaluation of the subclavian artery and distal vessels. If indicated, exploration and vascular repair are undertaken, combined with open reduction and internal fixation of the fracture. If impingement of the brachial plexus by a highly displaced

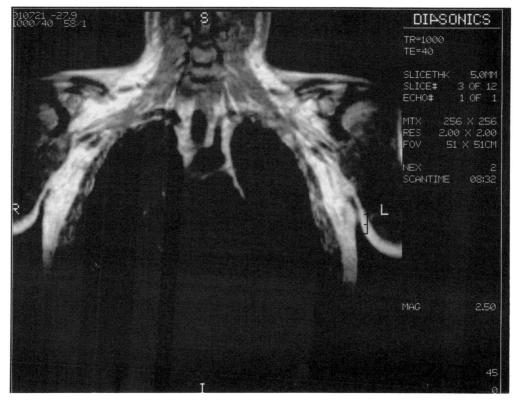

Fig. 17-4. MRI of brachial plexus.

fragment of bone is suspected, exploration of the plexus may be indicated to reduce the fragment and fix the fracture internally.

Early treatment of acute closed clavicle fractures with a figure-of-eight harness can also contribute to brachial plexus compression. If neurovascular compromise is suspected, adjustment or elimination of the offending device is immediately carried out. If improvement in the neurologic or vascular examination does not occur, an appropriate workup is performed and surgery, if indicated, carried out to repair injured vascular structures or remove compression on the brachial plexus from fracture fragments.[40,88] Stabilization of the fracture with internal fixation is important.

Compression Lesions

Although compression is not a common cause of brachial plexus injury, several entities have been described. Backpack paralysis is a well-recognized cause of brachial plexus injury in mountain climbers (Fig. 17-5). Prolonged compression from the axillary strap of a heavy knapsack leads to compression injury of the plexus against the clavicle. The shoulder girdle is also pulled posteriorly, perhaps adding a component of traction. Excellent results have been reported with conservative treatment[37] including a period of rest followed by physical therapy. Equipment modification is mandatory if the individual is to return to hiking.

Exhuberant callus formation during clavicle fracture healing has also been implicated in compression of the plexus. This may present as a progressive neurologic lesion during the latter stages of fracture healing. Kay and Eckardt[42] observed that the medial cord can be affected in delayed union, producing ulna nerve symptoms. Treatment may require resection of the callus with open reduction and internal fixation of the fracture to achieve union.

Burners/Stingers

The burner syndrome is a common football injury. It denotes a brief episode of burning and stinging (hence the name) and occasional weakness involving the upper extremity after a tackle or block to the neck and shoulder-girdle region.

In 1965 Chrisman et al.[17] originally described the entity as *cervical nerve pinch syndrome* from their analysis of 22 cases (17 football, 2 basketball, 1 wres-

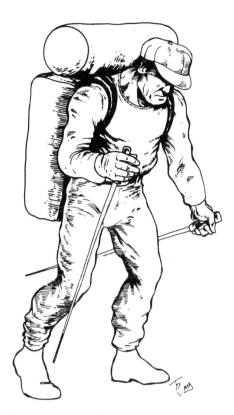

Fig. 17-5. Heavy backpacks can lead to combined compressive and traction lesions at the plexus.

tling, 1 pit fall in track, and 1 squash-wall collision). In the cases in which the mechanism could be determined, they described the injury as occurring when force was applied to the shoulder and the neck flexed laterally away from the contact point. In one-half the cases, the mechanism of injury could not be determined. Poindexter and Johnson[60] reported that both flexion and hyperextension of the spine in a violent fashion were the mechanisms of injury. Clancy[18] also noted several athletes who reported that the head and neck were laterally flexed toward the side of injury. Bergfeld[5] postulated a different mechanism of injury from that which produces acromiclavicular sprains. In the acromioclavicular joint injury, the point of contact is lateral, over the acromium. In a burner, the point of contact is over the clavicle (Fig. 17-6). This may explain why concomitant acromioclavicular joint sprains and burners are rare. It thus appears that a variety of positions may be associated with a burner, but that the most common is a blow occurring with the neck hyperextended forcibly in lateral flexion, with

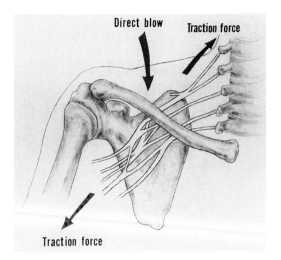

Fig. 17-6. Potential location of contact in brachial plexus stretch injuries.

the chin pointing away from the side of contact. The point of contact is over the clavicle, depressing the shoulder girdle in the athlete with a burner. The point of contact in acromioclavicular injuries is the acromion, a more lateral site of compression.

The pain in a burner radiates from the shoulder down to the arm. The distribution is circumferential and does not necessarily correspond to a specific dermatome.[35] Often the athlete will try to shake the arm to get the feeling back. The player can be easily spotted because the arm hangs down at the side, and the athlete is often holding the affected arm with the contralateral arm (Fig. 17-7). The symptoms usually only last for a few minutes, but may persist for as long as 2 weeks. Persistent sensory deficit is very unusual with burners and should alert the physician to the possibility of other injuries. Maroon[50] reported on two cervical central spinal cord injuries presenting as "burning hands." Failure to recognize a cervical injury can be catastrophic. Bilateral symptoms should alert the examiner to the possibility of a neck injury. Once the diagnosis is clear, repeated examinations are critical in evaluating these athletes, as weakness may not develop for hours to days following this injury.[59] Muscles commonly affected include those innervated by the upper plexus, in particular the external rotators of the shoulder, the deltoid, and the biceps.

The anatomic site of the injury that is consistent with the burner syndrome is generally believed to be at the level of the upper trunk. However, some authors believe that the injury occurs at the level of the C5 and

C6 root.[68] Clancy et al.[19] concluded that the upper trunk of the brachial plexus was the site of the lesion. Di Benedetto and Markey[24] used electrodiagnostic studies to localize the abnormality as compression of the most superficial fibers at Erb's point. Wilbourn[85] fuels the debate with electrodiagnostic findings consistent with injury either at the root level or the upper trunk of the plexus. Nevertheless, Wilbourn[85] suggests that the lesion is probably in the plexus, rather then the root, since fibrillation potentials in the paraspinal muscles are seldom found.

Other mechanisms of injury producing the burner syndrome have been proposed. These include direct contact at Erb's point by the medial border of the shoulder pad[49a] and acute or chronic root irritation in the neural foramen as the head is driven backward and toward the side of the injury (extension-compression).[71] Modification of the shoulder pads to include additional padding between the hard shell and Erb's point will help prevent the direct contact type of burner (Fig. 17-8B). Extension compression type burn-

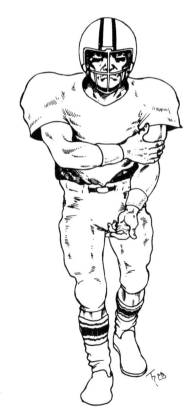

Fig. 17-7. Typical appearance of a football player following a "burner."

ers are often seen in athletes with cervical spinal steno-sis.[71] Neck padding to reduce hyperextension of the neck is often helpful in athletes with these injuries.

Once the diagnosis has been made and the possibility of cervical injury has been ruled out, the athlete should be removed from competition. Only after the burner has resolved and full strength can be elicited is the athlete permitted to return to competition.[6,75] Re-examination following competition and at regular intervals during the following week should be undertaken, since weakness may develop some time after the original injury.[35] Weakness is treated with an appropriate rehabilitation program emphasizing both strength and endurance.

When weakness or pain persists for longer then 3 weeks, an EMG examination is in order to help identify the location of the lesion. EMG changes often remain abnormal even in asymptomatic, normal strength individuals long after the initial injury.[6] Large motor unit potentials, consistent with reinervation, will be present on EMB years after a significant burner. These changes can be present with normal strength. Thus persistent EMG changes are not appropriate criteria for exclusion from competition. Rather, the clinical examination should guide the return to competition.

Many athletes report recurrent burners. A neck and shoulder strengthening program is extremely valuable. Some athletes use neck rolls (Fig. 17-8A) and extra-high shoulder pads (Fig. 17-8B) to limit neck motion. The effectiveness of these pads has not been fully determined.[35]

Acute Brachial Neuropathy

Acute brachial neuropathy is a rare cause of shoulder pain and weakness. It has been described as many entities including localized neuritis of the shoulder girdle,[76] neuralgic amyotrophy,[58] and Parsonage-Turner syndrome,[82] among many others. Acute brachial neuropathy is probably often misdiagnosed as cervical radiculopathy or traumatic neuropathy (supra-scapular, dorsal scapular, and long thoracic nerves most often).[85] The diagnosis should be entertained in any athlete complaining of unexplained shoulder pain or weakness, or both).

Understanding the presentation and clinical course of acute brachial neuropathy is important so that effective therapy and counseling can be offered. The condition arises as an acute, painful episode of shoulder and scapular pain extending into the arm or hand. The

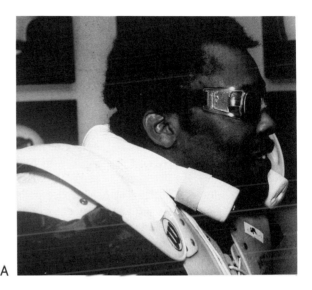

A

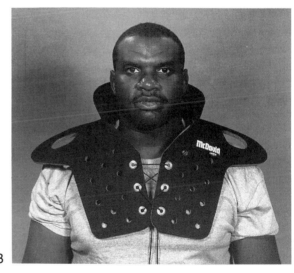

B

Fig. 17-8. (A) Neck roll. **(B)** Shoulder/neck pad. (From Pianka and Hershman,[59] with permission).

pain is often severe and may persist for days. Weakness generally follows. It most commonly occurs in men aged 18 to 40 but can occur in any age group from 3 months to 74 years.[81] Classically, no recent trauma or related injury can be recalled. The serratus anterior is the single most commonly affected muscle, with persistent scapular winging noted as a possible complication.[72] Rarely, the entire extremity and ipsilateral hemidiaphragm are affected, with wasting of the shoulder-girdle muscles.[81]

The pathogenesis of acute brachial neuropathy is unclear. Antecedent infections and recent immunizations have been most often implicated in the development of this entity. In addition, a hereditary form of brachial plexus neuropathy has been described infrequently.[87] The diagnosis rests on a careful examination of the shoulder and upper extremity. Laboratory studies (sedimentation rate, complete blood count, and cerebrospinal fluid) are generally normal.[36] Wilbourn[84] reviewed the EMG examination and found changes consistent with axon degeneration. Fibrillation potentials and decreased amplitude with motor nerve conduction were typically seen in affected nerves.[85] In addition, subclinical EMG abnormalities are often present in the unaffected upper extremity.

Tsairis et al.[81] reported on the outcome of 84 patients with brachial plexus neuropathy and gave an optimistic overall prognosis, despite the variable severity and extent of the initial lesion. Dillin et al.[25] also confirmed complete recovery in 90%.

Hershman et al.[36] divided the treatment of acute brachial neuropathy into two phases. In phase I, support for the affected extremity, rest, and analgesics are indicated for the acute period of symptoms. During this time, gentle range of motion exercises are important to maintain joint mobility. Once the severe pain resolves, the athlete enters phase II (rehabilitation) to regain strength. Emphasis must be placed on strengthening the entire shoulder girdle, since subclinical muscle involvement is common. Hershman et al.[36] recommended that return to competition should be guided by strength recovery. Athletes may consider return to sport when a plateau in their recovery has occurred only if sufficient strength to control the extremity is obtained. Corticosteroids have no demonstrated value in this disease entity. Recurrences, although extremely rare, have been reported.[13,71]

PERIPHERAL NERVE LESIONS
Long Thoracic Nerve

The long thoracic nerve, a pure motor nerve, lies on the medial wall of the axilla. Its superficial course and length render it prone to injury. Injury to the long thoracic nerve results in paralysis of the serratus anterior muscle. The serratus anterior muscle anchors the vertebral border of the scapula to the thoracic cage and acts to protract and rotate the scapula. Denervation of the muscle leads to "winging" of the scapula. Winging of the scapula is accentuated when the patient pushes against a wall with both hands since absence of serratus anterior function allows the scapula to move out like a wing. Patients also complain of difficulty flexing or abducting the arm above 45 degrees because of the action of the serratus anterior muscle on the scapula.[54]

Injury to the long thoracic nerve can occur from blows to the lateral thoracic wall, excessive use of the shoulder, or prolonged traction on the nerve.[49] It may also be susceptible to compression as it passes over the second rib.[86] The long thoracic nerve is also frequently involved in cases of acute brachial neuropathy, with scapula winging accompanying diffuse upper extremity weakness. Many sports have been implicated in injury to the long thoracic nerve including tennis, golf, cycling, gymnastics, soccer, bowling, weight lifting, ice hockey, wrestling, archery, basketball, football, and target shooting.[32,41,86]

Diagnosis of injury is confirmed by electromyographic evidence of isolated long thoracic nerve injury. If other upper extremity or cervical paraspinal muscle EMG abnormalities are present, then other diagnoses such as acute brachial neuropathy must be considered. Treatment involves restriction of activity involving the extremity if pain is a predominant feature. Physical therapy may be useful in strengthening adjacent muscle groups while recovery of the long thoracic nerve occurs. Recovery may take up to 2 years, although some winging may persist.[29] If associated with acute brachial neuropathy, resolution of winging is less likely. In all cases, athletic endeavor can be resumed when the individual can participate without pain and with acceptable function.

SUPRASCAPULAR NERVE

The suprascapular nerve supplies motor innervation to the supraspinatus and infraspinatus muscles and also has fibers extending into the capsule of the glenohumeral joint. It has no cutaneous sensory distribution, so sensory evaluation in suprascapular nerve injury will be unremarkable. The nerve originates from the upper trunk of the brachial plexus and runs in the posterior triangle of the neck, passing under the anterior border of the trapezius. It continues through the suprascapular notch, inferior to the transverse scapular ligament, and gives off a motor branch to the supraspinatus within 1 cm of the notch.[9] The nerve then courses obliquely and laterally around the lateral border of the scapula spine and through the spinoglenoid notch to innervate the infraspinatus muscle.

Injury of the suprascapular nerve can occur at the suprascapular notch or at the spinoglenoid notch. Both supraspinatus and infraspinatus muscles will be affected by proximal nerve injury at the suprascapular notch, while infraspinatus muscle function alone will be affected if the lesion is at the spinoglenoid notch.

Mechanisms of injury include repetitive trauma due to sports such as volleyball or weight lifting, to ganglion cyst or other mass phenomena compressing the nerve or to prolonged compression such as that occurring in backpacking.[1,2,10,28,30,57,80] Fractures of the scapula through the suprascapular notch[26] and glenohumeral dislocation[91] can also lead to injury.

Patients complain of poorly localized shoulder pain. Onset is usually insidious but can be associated with repetitive sports. At times, the only finding will be painless weakness of the external rotators.[28,43] Physical examination may disclose atrophy of the spinati and weakness at abduction or external rotation, or at both. Symptoms and findings are often similar to those of a rotator cuff tear. If an MRI for evaluation of a rotator cuff injury is performed, suprascapular nerve injury can be suspected if an intact but atrophic cuff is identified.[90] EMG will confirm the lesion and identify the site of compression. MRI is indicated in the evaluation of this entity to rule out the presence of a soft tissue mass as the etiology.

Treatment is directed at the specific etiology. If repetitive activity such as volleyball is the source of injury, a conservative trial of rest, anti-inflammatory medication, and strengthening is indicated. This is particularly true of lesions of the spinoglenoid notch. For mass lesions compressing the nerve, excision is often necessary. Occasionally, lesions at the suprascapular notch will not respond to conservative care, and surgical resection of the transverse scapular ligament can be performed with good results.[31,56,63]

AXILLARY NERVE

The axillary nerve passes through the quadrangular space, and its anterior branch winds around the surgical neck of the humerus (Fig. 17-9). It may be injured during fracture of the proximal humerus or during dislocation of the shoulder joint. Injury can also occur from a direct blow and has been reported in football, wrestling, and rugby.[37] Injury to the axillary nerve results in paralysis (Fig. 17-10), subsequent atrophy of the deltoid muscle, and a loss of sensation over the

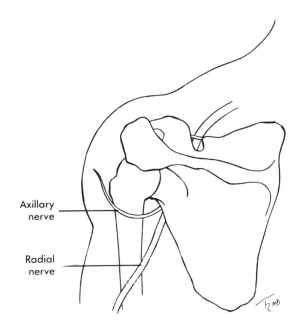

Fig. 17-9. Course of the axillary nerve.

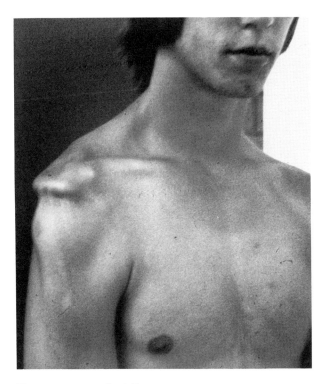

Fig. 17-10. Atrophy following severe axillary nerve lesion. (From Pianka and Hershman,[59] with permission).

lateral side of the proximal arm (deltoid patch). Weakness of shoulder abduction is present.

EMG evaluation is useful for identifying the site of injury along the course of the nerve. Incomplete lesions are treated conservatively, and recovery is likely. Complete lesions can be observed for 3 to 4 months. If no evidence of recovery is noted, exploration and surgical nerve reconstruction are appropriate.

PROGNOSIS

Most authors report better functional results in those patients with infraclavicular versus supraclavicular lesions (Bonney,[12] Leffert and Seddon,[48] and Leffert[45,46]). Yeoman[89] thought that prognosis was related to myelogram results. He correlated poor prognosis with a positive axon response to histamine in the root injured at the level of a pseudomeningocele. Bufulini and Pescatore[15] demonstrated that a posterior cervical EMG was particularly helpful in predicting and localizing plexus lesions. They showed that the presence of denervation potentials on the posterior cervical musculature implied a preganglionic lesion and therefore a bad prognosis. Hoffer et al.[38] believed that serial clinical examination results were more reliable then EMG or myelogram (which are helpful in localizing lesions) for obtaining prognostic information. They also noted return of strength as late as 21 months.

Rorabeck et al.[70] demonstrated that isolated injuries to the upper trunk have a better prognosis than isolated injuries to the cords, upper roots, and lower trunk. They also showed that pain persisting for more than 6 months, regardless of location, was a bad prognostic sign for neurologic recovery.

Bonney[11,12] noted that a poor prognosis for recovery was associated with a triple response to subcutaneous histamine injection into anesthetized skin. The findings of the histamine reflex can be difficult to interpret, especially with the seventh cervical root. In addition, some patients exhibit reactions to the histamine. For these reasons, and because other tests are available, many physicians no longer use this test.[47]

Controversy exists as to whether the presence of Horner syndrome is a prognostic indicator of recovery. Early studies have shown that this syndrome is a poor prognostic indicator of motor recovery.[4,48] However, Horner syndrome may not always be present at the time of injury and may in fact become evident several weeks later.[14] Still other authors have shown that Horner syndrome is not always accompanied by irreparable damage to the first thoracic root.[70] For example, fracture of the first rib may cause injury to the stellate ganglion or to the white rami communicantes. A myelogram should be performed in all cases of Horner syndrome to address injury to the first thoracic root.

TREATMENT

Indications for surgical exploration of closed brachial plexus injuries remain controversial. Bonney[12] originally recommended exploration for all postganglionic injuries if no recovery had been obtained after 8 weeks. Rorabeck and Harris[20] concluded that operation may be indicated in those patients with a postganglionic injury to the upper or lower trunk in whom no recovery occurred within 6 and 8 months of the injury, respectively; and in patients with closed cord injuries in whom no recovery occurred within 8 months. Results of surgery are poor in patients with two or more pseudomeningoceles, since this condition implies irreversible damage to the root.

In general, brachial plexus injuries in athletes are mild, and recovery is likely. Rehabilitation measures are appropriate to facilitate return to sports. Active athletic participation can resume when strength has recovered following these injuries.

REFERENCES

1. Agre JL, Ash N, Careon MC, House J: Suprascapular neuropathy after intensive progressive resistive exercise: case report. Arch Phys Med Rehabil 68:236–238, 1987
2. Aiello I, Serra G, Traina GC, Tugnoli V: Entrapment of the suprascapular nerve at the spinoglenoid notch. Ann Neurol 12:314–316, 1982
3. Archambault JL: Brachial plexus stretch injury. Injury. 31:1983
4. Barnes R: Traction injuries of the brachial plexus in adults. J Bone Joing Surg [Br] 31B:1949
5. Bergfeld J: Brachial plexus injuries. Presented at the American Association of Orthopaedic Surgeons Winter Sports Injuries Course, Steamboat Springs, CO, March 27, 1987
6. Bergfeld JA, Hershman EB, Wilbourn AJ: Brachial plexus injury in sports: a five-year follow-up. Orthop Trans 12:743–744, 1988
7. Bigliani LU, Perez-Sanz JR, Wolfe IN: Treatment of trapezius paralysis. J Bone Joint Surg [Am] 67A:871–877, 1985

8. Bigliani LU, Sakellarides HT: Paralysis of the trapezius. Orthop Consult 10:9, 1989

9. Bigliani LU, Dalsey RM, McCann PD, April EW: An anatomical study of the suprascapular nerve. Arthroscopy 6:301–305, 1990

10. Black KP, Lombardo JA: Suprascapular nerve injuries with isolated paralysis of the infraspinatus. Am Sports Med 18:225–228, 1990

11. Bonney G: The value of axon responses in determining the site of the lesion in traction injuries of the brachial plexus. Brain 77:588–609, 1954

12. Bonney G: Prognosis in traction lesions of the brachial plexus. J Bone Joint Surg [Br] 41B:4–35, 1959

13. Bradley WG, Madrid R, Thrush DC, Campbell MJ: Recurrent brachial plexus neuropathy. Brain 98:381–398, 1975

14. Brooks DM: Open wounds of the brachial plexus. Med Res Council Special Rep Ser (Lond) 282:418–428, 1954

15. Bufalini C, Pescatori G: Posterior cervical electromyography in the diagnosis and prognosis of brachial plexus injuries. J Bone Joint Surg [Br] 51:627–631, 1969

16. Castagno AA, Shuyman WP: MR imaging in clinically suspected brachial plexus tumor. AJR 149:1219–1222, 1987

17. Christman OD, Snook GA, Stanitis JM et al: Lateral flexion neck injuries in athletics. JAMA 192:117–119, 1965

18. Clancy WG: Brachial plexus and upper extremity peripheral nerve injuries. p. 215. Torg JS (ed): Athletic Injuries to the Head, Neck, and Face. Lea & Febiger, Philadelphia, 1982

19. Clancy WG, Brand RL, Bergeld JA: Upper trunk brachial plexus injuries in contact sports. Am J Sports Med 5:209–216, 1977

20. Crafts RC: A Textbook of Human Anatomy. p. 32. 3rd Ed. John Wiley & Sons, New York, 1985

21. Date ES, Rappaport M, Ortega HR: Dermatomal somatosensory evoked potentials in brachial plexus injuries. Clin Electroencephalography 22:236, 1991

22. Davis DH, Onofrio BM, MacCarty S: Brachial plexus injuries. Mayo Clinic Proc 53:799–807, 1978

23. Denny-Brown D, Doherty M: Effects of transient stretching of peripheral nerve. Arch Neurol Psychiatr 54:116-129, 1945

24. Di Benedetto M, Markey K: Electrodiagnostic localization of traumatic upper trunk brachial plexopathy, Arch Phys Med Rehabil 65:1984

25. Dillin, Linden, Hoaglund et al: Brachial neuritis, J Bone Joint Surg [Am] 67A:6, 1985

26. Edeland HG, Zachrisson BE: Fracture of the scapular notch associated with lesion of the suprascapular nerve. Acta Orthop Scand 46:758–763, 1975

27. Enker SH, Murphy KK: Brachial plexus compression by excessive callus formation secondary to a fractured clavicle. A case report. Mt Sinai J Med 37:678–682, 1972

28. Ferretti A, Andrea, Cerullo et al: Suprascapular neuropathy in volleyball players. J Bone Joint Surg 69:260, 1987

29. Foo CL, Swann M: Isolated paralysis of the serratus anterior: a report of 20 cases. J Bone Joint Surg [Br] 65B:552–556, 1983

30. Ganzhorn RW, Hocker JT, Horowitz M, Switzer E: Suprascapular-nerve entrapment: a case report. J Bone Joint Surg [Am] 63A:492–494, 1981

31. Garcia, Guillermo, McQueen D: Bilateral suprascapular-nerve entrapment syndrome. Case report and review of the literature. J Bone Joint Surg [Am] 63A:491–492, 1981

32. Gregg JR, Labosky D, Harty M: Serratus anterior paralysis in the young athlete. J Bone Joint Surg [Am] 61A:825–832, 1979

33. Gupta RK, Mehta VS, Banerji AK, Jain RK: MR evaluation of brachial plexus injuries. Neuroradiology 31:377–381, 1989

34. Heon M: Myelogram a questionable aid in diagnosis and prognosis in avulsion of brachial plexus components by traction injuries. Conn Med 29:260–262, 1965

35. Hershman B: Brachial plexus injuries. Clin Sports Med 9:311–329, 1990

36. Hershman EB, Wilbourn AJ, Bergfeld JA: Acute brachial neuropathy in athletes. Am J Sports Med 17:655–659, 1989

37. Hirasawa Y, Sakakida K: Sports and peripheral nerve injury. Am J Sports Med 11:420–426, 1983

38. Hoffer MM, Braun R, Hsu J et al: JAMA 27:2467–2470, 1981

39. Hoppenfeld, S. Physical Examination of the Spine and Extremities. p. 3. Appleton-Century-Crofts, Norwalk, CT, 1976.

40. Howard FM, Shafer SJ: Injuries to the clavicle with neurovascular complications: a study of fourteen cases. J Bone Joint Surg [Am] 47A:1335–1346

41. Johnson JTH, Kendall HO: Isolated paralysis of the serratus anterior muscle. J Bone Joint Surg [Am] 37A:567–574, 1955

42. Kay SP, Eckardt JJ: Brachial plexus palsy secondary to clavicular nonunion. Case report and literature survey. Clin Orthop 206:219–222, 1986

43. Kukowski B: Suprascapular nerve lesion as an occupational neuropathy in a semiprofessional dancer. Arch Phys Med Rehabil 74:768–769, 1993

44. Landi A, Copeland SA, Parry CB, Jones SJ: The role of somatosensory evoked potentials and nerve conduction studies in the surgical management of brachial plexus injuries. J Bone Joint Surg [Br] 62B:492–496, 1980

45. Leffert RD: Orthop Clin North Am 1:399–417, 1970

46. Leffert RD: Brachial plexus injuries. N Engl J Med 291:1059–1067, 1974

47. Leffert RD. Lesions of the brachial plexus revisited. p. 245. In: American Academy of Orthopaedic Surgeons,

Instructional Course Lectures. Vol. 38. CV Mosby, St Louis, 1989

48. Leffert RD, Seddon H: Infraclavicular brachial plexus injuries J Bone Joint Surg [Br] 47B:9–22, 1965

49. Lorei MP, Hershman EB: Peripheral nerve injuries in athletes: treatment and prevention. Sports Med 16:130–147, 1993

49a. Markey KL et al: Upper trunk brachial plexopathy: the stinger syndrome. Am J Sports Med 21(5):650, 1993

50. Maroon JC: 'Burning hands' in football spinal cord injuries. JAMA 238:1977

51. Marshall RW, De Silva RDD: Computerised axial tomography in traction injuries of the brachial plexus. J Bone Joint Surg [Br] 68-B:1986

52. Matz SO, Welliver PS, Welliver DI: Brachial plexus neuropraxia complicating a comminuted clavicle fracture in a college football player. Am J Sports Med 17:581–583, 1989

53. Miller DS, Boswick JA Jr: Lesions of the brachial plexus associated with fractures of the clavicle. Clin Orthop 64:144–149, 1969

54. Moore KL: Clinically Oriented Anatomy. pp. 608, 640, 641, 642, 651, 1022. Williams & Wilkins, Los Angeles, 1985

55. Murphey F, Hartung W, Kirklin JW: Myelographic demonstration of avulsing injury of the brachial plexus. AJR 58:102, 1947

56. Murray JWG: A surgical approach for entrapment neuropathy of the suprascapular nerve. Orthop Rev 3:33–35, 1974

57. Neviaser TJ, Ain BR, Neviaser RJ: Suprascapular nerve denervation secondary to attenuation by a ganglionic cyst. J Bone Joint Surg 68A:627–628, 1986

58. Personage MJ, Turner JWA: Neuralgic amyotrophy: shoulder-girdle syndrome. Lancet 1:973–978, 1948

59. Pianka G, Hershman EB: Neurovascular injuries. p. 691. In: The Upper Extremity in Sports Medicine. CV Mosby, St Louis, 1990

60. Poindexter DP, Johnson EW: Football shoulder and neck injury: a study of the stinger. Arch Phys Med Rehabil 65:601, 1984

61. Posner MA: Compressive neuropathies of the median and radial nerves. Clin Sports Med 343–363, 1990

62. Rapoport S, Blair DN, McCarthy SM et al: Brachial plexus: correlation of MR imaging with CT and pathologic findings. Radiology 167:161–165, 1988

63. Rask MR: Suprascapular nerve entrapment. A report of two cases treated with suprascapular notch resection. Clin Orthop 123:73–75, 1977

64. Rayan, Ghazi M: Lower trunk brachial plexus compression neuropathy due to cervical rib in young athletes. Am J Sports Med 16: 1988

65. Roaf R: Lateral flexion injuries of the cervical spine. J Bone Joint Surg [Br] 45B:36–38, 1963

66. Robles J. Brachial plexus avulsion: a review of diagnostic procedures and report of six cases. J Neurosurg 28:434–439, 1968

67. Robertson WC Jr, Eichman PL, Clancy WG: Upper trunk brachial plexopathy in football players. JAMA 241:1480, 1979

68. Rockett FX: Observations on the "burner:" traumatic cervical radiculopathy. Clin Orthop 1982:164:18–19

69. Roger B, Travers V, Laval-Jeantet M: Imaging of posttraumatic brachial plexus injury. Clin Orthop 237:57–61, 1988

70. Rorabeck CH, Harris RW: Factors affecting the prognosis of brachial plexus injuries J Bone Joint Surg [Br] 63B:3;404–407, 1981

71. Meyer SA: Cervical spinal stenosis and stingers in collegiate football players. Am J Sports Med 22(2):158, 1984

72. Schaumburg HH: Bell's palsy, brachial neuritis, and trigeminal neuropathy. In Wyngaarden and Smith (eds): Cecil Textbook of Medicine. WB Saunders, Philadelphia 1985

73. Seddon HJ: Three types of nerve injury. Brain 66:237–287, 1943

74. Sherrier RH, Sostman H: Magnetic resonance imaging of the brachial plexus. J Thorac Imaging 8; 1993

75. Speer KP, Bassett H III: The prolonged burner syndrome. Am J Sports Med 18: 1990

76. Spillane JD: Localized neuritis of shoulder girdle: report of 46 cases in MEF. Lancet 2:532–535, 1943

77. Sunderland S: Nerves and Nerve Injuries. Churchill Livingstone, London, 1972

78. Tarlov IM, Day R: Myelography to help localized traction lesions of the brachial plexus. Am J Surg 88:266, 1954

79. Taylor PE: Traumatic intradural avulsion of the nerve roots of the brachial plexus. Brain 85:579–602, 1962

80. Thompson RC Jr, Schneider W, Kennedy T: Entrapment neuropathy of the inferior branch of the suprascapular nerve by ganglia. Clin Orthop 166:185–187, 1982

81. Tsairis P, Dyck PJ, Mulder DW: Natural history of brachial plexus neuropathy: report of 99 patients. Arch Neurol 27:109, 1972

82. Turner JWA, Parsonage MJ: Neuralgic amyotrophy (paralytic brachial neuritis): with special reference to prognosis. Lancet 2:209–212, 1957

83. de Verdier HJ, Colletti M, Terk MR: MRI of the brachial plexus: a review of 51 cases. Comput Med Imaging Graphics. 17:45–50, 1993

84. Wilbourn AJ: Electrodiagnosis of plexopathies. Neurol Clin 3:511–529, 1985

85. Wilbourn AJ: Electrodiagnostic testing of neurologic injuries in athletes. Clin Sports Med 229–245, 1990

86. Woodhead AB III: Paralysis of the serratus anterior in a world class marksman: a case study. Am J Sports Med 13:359–362, 1985

87. Yang SS, Hershman EB: Idiopathic brachial plexus neuropathy: a review. Crit Rev Phys Rehabil Med 5:193–201, 1993

88. Yates DW: Complications of fractures of the clavicle. Injury 7:881–883, 1976

89. Yeoman PM: Cervical myelography in traction injuries of the brachial plexus. J Bone Joint Surg 50B:253–260, 1968

90. Zeiss J, Woldenberg JS, Saddami SR, Ebraheim NA: MRI of suprascapular neuropathy in a weight lifter. J Comput Assist Tomogr 17:303–308, 1993

91. Zoltan JD: Injury of the suprascapular nerve; association with anterior dislocation of the shoulder: case report and review of the literature. J Trauma 19:203–206, 1979

18

Neurovascular Syndromes

CHAMP L. BAKER, JR.

INTRODUCTION

Shoulder injuries in athletes most often involve soft tissue structures. They may also cause injury to neurovascular structures within the shoulder complex, as a result of local trauma or the repetitive overhead activities of throwing athletes. Because of the unusual demands placed on the shoulder of the throwing athlete, normal anatomic structures can become pathologic, compressing nerves and blood vessels. Signs and symptoms can be neurologic or vascular, or both, depending on the nerves or vessels being compressed and on the site of the compression. Diverse clinical presentations can make the diagnosis difficult at times.

Distinct syndromes occur because of compression of specific neurovascular structures at particular anatomic sites. The most commonly recognized neurovascular compression syndromes of the shoulder are

Thoracic outlet syndrome—compression of adjacent neurovascular structures by the clavicle, the first rib, or the scalene anticus muscle

Axillary artery occlusion, by the pectoralis minor muscle

Effort thrombosis—venous thrombosis of the subclavian or axillary veins due to constriction by the clavicle or the first rib

Quadrilateral space syndrome—occlusion of the posterior humeral circumflex artery or axillary nerve in the quadrilateral space.

The first reports on neurovascular compression in the shoulder focused on thoracic outlet syndromes: in 1743 Hunald noted that cervical ribs were a cause of thoracic outlet compression.[44] Coote[13] reported on a successful thoracic decompression after he excised the cervical rib. Stopford and Telford[38] showed that surgical removal of the first thoracic rib alleviated symptoms associated with compression of thoracic outlet structures compressed by the rib. Similar findings were reported by Wheeler,[48] Brickner and Milch,[6] and Telford and Mottershead.[41] Adson and Coffey[2] reported success in relieving thoracic outlet compression by sectioning the scalenus anticus muscle. Their results were supported by Ochsner and associates[26] and Naffiziger and Grant.[24]

Costoclavicular compression of neurovascular structures, as a result of hyperabduction of the arm, was reported by a number of different authors in the 1930s and 1940s.[15,16,21] In 1945, Wright[49] described a hyperabduction syndrome, in which the middle portion of the axillary artery became occluded due to external pressure by the pectoralis minor muscle when the arm was brought overhead.

Thrombosis of the subclavian vein was described by Sir James Paget[27] in 1875 and Von Schroetter[47] in 1884 (known as the Paget-Schroetter syndrome). Matas[23] reported on its existence in 1934. The condition is currently termed *effort thrombosis* because of the associated physical activity that produces direct or indirect trauma to the vein.

While studying treatment failure of thoracic outlet syndrome, Cahill[10,11] noted that a high percentage was due to occlusion of the posterior humeral circumflex artery. Further investigation led to the recognition of quadrilateral space syndrome.

SPECIFIC SYNDROMES
Thoracic Outlet Syndrome

The thoracic outlet is bounded superiorly by the lower border of the clavicle and inferiorly by the upper border of the first rib. This space is divided by the scalene muscles. The anterior scalene muscle originates from the transverse process of the third, fourth, fifth, and sixth cervical vertebrae and inserts posterior to the subclavian vein into the first rib. The middle scalene muscle, which originates from the transverse process of the second through the seventh cervical vertebrae, inserts behind the subclavian artery into the first rib. The subclavian artery and the brachial plexus enter between the anterior and midline scalene muscles (Fig. 18-1). The neurovascular bundle (including the axillary artery) courses more distally underneath the pectoralis minor muscle.

Thoracic outlet syndrome is an ill-defined term that encompasses the signs and symptoms attributed to compression of the neurovascular structures as they traverse from the neck to the axilla. Because of the proximity to one another of nerves and vessels in the thoracic outlet, varying degrees of compression of the brachial plexus and subclavian vessels can occur. Proximal compression may occur as they pass between the anterior and middle scalene muscle; more distally, compression may occur through the costoclavicular space; and most distally, compression proximal to the axilla may occur as they pass underneath the pectoralis minor muscle.

Numerous causes have been suggested for thoracic outlet syndromes. Cervical ribs are the most commonly noted bony abnormality associated with the syndrome, although less than 10% of the individuals who have cervical ribs have symptoms related to thoracic outlet compression.[8] Fibrous bands originating from the end of a prominent C7 transverse process or from the end of a short cervical rib can also cause mechanical compression within the thoracic outlet.[19] When present, anomalous fibromuscular bands within the scalene muscles can entrap the upper trunk of the brachial plexus.[31,37] Following clavicular fracture, excessive callus formation or malunion may decrease the costoclavicular space.[5]

Thoracic outlet syndrome has also been associated in recent years with the trauma and anatomic changes that can occur as a result of the mechanics of throwing.[19,25,30,39] Injury to the shoulder muscles may cause hemorrhage and abnormal shoulder mechanics, which can result in subsequent functional impairment and secondary neurovascular compression.

Axillary Artery Occlusion

Anatomically, the axillary artery is the main artery of the upper extremity. It originates as a continuation of the subclavian artery at the lateral border of the first rib and is divided into three segments: the first, proximal to the pectoralis minor muscle; the second, deep to the muscle; and the third, distal to the muscle (Fig. 18-2). It has six primary branches: the superior thoracic artery, medial to the pectoralis minor muscle; the thoracoacromial artery and lateral thoracic artery, at the level of the pectoralis minor muscle; and the subscapular artery and posterior and anterior circumflex humeral arteries, prior to the origin of the brachial artery.

Wright[49] described a hyperabduction syndrome, whereby the middle portion of the axillary artery became occluded secondary to pressure from the overlying pectoralis minor muscle when the arm was brought overhead. This movement of the arm became the classic hyperabduction maneuver of Wright. Tullos and associates[43] were the first to report this syndrome in baseball pitchers. Transient occlusion of the axillary

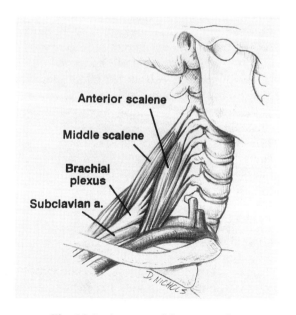

Fig. 18-1. Anatomy of thoracic outlet.

Anterior scalene

Middle scalene

Brachial plexus

Subclavian a.

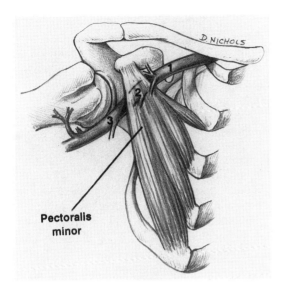

Fig. 18-2. Anatomy of axillary artery.

artery, secondary to pressure from the pectoralis minor muscle, was noted during the cocking phase of each pitch when the arm was abducted, externally rotated, and extended. The syndrome has since been reported in other throwing athletes and a windsurfer, in whom injury was caused by repetitive overhead activities requiring hyperabduction and external rotation of the shoulder joint.[25,30,32]

Effort Thrombosis

The axillary vein, located medial to the axillary artery, originates as a continuation of the basilic vein at the lower border of the teres major muscle. It becomes the subclavian vein at the lateral border of the first rib (Fig. 18-3). The subclavian vein follows the same general course as the subclavian artery; the two are separated by the anterior scalene muscle near its insertion into the first rib.

The axillary vein can become compressed at various sites along its track, the most significant being in the costoclavicular space.[42] Compression here most often occurs when patients hyperextend their neck and hyperabduct their arm at the same time, or when they assume a military brace position with a backward thrust of the shoulders. Other areas where compression can occur are between the clavicle and first rib, the costo-

cortacoid ligament and first rib, or the subclavian muscles and first rib.

The term effort thrombosis is used because of the frequent association with repetitive, vigorous activities or blunt trauma that results in direct or indirect injury to the vein.[46] However, this clinical entity has been noted in healthy individuals with no apparent predisposing causes.[36] Even though effort thrombosis is rare—it comprises just 2 percent of all venous thromboses and only 53 sports-related cases have been reported—athletes who perform repetitive and vigorous upper extremity activities are clearly at risk of developing the condition.[1,34] Sports activities that have been linked with effort thrombosis include swimming, basketball, tennis, golf, rowing, handball, volleyball, weightlifting, football, baseball, gymnastics, and hockey.[14,20,25,30,34,36,40,46]

Quadrilateral Space Syndrome

The quadrilateral space is located over the posterior scapula and subdeltoid area. It is bounded superiorly by the teres minor muscle, inferiorly by the teres major muscle, medially by the long head of the triceps muscles, and laterally by the surgical neck of the humerus (Fig. 18-4). Quadrilateral space syndrome, first described by Cahill and Palmer in 1967, involves compression of the axillary nerve (or one of its major branches) and the posterior humeral circumflex artery, which pass through this area.[10,11] Fibrous bands located in the quadrilateral space can also compress the nerves and vessels when the arm is abducted and externally rotated. Recent reports have noted this syndrome in throwing athletes.[25,28,30]

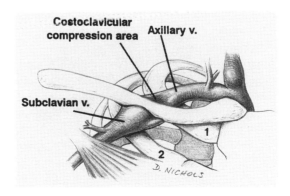

Fig. 18-3. Anatomy of subclavian and axillary vein.

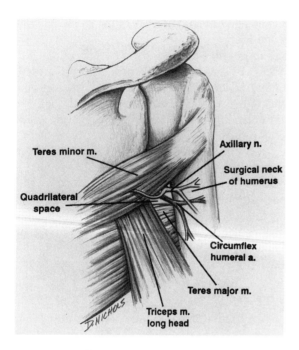

Fig. 18-4. Anatomy of quadrilateral space.

CLINICAL PRESENTATION

Signs and Symptoms

Thoracic Outlet Syndrome

Signs and symptoms depend on the degree to which particular neurovascular structures are compromised and are similar to those of any compression of the nerves, arteries, or veins in the thorax. If nerves and vessels are both being compressed, a mixed pattern of neurologic and vascular symptoms may be present. In athletes, symptoms usually are associated with specific throwing or overhead activities and can be elicited by repeating the movement.

Primary compression of the lower trunk of the brachial plexus usually causes pain and paresthesia from the patient's neck and shoulder down to the medial aspect of the hand, with associated weakness of grasp and difficulty with fine finger movements. Compression of the upper trunk of the brachial plexus causes more obscure symptoms, with pain more proximal in the neck and shoulder region. The symptoms are frequently similar to those of cervical disk herniation.

Signs and symptoms of vascular compression will vary depending on the degree of arterial and venous compromise. Arterial insufficiency usually produces symptoms of claudication, coolness, numbness, and exertional fatigue. Venous obstruction causes venous engorgement, upper limb edema, heaviness, and cyanosis. Discoloration, ulceration, and, infrequently, symptoms of Raynaud syndrome also may be present.[22]

Axillary Artery Occlusion

Patients may present with pain, tenderness over the pectoralis minor area, claudication, fatigue, cool skin, diminished or absent distal pulses, and cyanosis. These symptoms can often be reproduced when the patient's arm is hyperabducted and externally rotated. Definitive diagnosis, however, usually depends on angiography and demonstration of thrombosis with complete occlusion of the axillary artery or an aneurysmal dilation of the artery secondary to partial occlusion.

Effort Thrombosis

Symptoms usually occur within 24 hours after the preceding trauma or precipitating activity and are limited to the upper extremity involved. Most often the patient will complain of a dull aching pain, numbness, and "heaviness" of the upper arm and shoulder, along with fatigue following activities involving the extremity. The entire upper extremity will be edematous, the skin may be mottled and cold, and superficial veins may be prominent. Pulses most often are normal, although hyperesthesia in a nondermatomal pattern may be present. Occasionally, a tender, cord-like structure may be palpated in the axilla. These physical signs may become more pronounced when the patient is instructed to perform overhead arm activities or exercise tests.

Quadrilateral Space Syndrome

Patients usually complain of poorly localized pain and paresthesia in the upper extremity, without associated trauma. The pain is exacerbated when the arm is abducted and externally rotated, and it often interferes with overhead arm or throwing activities. Although point tenderness may be elicited over the affected quadrilateral area, the physical and neurologic examinations usually are normal.

Physical Examination

The physical examination should emphasize the shoulder girdle and cervical spine as well as three particular tests (Adson's test, costoclavicular maneuver, and hyperabduction maneuver) to localize the anatomic site of compression. During patient inspection, the examiner should pay special attention to the presence of shoulder asymmetry, poor muscular development, or unusually large breasts. These findings may indicate developmental or postural abnormalities that can predispose a patient to neurovascular compression syndromes.[19]

In *Adson's test*, as described by Alford Adson,[2] the patient is instructed to inhale deeply, extend the neck, and turn the chin toward the involved shoulder (Fig. 18-5). Diminished or absent radial pulse or change in blood pressure during this maneuver demonstrates compression of the subclavian artery by the scalene anticus muscle, indicating thoracic outlet syndrome.

For the *costoclavicular maneuver*, the patient thrusts the shoulders backward and downward, similar to a military brace position[4] (Fig. 18-6). Doing so decreases the space between the clavicle and the first rib and compresses the neurovascular structures located in this area.

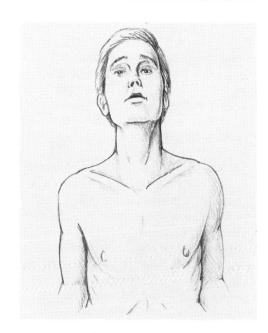

Fig. 18-6. Costoclavicular maneuver.

In the *hyperabduction maneuver*, as described by Wright,[49] the patient inhales deeply and turns the head to the side opposite the affected shoulder, as the involved arm is abducted and externally rotated (Fig. 18-7). This test is most specific for neurovascular compression in the subcoracoid area, especially compres-

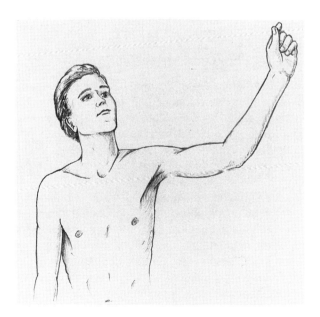

Fig. 18-5. Adson's test.

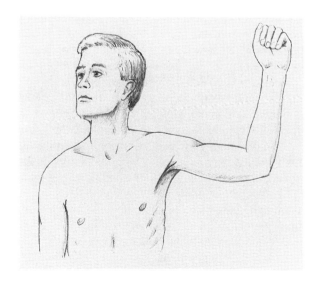

Fig. 18-7. Hyperabduction maneuver.

sion of the middle portion of the axillary artery under the pectoralis minor muscle.

It must be remembered that all these tests can produce false-positive or false-negative results. Several authors have reported that up to 50 percent of normal asymptomatic individuals have a positive Adson's test.[29,33] Therefore a test should only be considered truly positive when the maneuver reproduces the patient's symptoms.

Some additional physical findings may help the examiner establish the diagnosis of neurovascular compression syndrome. Pain or paresthesia elicited by firm pressure on or percussion over the brachial plexus in the supraclavicular fossa may indicate nerve irritation at the site of compression. The presence of bruits during provocative testing is a sign of vascular compromise. The overhead exercise test, performed with the patient sitting down, rapidly flexing and extending the fingers while keeping the arms elevated overhead, is considered positive when the symptoms are reproduced.[19]

ANCILLARY DIAGNOSTIC STUDIES

The presence of cervical or first thoracic ribs, or irregularities of the clavicle or first rib, should be determined with plain radiographs of the cervical spine. Cervical ribs, the most common bony abnormalities associated with neurovascular compression, originate from the transverse process of C7 and normally attach directly or by ligaments to the first rib. Fewer than 10 percent of patients with cervical ribs have symptoms of neurovascular compression.[8] Abnormalities or fractures of the clavicle or first rib, which can result in compression of nerves and vessels depending on the position of the bones, may be seen on an anteroposterior view. Arthritic changes of the cervical spine may cause nerve root compression, resulting in symptoms similar to those found in neurovascular compression syndromes. Chest radiographs can rule out conditions that may refer pain to the shoulder.

Although differences of opinion exist on the usefulness or reliability of electrodiagnostic tests (e.g., nerve conduction studies and evoked potential stimulation) in confirming the diagnosis of neurovascular compression syndromes, they can be helpful in ruling out more peripheral lesions at the elbow or wrist (e.g., carpal tunnel syndrome or ulnar nerve neuropathy),

or in the differential diagnosis of cervical radiculopathy with referred shoulder pain.[4,18,29,31,33,37,45]

Noninvasive and invasive vascular studies can also be used to assist in the diagnosis of neurovascular compression.[4,10,43,49] Doppler ultrasound, an effective modality for measuring arterial blood flow in the arm, has been successfully used to screen throwing athletes.[25] Digital subtraction angiography may be used in place of arteriograms in certain patients. Definitive diagnosis of vascular compromise, however, depends on venogram and angiogram studies of the subclavian and axillary vessels. It is important to perform these studies with the patient's involved arm in both the normal anatomic position and the position in which the symptoms are produced.

The presence of thrombi occluding the axillary or subclavian veins is the typical finding in cases of effort thrombosis. Extensive collateralization and recanalization of the thrombosed vein may be seen.[36,46] The diagnosis of quadrilateral space syndrome is based on a subclavian arteriogram performed with the arm held both at the patient's side and in an abducted, externally rotated position. In affected patients, the subclavian arteriogram will show a patient posterior humeral circumflex artery with the arm at its side, but occlusion of the artery when the arm is hyperabducted and externally rotated.

TREATMENT
Thoracic Outlet Syndrome

Initial treatment is directed toward alleviating the pain, usually with nonsteroidal anti-inflammatory drugs, local trigger-point injections, and by having the patient refrain from the precipitating activity until the symptoms resolve. Patients with vascular problems need to have appropriate invasive studies and follow-up treatment.

As the pain and inflammation subside, a rehabilitative exercise program should be established to correct any postural abnormalities (rounded shoulders and a head-forward position can contribute to neurovascular compression) and to strengthen the shoulder girdle and scapular musculature.[1] It is important, though, not to exacerbate the patient's symptoms with the exercises.

The trapezius muscle group (the suspension structure for the shoulder girdle) and the parascapular muscles (which assist in correct shoulder alignment) can be strengthened by having the patient perform shoulder shrugs with scapular abduction exercises. The scapular rotators can be strengthened by having the patient perform abduction in the plane of the scapula, sitting dips, bent rows, and push ups with protraction of the shoulder girdle. Each exercise should be performed 10 times with 0 to 5 lb for three to five sets at least twice a day.

Pulling the patient's head forward and to the opposite side while rotating toward the tight side may help stretch the levator scapulae if it is tight. It may be possible to relieve symptoms secondary to scalene muscle involvement by extending and rotating the patient's head and neck toward the affected side to stretch the anterior muscles, and laterally flexing and rotating the head and neck away from the affected side to stretch the posterior muscles. Stretching should be done 15 to 25 times at least three times a day. Although symptoms caused by congenital abnormalities (e.g., cervical ribs or fibrous bands at C7) are difficult to treat with exercises, increasing spinal flexibility with various stretching exercises may help to decrease compression. In addition to these exercises, having the patient sleep supine or in the semi-side-lying position with a small pillow supporting the thoracic spine may help to "open" the thoracic outlet.

Surgery is indicated only if well-directed rehabilitation fails to relieve the patient's pain and improve functional impairment. Occasionally, surgical decompression is recommended in cases of acute vascular insufficiency or progressive neurologic symptoms. Surgical intervention depends on the particular cause of the syndrome and includes excision of the cervical rib, scalenotomy of the scalene anticus muscle, and release of fibromuscular bands located in the thorax at the site of occlusion.[4] Good to excellent results have been reported by many surgeons, with unsatisfactory outcomes usually due to poor patient selection or a coexisting medical condition.[17]

Axillary Artery Occlusion

Increasing flexibility of the pectoralis minor muscle is important when it is causing compression of the axillary artery. Overhead stretching may help loosen the muscle, and light strengthening exercises (e.g., sitting dips) may alleviate spasms in the area. These stretching exercises may not be effective, though, since the compression is caused by hyperabduction and external rotation of the arm. Strengthening the posterior rotator cuff may protect against added stress on the anterior shoulder neurovascular structures by minimizing subluxation of the humeral head during the acceleration phase of throwing. The patient should be instructed to perform prone horizontal abduction, prone external rotation, and external rotation exercises with the arm at 0 degrees abduction.

Although stretching and strengthening exercises may help reduce symptoms, surgery usually is required to treat axillary artery occlusion effectively. Commonly used operative procedures include thrombectomy, sympathectomy, segmental excisions, bypass with vascular graft, anastomosis, and angioplasty.[25,30,43]

Effort Thrombosis

Initial treatment is directed toward relieving patient symptoms and enabling the individual to resume previous athletic activities. Rest and elevation of the affected extremity usually decrease the acute pain and swelling within 3 to 4 days; however, many conservatively treated patients suffer continuing symptoms due to continuing venous occlusion and inadequate collateral flow, resulting in possible long-term disability.[1]

Anticoagulation therapy with heparin, followed by warfarin, is often used in the acute phase to inhibit progression of the thrombus.[1,36,46] Some authors, however, have reported that up to 50 percent of their patients treated with anticoagulation therapy continued to have symptoms and that some developed pulmonary embolism despite the use of anticoagulation medication.[1,12] Recently, streptokinase has been found effective for the lysis of acute intravenous clots, but not for chronic clots.[35,40]

Good long-term results with no residual symptoms have been reported with surgical intervention, including early thrombectomy with simultaneous decompression of the thoracic outlet and first rib resection following fibrinolytic therapy.[1,3,12,40]

Although athletic activities requiring repetitive and vigorous shoulder activities have been implicated as causes of effort thrombosis, few reports exist on the return-to-play status of patients treated for this condition. In a study of hockey players, one player who had developed both subclavian vein thrombosis and pulmonary embolism was able to return to professional hockey 8 weeks after anticoagulation therapy.[9]

He was still playing 4 years later. In another report, two athletes (a quarterback and a swimmer) were able to resume college competition after thrombolytic treatment and first rib resection.[14] One high school athlete (a football quarterback and baseball pitcher) returned to pitching after anticoagulation therapy but his subclavian vein rethrombosed 5 months later.[34]

Quadrilateral Space Syndrome

Treatment of quadrilateral space syndrome includes symptomatic care, reassurance, and surgical decompression if conservative methods fail to alleviate the symptoms. A baseball pitcher was reported to have obtained symptomatic relief by altering his pitching delivery from overhead to three-quarters.[28] Physical therapy consisting of gentle internal rotation stretching of the shoulder joint, horizontal stretching into adduction, and strengthening of the posterior rotator cuff may help relieve patient symptoms. For patients who continue to be symptomatic, surgical decompression of the quadrilateral space via a posterior approach has been recommended.[10]

DIFFERENTIAL DIAGNOSIS

Other conditions of the shoulder and arm can produce symptoms similar to those resulting from compression of neurovascular structures. These include (1) diseases of the cervical spine, (2) acute brachial neuropathy, (3) carpal tunnel syndrome, (4) cubital tunnel syndrome, and (5) peripheral nerve injuries of the shoulder involving the suprascapular nerve, axillary nerve, long thoracic nerve, musculocutaneous nerve, spinal accessory nerve, or dorsal scapular nerves. These lesions may occur as isolated entities. A thorough history and physical examination, along with electromyographic and nerve conduction studies, can help in the diagnosis of these conditions and can distinguish them from neurovascular compression syndromes.

CONCLUSIONS

Recent interest in injuries of the throwing athlete has led to a better understanding of neurovascular compression syndromes of the shoulder. However, because the signs and symptoms are often vague and obscure (ranging from exertional fatigue to frank anesthesia and loss of blood supply), recognizing these conditions can be difficult. Accurate diagnosis requires (1) a thorough history and detailed physical examination with emphasis on Adson's test, the costoclavicular maneuver, and Wright's hyperabduction maneuver; and (2) ancillary diagnostic studies including cervical and chest radiographs, Doppler measurements, venography, arteriography, and possibly electromyelograms and nerve conduction studies.

Initial treatment usually is conservative, including postural and shoulder girdle strengthening exercises and avoidance of precipitating activities until symptoms are resolved. Anticoagulation or thrombolytic therapy may be indicated in cases of vascular occlusion. Surgery usually is reserved for patients in whom nonoperative treatment fails and includes thrombectomy, sympathectomy, segmental excisions, and vascular bypass grafts. Surgical decompression to enlarge the floor of the thoracic outlet may be indicated for chronic symptomatic patients. With proper treatment, most patients are able to resume their athletic activities in a timely fashion with minimal disability.

REFERENCES

1. Adams JT, DeWeese JA: 'Effort' thrombosis of the axillary and subclavian veins. J Trauma 11:923–930, 1971
2. Adson AW, Coffey JR: Cervical rib: method of anterior approach for relief of symptoms by division of scalenus anticus. Ann Surg 85:839–857, 1927
3. Aziz S, Straehley CJ, Whelan TJ: Effort related axillosubclavian vein thrombosis. A new theory of pathogenesis and a plea for direct surgical intervention. Am J Surg 152:57–61, 1986
4. Baker CL, Thornberry R: Neurovascular syndromes. pp. 176–188. In Zarins B (ed): Injuries to the Throwing Arm. WB Saunders, Philadelphia, 1985
5. Bateman JE: Nerve injuries about the shoulder in sports. J Bone Joint Surg [Am] 49A:785–792, 1967
6. Brickner WM, Milch H: First dorsal, simulating cervical rib by maldevelopment or by pressure symptoms. Surg Obstet Gynecol 40:38–44, 1925
7. Britt LP: Nonoperative treatment of thoracic outlet syndrome symptoms. Clin Orthop 51:45–48, 1967
8. Brown C: Compressive, invasive referred pain to the shoulder. Clin Orthop 173:55–62, 1983
9. Butsch JL: Subclavian thrombosis following hockey injuries. Am J Sports Med 11:448–450, 1983
10. Cahill BR: Quadrilateral space syndrome. pp. 602–606.

In Omer GE, Spinner M (eds): Management of Peripheral Nerve Problems. WB Saunders, Philadelphia, 1980

11. Cahill BR, Palmer RE: Quadrilateral space syndrome. J Hand Surg 8:65–69, 1983

12. Campbell CB, Chandler JG, Tegtmeyer CJ et al: Axillary, subclavian and brachiocephalic vein obstruction. Surgery 82:816–826, 1977

13. Coote H: Pressure on the axillary vessels and nerve by an exostosis from a cervical rib; interference with the circulation of the arm, removal of the rib and exostosis; recovery. Med Times 2:108, 1861

14. Donayre CE, White GH, Mehringer SM, Wilson SE: Pathogenesis determines later morbidity of axillosubclavian vein thrombosis. Am J Surg 152:179–184, 1986

15. Eden KC: The vascular complications of cervical ribs and first thoracic rib abnormalities. Br J Surg 27:111–139, 1939

16. Falconer MA, Weddell G: Costoclavicular compression of the subclavian artery and vein. Relation to the scalenus anticus syndrome. Lancet 2:539, 1943

17. Hawkes CD: Neurosurgical considerations in thoracic outlet syndrome. Clin Orthop 207:24–28, 1986

18. Huffman JD: Electrodiagnostic techniques for and conservative treatment of thoracic outlet syndrome. Clin Orthop 207:21–23, 1986

19. Karas SE: Thoracic outlet syndrome. Clin Sports Med 9:297–310, 1990

20. Kleinsasser LJ: Effort thrombosis of the axillary and subclavian vein. Arch Surg 59:258–274, 1949

21. Lewis T, Pickering G: Observations upon maladies in which the blood supply to digits ceases intermittently or permanently. Clin Sci 1:327–366, 1934

22. Lord JW, Rosati LM: Thoracic-outlet syndrome. Clin Symp 23:3–34, 1971

23. Matas R: Primary thrombosis of the axillary vein caused by strain. Am J Surg 24:642–666, 1934

24. Naffziger HC, Grant WT: Neuritis of the brachial plexus, mechanical in origin: the scalenus syndrome. Surg Obstet Gynecol 67:722–730, 1938

25. Nuber GW, McCarthy WJ, Yao JST, et al: Arterial abnormalities of the shoulder in athletes. Am J Sports Med 18:514–519, 1990

26. Ochsner A, Gage M, DeBakey M: Scalenus anticus (Naffziger) syndrome. Am J Surg 28:669–695, 1935

27. Paget J: Clinical Lectures and Essays. Longman's Green, London, 1875

28. Redler MR, Ruland LJ, McCue FC: Quadrilateral space syndrome in a throwing athlete. Am J Sports Med 14:511–513, 1986

29. Riddell DH, Smith BM: Thoracic and vascular aspects of the thoracic outlet syndrome, 1986 update. Clin Orthop 207:31–36, 1986

30. Rohrer MJ, Cardullo PA, Pappas AM et al: Axillary artery compression and thrombosis in throwing athletes. J Vasc Surg 11:761–769, 1990

31. Roos DB: The place for scalenectomy and first rib resection in thoracic outlet syndrome. Surgery 92:1077–1085, 1982

32. Sadat-Ali M, Al-Awami SM: Wind-surfing injury to the axillary artery. Br J Sports Med 19:165–166, 1985

33. Sellke FW, Kelley TR: Thoracic outlet syndrome. Am J Surg 156:54–57, 1988

34. Skerker RS, Flandry FC: Painless arm swelling in a high school football player. Med Sci Sports Exerc 24:1185–1189, 1992

35. Smith-Behn J, Althar R, Katz W: Primary thrombosis of the axillary/subclavian vein. South Med J 79:1176–1178, 1986

36. Sotta RP: Vascular problems in the proximal upper extremity. Clin Sports Med 9:379–388, 1990

37. Stallworth JM, Horne JB: Diagnosis and management of thoracic syndrome. Arch Surg 119:1149–1151, 1984

38. Stopford JSB, Telford ED: Compression of the lower trunk of the brachial plexus by a first dorsal rib. Br J Surg 7:168–177, 1919

39. Strukel RJ, Garrick JG: Thoracic outlet compression in athletes. A report of four cases. Am J Sports Med 6:35–39, 1978

40. Taylor LM, McAllister WR, Dennis DL, Porter JM: Thrombolytic therapy followed by first rib resection for spontaneous "effort" subclavian vein thrombosis. Am J Surg 149:644–647, 1985

41. Telford ED, Mottershead S: Pressure at the cervicobrachial junction. J Bone Joint Surg 30B:249–265, 1948

42. Tilney NL, Griffiths HJG, Edwards EA: Natural history of major venous thrombosis of the upper extremity. Arch Surg 101:792, 1970

43. Tullos HS, Erwin WD, Woods GW et al: Unusual lesions of the pitching arm. Clin Orthop 88:169–182, 1972

44. Tyson RR, Kaplan GF: Modern concepts of diagnosis and treatment of the thoracic outlet syndrome. Orthop Clin North Am 6:507–519, 1975

45. Urschel HC Jr, Razzuk MA: Management of thoracic outlet syndrome. N Engl J Med 286:1140–1143, 1972

46. Vogel CM, Jensen JE: 'Effort' thrombosis of the subclavian vein in a competitive swimmer. Am J Sports Med 13:269–272, 1985

47. Von Schroetter L: Erkrankungen der Gefasse. In: Nothnagel Handbuch der Pathologie und Therapie. Holder, Wien, 1884

48. Wheeler WI: Compression neuritis due to the normal first dorsal rib. Practitioner 104:409, 1920

49. Wright IS: The neurovascular syndrome produced by hyperabduction of the arms. Am Heart J 29:1, 1945

19

Athletic Training of the Upper Extremity

JAMES J. IRRGANG
DAVE PEZZULLO
MARNIE ALLEGRUCCI

INTRODUCTION

Injury to the upper extremity results in pain and disuse, accompanied by loss of motion, muscle atrophy, and loss of neuromuscular control and coordination. Rehabilitation following injury is used to restore range of motion (ROM) and muscle function. Once these have been restored, specific exercises and activities need to be performed to recondition and prepare the athlete for return to sports. These activities must condition the athlete to withstand the demands imposed by the sport. The reconditioning and return to sport activities must be designed specifically for the sport that the athlete is involved in to allow the athlete to withstand the stresses and strains inherent in the particular sport. Additionally, the conditioning program should allow for development of neuromuscular control and skill to enhance performance and prevent recurrence of the injury. Failure to prepare the athlete adequately for return to sport may result in pain and reinjury as well as diminished performance. The purpose of this chapter is to describe the exercises and activities used to progress the athlete from rehabilitation to reconditioning and return to sport following sport-related injuries to the upper limb. The theoretic basis for these activities and guidelines for progression are discussed.

BIOMECHANICAL CONSIDERATIONS FOR UPPER EXTREMITY SPORTS

Overhead Throwing Sports

Overhead throwing sports include baseball, volleyball, and tennis. The throwing mechanism for baseball, in particular for pitchers, has been described in detail.[9,9a,14,15,23,26,28,30,37] The biomechanics of tennis and volleyball have been less well described; however, they are similar to those involved in throwing a baseball. The throwing mechanism is characterized by an extreme ROM at the shoulder and joint velocities in excess of 6,000 degrees/sec for the shoulder and 4,500 degrees/sec for the elbow.[28] This motion is produced and controlled by concentric and eccentric contraction of muscles to accelerate and decelerate the arm, respectively. These contractions produce high loads on the musculotendinous unit and joint structures. Injury may result if the arm is not adequately conditioned to accept these stresses.

The throwing mechanism can be divided into four stages: wind-up, cocking, acceleration, and deceleration and follow-through[14,15,28] (Fig. 19-1). Wind-up begins with both feet on the ground and the throwing arm shifted away from the direction of the throw. During wind-up the contralateral leg is raised. The player

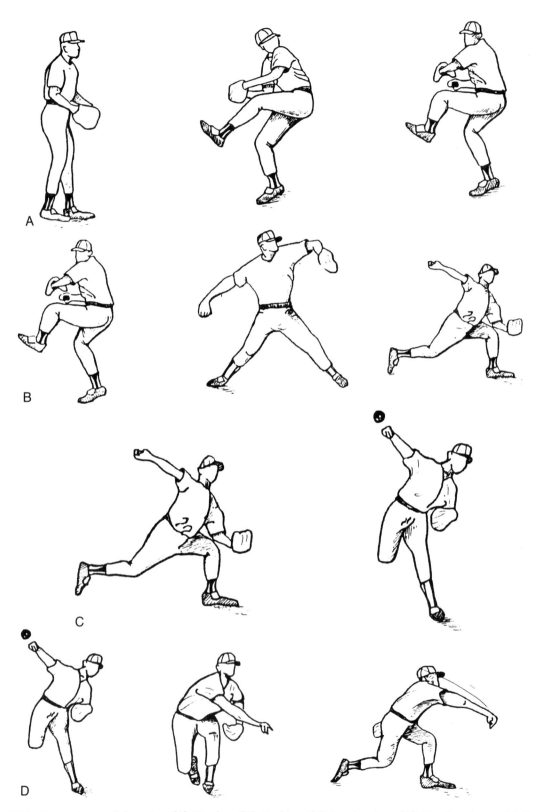

Fig. 19-1. Four phases of throwing. **(A)** Windup. **(B)** Cocking. **(C)** Acceleration. **(D)** Deceleration and follow-through.

should be balanced at the top of the leg kick. Wind-up ends with removal of the ball from the glove. The forces during wind-up are low and the muscle activity is minimal and quite variable.[14]

During cocking, the trunk and lower body move forward while the arm and ball lag behind. The shoulder is abducted to 90 degrees and by the end of this stage the arm is maximally externally rotated to 160 degrees.[28] This is not pure glenohumeral rotation, but rather a composite of glenohumeral and scapulothoracic rotation combined with trunk extension. At the end of cocking, the anterior and inferior capsule and internal rotators are maximally stretched. This preloading of the internal rotators prepares the muscles for the subsequent maximum contraction, which allows for acceleration of the ball during the next phase of throwing. At the end of cocking, the internal rotators are eccentrically loaded to decelerate further external rotation. This eccentric contraction facilitates the stretch reflex and stores energy in the elastic component of the muscle, both of which contribute to the force of the concentric contraction that follows. Training to recondition the throwing athlete must include eccentric exercise for the internal rotators at the end range of external rotation. At the end of cocking, the elbow is flexed to 90 degrees and the wrist is slightly extended.

Cocking can be further divided into an early and late phase. The early phase of cocking begins when the ball leaves the glove and ends when the contralateral foot makes contact with the ground.[14] At the end of early cocking, the shoulder has reached a position of 90 degrees of abduction, 30 degrees of horizontal abduction, and 90 to 120 degrees of external rotation.[28] Additionally, the elbow has reached 90 degrees of flexion and the wrist is in the neutral position. Late cocking occurs from ground contact of the contralateral foot until maximum external rotation has been reached.

During the early phase of cocking, peak electromyographic (EMG) activity develops in the anterior, middle, and posterior deltoid, allowing the arm to be elevated to 90 degrees. At the end of the early phase of cocking, the supraspinatus, infraspinatus, and teres minor begin to contract. Activity in these muscles increases during the late phase of cocking. Contraction of the posterior rotator cuff muscles during this period of time assists in producing maximum external rotation while at the same time controlling anterior translation

of the humeral head.[28] Toward the end of cocking, the subscapularis becomes active to decelerate external rotation and to prepare for rapid acceleration of the arm and ball. In the late phase of cocking peak activity also occurs in the serratus anterior and pectoralis major. Activity in the serratus anterior initiates protraction of the scapula, and contraction of the pectoralis major decelerates external rotation of the shoulder.[26] Throughout cocking, moderate activity occurs in the biceps muscle,[15,37] which serves to flex the elbow. The wrist flexors and forearm pronators demonstrate activity throughout cocking that reaches a peak just prior to maximum rotation.[36] Contraction of these muscles during cocking protects the elbow from excessive valgus stress.[37]

Acceleration begins with forward movement of the shoulder and arm and ends with release of the ball. This stage is very short, comprising less than 1/20 of a second, during which the ball must be accelerated to more than 80 miles an hour.[28] Ball release occurs with the shoulder between 40 and 60 degrees of external rotation, and the arm is abducted to approximately 90 degrees. Individuals who throw "over the top" do so through a greater degree of side bending of the trunk to the contralateral side. Individuals with a side arm delivery do so with less lateral trunk flexion.[28] During acceleration the scapula protracts and the glenohumeral joint internally rotates and horizontally adducts. The muscles responsible for internal rotation and horizontal adduction show strong activity; these muscles include the subscapularis, pectoralis major, and latissimus dorsi. Strong activity in the serratus anterior produces protraction of the shoulder. During acceleration the elbow rapidly extends and ball release occurs with the elbow in approximately 20 to 25 degrees of flexion.[28,37] Peak angular velocity for elbow extension during acceleration was reported to average 4,500 degrees/sec by Pappas et al.[28] and 2,300 degrees/sec by Werner et al.[37] During this period, the triceps show increased EMG activity, accompanied by a decrease in biceps activity.[37] During acceleration, the wrist flexes from a position of extension to neutral at ball release. The forearm is pronating during this time, and ball release occurs with the forearm pronated 90 degrees.[28] Movement of the forearm and wrist during acceleration is accompanied by continued activity in the wrist flexors and forearm pronators.[37]

After the ball is released from the hand, the shoulder continues to rotate internally and to adduct horizontally across the body. The elbow undergoes a rebound effect and flexes to approximately 45 degrees. The forearm remains pronated.[28] During deceleration and follow-through the arm motion, which has been accelerated to its maximum velocity at ball release, must now be decelerated. During follow-through the body continues to move forward with the arm, which reduces the distraction forces applied to the shoulder. The planted contralateral leg is critical at this time, as it allows for balance and a smooth transition during deceleration of the body. During deceleration and follow-through, the forces are approximately two times as great as the forces during acceleration and are produced as the muscles contract eccentrically to slow the arm down.[22] The greatest muscle activity during throwing occurs in the shoulder muscles during this period. Strong muscle activity during deceleration and follow-through has been identified in the deltoid, supraspinatus, infraspinatus, and teres minor muscles.[26] Perry[30] indicated that the posterior musculature of the shoulder was responsible for decelerating the arm. Jobe and Moynes[13] demonstrated strong activity in the subscapularis and latissimus dorsi during deceleration and follow-through. It is postulated that activity in these muscles allows for continued internal rotation and horizontal adduction of the arm across the body. Additionally, activity in these muscles may also lend stability to the glenohumeral joint by contributing to the joint compressive forces. During this period, strong activity also occurs in the scapular retractors including the trapezius and rhomboids. Elbow extension is decelerated by strong contraction of the biceps, which produces recoil flexion of the elbow.[37] After release of the ball, maximum activity occurs in the wrist extensors to decelerate wrist flexion.[36]

During throwing, the arm undergoes an extreme ROM and the muscles undergo forceful concentric and eccentric contractions. This results in high loading of joint and musculotendinous structures. Prior to return to overhead throwing activities the arm must be reconditioned to be able to withstand the stresses imposed by the act of throwing; if it is not, the risk of reinjury will be increased and the athlete's performance will suffer. Rehabilitation and reconditioning of the throwing athlete must include specific activities that will stress the arm in a systematic and progressive manner to allow safe resumption of throwing. Additionally, reconditioning of the throwing athlete must also include

the trunk and lower extremity. The trunk and legs contribute to the development and dissipation of the forces used to propel an object. If these areas are not fully reconditioned, excessive stress will be placed on the upper extremity when the athlete returns to throwing. This will result in reinjury, decreased performance, or both.

Swimming

Swimming is a sport in which speed is equated with success. Limb velocities during swimming have not been documented; speeds may vary depending on the event (i.e., sprint versus long distance). Swimming does not appear to involve the same violent eccentric contraction of the posterior rotator cuff muscles that occurs during the deceleration and follow-through phase of throwing. Injuries in swimmers appear to develop as a function of excessive use of the upper extremity. Swimmers average 8,000 to 20,000 yards a day and may practice up to twice a day 5 to 7 times a week.[4,10,33] An average of 4,000 revolutions/shoulder occur daily in swimming, which is the highest frequency of use reported for any upper extremity sport.[31] Minimal time is available for recovery during the stroke, particularly for long-distance swimmers, who swim for minutes at a time without a rest. The biomechanics of swimming places the shoulder in vulnerable positions and does so on a repetitive basis.

The freestyle swimming stroke is divided into the recovery and pull-through phase. The pull-through phase is that portion of time when the arm is in the water. The recovery phase occurs when the arm is above the water (Fig. 19-2). The pull-through phase is when most swimmers report pain.[8,33]

The pull-through phase is subdivided into early, mid, and late stages. Mid-pull-through occurs when the arm is perpendicular to the body. Early pull-through occurs from hand entry into the water until the arm is perpendicular to the body. Late pull-through begins when the arm is perpendicular to the body and ends when the hand exits the water. The arm moves in an S-shaped pattern during pull-through.[24] Upon hand entry, the shoulder is internally rotated and abducted with the palm turned outward and the elbow slightly flexed. The upper trapezius, rhomboids, supraspinatus, serratus anterior, and anterior and middle deltoids are active

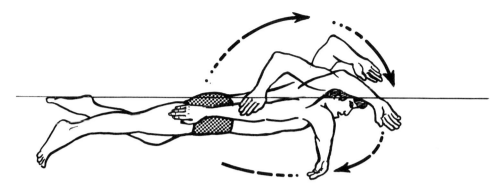

Fig. 19-2. Freestyle swimming stroke is divided into recovery and pull-through phase.

to abduct the shoulder and rotate the scapula upward during early pull-through.[31]

From hand entry the hand moves down and out from the body while the shoulder appears to extend and abduct horizontally in the initiation of the S-shaped curve.[24] Mid-pull-through begins when the arm is deepest in the water. At mid-pull-through the shoulder is internally rotated and horizontally adducted with the elbow flexed. In some instances the hand may cross the midline of the body.[24,31] The pectoralis major, teres minor, subscapularis, and serratus anterior are all active to internally rotate and extend the shoulder, pulling the body forward over the arm.[31] The latissimus dorsi begins to fire when the arm becomes perpendicular to the body. The shoulder will move from internal rotation and horizontal abduction to adduction with full internal rotation by the end of mid-pull-through.[7,27] The highest incidence of shoulder pain is reported in mid-pull-through,[8] possibly caused by the combination of internal rotation and horizontal adduction, which is similar to the test used to elicit subacromial impingement.

Late pull-through begins when the arm is perpendicular to the body and ends when the hand exits the water with the palm facing the thigh.[24] Muscle activity of the shoulder during late pull-through involves sequential firing of the posterior, middle, and anterior deltoid muscles.[31]

Recovery occurs when the arm is above the water and is divided into early and late phases. Early recovery begins when the arm exits the water. The shoulder internally rotates, extends, and abducts and the scapula retracts. During early recovery, activity occurs in the deltoid, supraspinatus, subscapularis, and infraspinatus. Maglischo[24] suggests that the arm internally rotates in order to reduce drag. The infraspinatus is the prime mover from midrecovery to hand entry, to control internal rotation as the hand meets the water.

The body should roll approximately 30 degrees to the horizontal in each direction. This allows optimum position for breathing and enhances the effectiveness of the arm in the water during mid-pull-through.[29]

PREREQUISITES FOR RECONDITIONING AND RETURN TO SPORT PHASE

Before initiating reconditioning and return to sport activities, sufficient tissue healing must take place to withstand the stresses that will be imposed by these activities. Basic scientific knowledge of soft tissue healing and the loads that healing tissues can withstand are incomplete. Additionally, the loads applied to the healing structures by these conditioning activities are unknown. Therefore, one cannot rely on healing time alone to determine when to initiate these activities.

Initiation of reconditioning and return to sport activities should be based on clinical examination of the athlete. The athlete should be without complaints of pain and signs of inflammation. Adequate ROM and muscle function is also necessary, to withstand the stresses imposed by these conditioning activities. These prerequisites can only be accomplished through a well-planned and -designed rehabilitation program.

Restoration of Range of Motion and Flexibility

Adequate ROM is necessary to perform sports that involve use of the upper extremity such as overhead throwing sports and swimming. Failure to achieve adequate ROM for these sports will result in use of substitute motion to perform the activities, accompanied by an increased risk of injury and decreased performance. Recovery of motion is particularly important for the shoulder, but care must be taken to avoid hypermobility of the shoulder, which may contribute to further problems. Hypermobility of the shoulder may contribute to eccentric overload of the rotator cuff and secondary impingement of the shoulder.[12]

The range of external and internal rotation with the arm abducted to 90 degrees is important for the throwing athlete. The range of external rotation with the shoulder abducted to 90 degrees in the normal population is considered to be 90 degrees, but this is inadequate for the throwing athlete.[2] The late cocking requires external rotation in excess of 90 degrees.

During deceleration and follow-through, the arm internally rotates and horizontally adducts across the body. Throwing athletes frequently lose internal rotation of the shoulder as a result of scarring and adaptive shortening of the posterior capsule and rotator cuff that is associated with repeated loading of the posterior structures during throwing. Inadequate flexibility of the posterior rotator cuff increases the athlete's susceptibility to injury as the cuff is eccentrically loaded to decelerate the arm during deceleration and follow-through. Posterior capsular tightness may lead to increased anterior and superior migration of the humeral head and may contribute to impingement.[11] We have found posterior glide of the glenohumeral joint with the shoulder flexed to 90 degrees to be useful for restoring internal rotation. Additionally, the posterior rotator cuff and capsule can be passively stretched by horizontally adducting the arm across the body with the arm elevated to 90 degrees (Fig. 19-3).

Although swimmers are often considered extremely flexible, recent research suggests that increased motion in one direction may be compensated for by limitations in motion in the opposite direction. Beach et al.[4] reported that swimmers had significantly greater external rotation at the expense of internal rotation. Limitation of internal rotation may be detrimental because the freestyle swimming stroke requires internal rota-

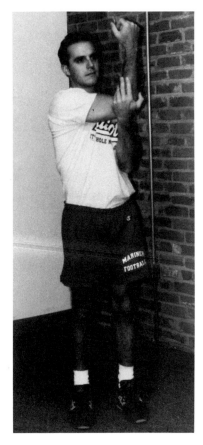

Fig. 19-3. Horizontal abduction of the arm across the body with the arm elevated to 90 degrees stretches the posterior rotator cuff and capsule.

tion during most of the stroke cycle. Limitation of internal rotation may result in increased anterosuperior migration of the humeral head with elevation of the arm. This may contribute to the high incidence of impingement in swimmers. Measurement of internal rotation at 90 degrees of abduction in swimmers may not accurately reflect the motion needed during freestyle swimming. During late recovery the shoulder is abducted and internally rotated in preparation for hand entry. During mid-pull-through a combination of horizontal adduction and internal rotation is needed. These combined movement patterns change the structures about the shoulder that are stressed. ROM of the swimmer's shoulder should be assessed in these combined movement patterns.

In addition to evaluating ROM in the cardinal planes and in the combined movement patterns described above, it is also important to assess flexibility of the anterior shoulder musculature in swimmers. Flexibility of the pectoralis minor, serratus anterior, and subscapularis should be addressed.

Motion at each joint and flexibility of all major muscle groups must be carefully assessed before initiation of reconditioning and return to sport activities. ROM and flexibility of the upper extremity can be developed by performing active and passive stretching exercises. Mobilization techniques can be used to increase motion when joint mobility (i.e., gliding and separation of joint surfaces) is limited. Mobilization techniques should not be used to increase motion when joint mobility is normal or hypermobile. Contract-relax and contract-relax-contract stretching techniques can be utilized to increase motion limited by muscular tightness. These techniques incorporate the neurophysiologic principles of autogenic inhibition and reciprocal inhibition.[20] Adequate ROM and flexibility must be developed for all segments of the upper extremity including the shoulder, elbow, wrist, and forearm. Particular emphasis should be placed on developing adequate internal and external rotation of the shoulder at 90 degrees of abduction and developing flexibility of the wrist flexors and extensors.

Development of Isolated Muscle Function

Injury and disuse result in muscle atrophy and loss of strength and endurance. In particular, we have seen weakness and loss of endurance of the scapular and rotator cuff muscles following injury to the upper extremity even if the pathology does not involve the shoulder. Weakness of these muscles will result in loss of dynamic control of the humeral head and can lead to secondary impingement of the shoulder. A detailed examination of muscle strength must be performed prior to initiation of reconditioning and return to sport activities. We prefer manual muscle testing over isokinetic testing so that isolated muscle weakness can be identified. Once identified, specific exercises to eliminate isolated muscle weakness must be performed. Muscle function must be restored prior to initiation of reconditioning and return to sport activities. Manual muscle testing should be strong and pain-free before these activities are initiated.

As noted above, we commonly find weakness of the rotator cuff and scapular muscles following injury to the upper extremity. In particular, we have noticed weakness of the supraspinatus, infraspinatus, teres minor, serratus anterior, and middle and lower portions of the trapezius. Specific exercises need to be performed to develop these muscles. Generally these are progressed from isometric to active exercises and finally to progressive resistive exercises (PREs), which emphasize development of both concentric and eccentric muscle function. Light resistance is used when performing PREs. Generally exercises are progressed to no more than 2.3 to 4.5 kg. Use of heavier resistance results in use of substitute muscle actions.

We have found resisted internal and external rotation of the shoulder with the arm at the side to be ineffective in improving isolated function for all the rotator cuff muscles. Jobe and Moynes,[13] Blackburn et al.,[6] and Townsend et al.[36] used fine-wire EMG analysis to identify optimum exercises for training specific rotator cuff muscles. Exercises for the supraspinatus include scapular plane abduction to 90 degrees with the shoulder internally rotated[13] (Fig. 19-4) and prone horizontal abduction with the arm externally rotated and abducted to 100 degrees in the frontal plane[6] (Fig. 19-5). Worrell et al.[40] utilized fine-wire EMG analysis of the supraspinatus and assessment of maximal voluntary isometric force to compare these two exercises. They found greater EMG activity during prone horizontal abduction with the arm externally rotated and abducted to 100 degrees in the frontal plane compared with scapular plane abduction with the arm internally rotated. However, they found greater force production with scapular plane abduction. Since supraspinatus EMG activity in this position was lower, it was hypothesized that greater substitution occurred. Substitution by the deltoid may have been responsible for the increased force of contraction with scapular plane abduction. Maximum EMG activity in the infraspinatus is produced during prone horizontal abduction with the arm externally rotated and abducted to 90 degrees in the frontal plane[6] (Fig. 19-6). Maximum EMG activity in the teres minor is developed during prone external rotation with the arm abducted to 90 degrees (Fig. 19-7) and during prone shoulder extension with the arm externally rotated[6] (Fig. 19-8). Our clinical experience indicates that these exercises can be used to strengthen the rotator cuff muscles effectively.

Strong scapular stabilizers are necessary to provide a stable base for the scapulohumeral muscles to act on. If the scapulohumeral muscles are weak, their effi-

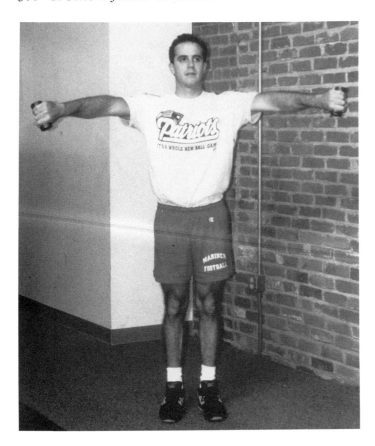

Fig. 19-4. Scapular plane abduction with the shoulder internally rotated is used to strengthen the supraspinatus.

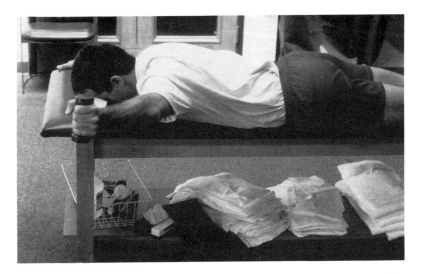

Fig. 19-5. Prone horizontal abduction with the arm externally rotated and abducted to 100 degrees in the frontal plane can also be used to strengthen the supraspinatus.

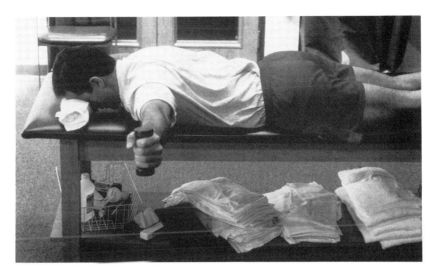

Fig. 19-6. The infraspinatus can be strengthened by performing prone horizontal abduction with the arm externally rotated and abducted to 90 degrees in the frontal plane.

ciency will be compromised.[18] Additionally, normal scapular rotation is important for maintaining inherent stability of the glenohumeral joint[21] and delaying subacromial impingement.[17,19] The scapular protractors function during the acceleration phase of throwing to assist in propelling the upper extremity forward. During the deceleration and follow-through phase of throwing, the scapular retractors function eccentrically to limit scapular protraction and provide a stable base from which the rotator cuff muscles can act to deceler-

ate the humeral head. In swimming the serratus anterior fires continuously to upwardly rotate, protract, and stabilize the scapula. Other scapular muscles probably assist in stabilizing the scapula during mid-pull-through and recovery.

Rehabilitation of upper extremity injuries in overhead throwing athletes and swimmers must include isolated exercises to improve the function of the serratus anterior, upper, middle, and lower trapezius, and rhomboids. Moseley et al.[25] used fine-wire EMG analy-

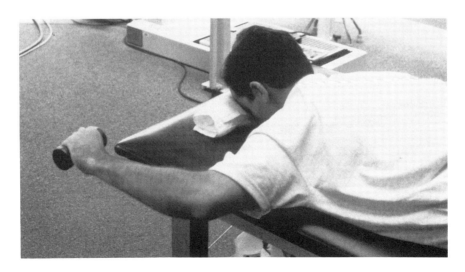

Fig. 19-7. Prone external rotation with the arm abducted to 90 degrees can be used to strengthen the teres minor.

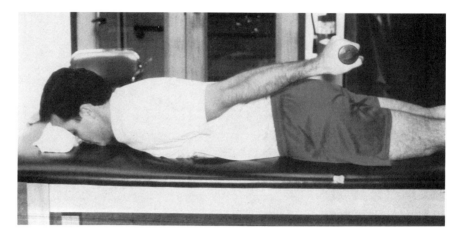

Fig. 19-8. Teres minor can also be strengthened by performing prone shoulder extension with the arm externally rotated.

sis to study activity in the scapular muscles during a variety of exercises. Based on their results, they recommended four exercises to develop the scapular muscles: scapular plane abduction for the upper and lower trapezius, levator scapulae, and middle and lower serratus anterior; rowing for the upper, middle, and lower trapezius, levator scapulae, and rhomboids (Fig. 19-9); push-ups with a plus for the middle and lower serratus anterior and pectoralis minor (Fig. 19-10); and seated press-ups for the pectoralis minor (Fig. 19-11). Kamkar[16] studied EMG activity of the lower serratus anterior using fine wires and found the greatest EMG activity with flexion of the shoulder above 90 degrees.

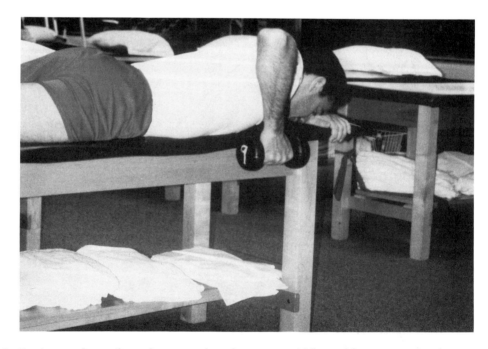

Fig. 19-9. Rowing can be performed to strengthen the upper, middle, and lower trapezius, levator scapulae, and rhomboids.

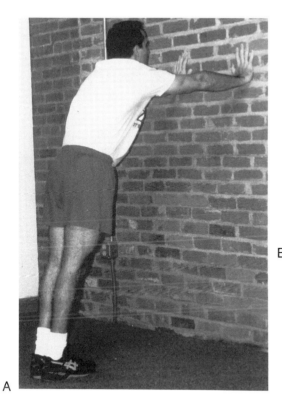

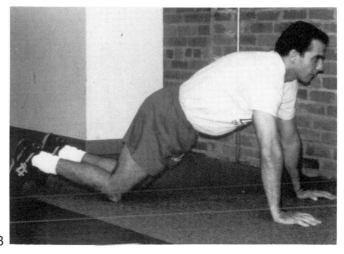

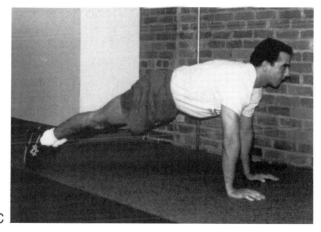

Fig. 19-10. Push-ups with a plus can be used to strengthen the middle and lower serratus anterior and pectoralis minor. The scapulae are protracted at the end of the range of the push-up. Push-ups with a plus are initially performed against the wall **(A)** and are progressed to push-ups on hands and knees **(B)** and then to regular push-ups **(C)**.

Clinically we use prone horizontal abduction with the arm externally rotated and abducted to 90 degrees in the frontal plane to develop the middle trapezius and prone horizontal abduction with the arm externally rotated and abducted to 150 degrees in the frontal plane to develop the lower trapezius (Fig. 19-12). To develop the serratus anterior we use serratus punches, push-ups with a plus, and forward flexion of the arm from 90 to 150 degrees. The serratus punch is a protraction of the scapula with the shoulder flexed to 90 degrees. Resistance can be provided by holding a dumbbell in the hand, use of elastic tubing, or performing the exercise on a chest press machine (Fig. 19 13). Push-ups with a plus are initially performed leaning against a wall and are progressed to push-ups on the knees and finally to regular push-ups.

GUIDELINES FOR RECONDITIONING AND RETURN TO SPORT PHASE

The athlete should be pain-free and should demonstrate the ROM and muscle function necessary to perform the sport activities before reconditioning begins.

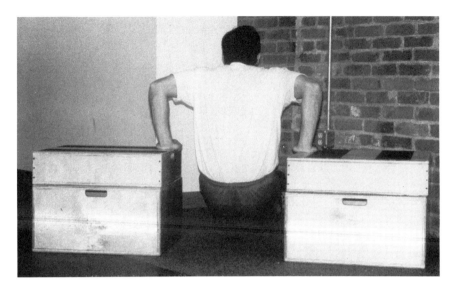

Fig. 19-11. The seated press-up can be used to strengthen the pectoralis minor.

Generally the athlete should have strong and pain-free resisted tests for all isolated muscles of the upper extremity. The tissues should have had sufficient time to heal, in order to withstand the stresses that will be imposed by the conditioning activities. When planning the reconditioning program, activities that are similar to the sport that the athlete is involved in should be selected.

Activities should be introduced in a systematic and progressive manner. Generally they are progressed from slow speed to fast speed, from low force to high force, from concentric to eccentric, and from controlled to uncontrolled activities. Sufficient time must be provided in the progression to allow the tissues to adapt to the new stresses imposed. Failure to provide sufficient time for adaptation will result in increased pain. Pain or soreness from the reconditioning activities should subside within several hours. Progressive increase in pain indicates that the athlete is progressing too rapidly and the program should be slowed down.

A factor often overlooked in the cause and treatment of athletic injuries to the upper extremity is the role of proprioception. Proprioception involves sensory input from mechanoreceptors located in the skin, muscles, and joints that is processed on the spinal, cerebellar, and cortical levels. Proprioceptive input includes infor-

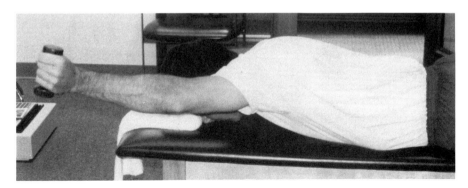

Fig. 19-12. Prone horizontal abduction with the arm abducted to 150 degrees in the frontal plane is used to develop the lower trapezius.

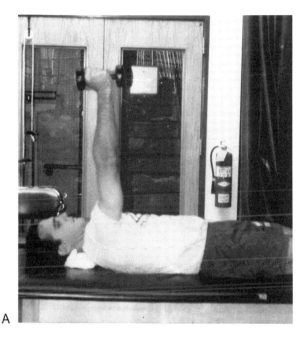

A

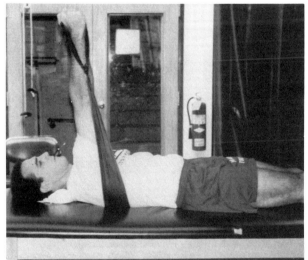

B

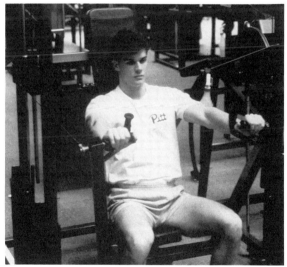

C

Fig. 19-13. The serratus punch is protraction of the scapula with the shoulder flexed to 90 degrees. Resistance can be provided by: **(A)** holding a dumbbell in the hand; **(B)** use of elastic tubing; **(C)** performing the exercise on a chest press machine.

mation on static and dynamic joint movement, joint position, velocity of movement, and forces of muscular contraction. Injury to joint or musculotendinous structures (or to both) may damage mechanoreceptors and may result in altered somatosensory feedback. Smith and Brunoli[34] demonstrated kinesthetic deficits in indi-

viduals following anterior dislocation of the glenohumeral joint. Their subjects had deficits in angular reproduction of midrange lateral rotation, threshold to detection of end-range lateral rotation, and end-range reproduction of lateral rotation. It was hypothesized that deficits in somatosensory input may adversely affect motor control. Loss of normal motor control may result in loss of dynamic stabilization of the joint and may contribute to repeated injury. Additionally, abnormal somatosensory input may result in substitute motor patterns, which could affect performance. Reconditioning and return to sport activities should be sport-specific, performed in a manner that will enhance proprioception and ensure use of correct motor patterns. This requires sport-specific activities to be performed repeatedly using correct technique to enhance awareness of joint position and movement sense and to develop proper timing, sequence, and coordination of muscle activity. Performing reconditioning and return to sport activities with poor technique will result in development of abnormal substitute motion patterns and may lead to reinjury and poor performance.

USE OF PLYOMETRIC AND ECCENTRIC EXERCISES

Plyometric and eccentric exercises are important in reconditioning and return to sport activities for the throwing athlete. Plyometric and eccentric activities are not as important for the swimming athlete since the muscles function concentrically during swimming. Plyometric exercises are stretch-shortening exercises characterized by a stretch of the muscle prior to concentric contraction. A quick stretch of the muscle will contribute to increased force of the subsequent concentric contraction. Increased force production with a stretch-shortening contraction is attributed to facilitation of the stretch reflex, which is mediated by the muscle spindle. Stretching the muscle spindle results in a monosynaptic reflex contraction of the muscle in which the spindle lies. Activation of the muscle spindle by a quick stretch results in increased contractile force generated by the muscle. Stretching of the muscle prior to contraction also results in lengthening of the series elastic component within the muscle, which stores elastic energy within the connective tissue component of the muscle. In the subsequent concentric contraction, this stored elastic energy is released and contributes to increased force produced by the musculotendinous unit.

Stretch-shortening exercises involve three phases: the eccentric phase, amortization phase, and concentric phase.[39] During the eccentric phase the muscle is elongated, which activates the muscle spindle and stores elastic energy in the connective tissue component of the muscle. The amortization phase is the time lag between the yielding eccentric phase and the concentric contraction. If the amortization phase is slow, elastic energy is wasted and the stretch reflex is not activated. A more powerful concentric response will occur as the amortization phase is shortened. The concentric phase is the resultant concentric contraction that results from prestretching of the muscle. This concentric contraction is more forceful than a concentric contraction that is not preceded by prestretching of the musculotendinous unit.

A stretch-shortening contraction of the internal rotators occurs during the late cocking and acceleration phases of throwing. The eccentric phase occurs as the shoulder externally rotates, resulting in lengthening of the internal rotators. This activates the stretch reflex and lengthens the series elastic component of the internal rotators. During acceleration the internal rotators undergo a powerful concentric contraction. The force of this contraction is increased reflexly by elongation of the muscle spindle and release of stored energy from the series elastic component.

During the reconditioning and return to sport phase for throwing athletes, activities should be included to enhance and develop the stretch-shortening contraction of the internal rotators of the shoulder as well as the wrist flexors. In tennis, plyometric exercises for the wrist extensors are necessary to prepare the athlete for the stresses imposed by the backhand. Plyometric training may result in improved muscle performance by increasing the speed of the monosynaptic stretch reflex, desensitizing or inhibiting the influence of the Golgi tendon organ, and/or enhancing neuromuscular coordination.[39]

The eccentric contraction of the posterior shoulder muscles during the deceleration and follow-through phase of throwing should not be confused with a stretch-shortening contraction. During this phase of throwing, the posterior deltoid, supraspinatus, infraspinatus, and teres minor contract eccentrically to decelerate the arm and maintain the humeral head in the glenoid cavity. During this period, the muscles lengthen to absorb the energy created during acceleration. Eccentric contraction of the posterior shoulder muscles is not preceded by stretching of the muscle nor do the muscles undergo a powerful concentric contraction after they have been lengthened. As a result, plyometric or stretch-shortening exercises for the

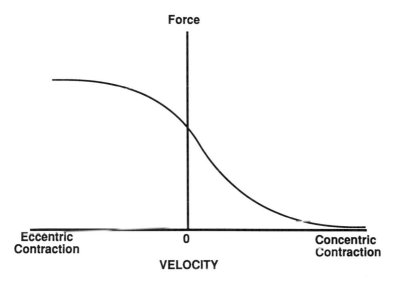

Fig. 19-14. Force-velocity relationship for a concentric and eccentric contraction. As the speed of a concentric contraction increases, force production decreases. Force increases as the speed of lengthening increases during an eccentric contraction.

posterior shoulder muscles are not needed for the throwing athlete. However, eccentric training of these muscles is still important.

For a given velocity of contraction, the force created by the musculotendinous unit during a maximal eccentric contraction is greater than the force created by a maximal concentric contraction (Fig. 19-14). Greater force during an eccentric contraction is related to increased contractile force due to facilitation of the stretch reflex as the muscle is lengthened. Additionally, stretching of the series elastic component as the muscle lengthens contributes to the noncontractile force generated by the musculotendinous unit. Force created by the musculotendinous unit is also dependent on the speed of contraction. For a concentric contraction the force generated by the musculotendinous unit decreases as the speed of shortening increases. During an eccentric contraction, force generated by the musculotendinous unit increases as the speed of lengthening increases, resulting in high loads on the musculotendinous unit. Failure to include eccentric exercise for the posterior shoulder musculature when reconditioning the throwing athlete will not fully prepare the athlete for the loads imposed on the shoulder when throwing activities are resumed; pain and reinjury will result. Eccentric exercise for the posterior shoulder muscles is important to prepare the throwing athlete fully for resumption of throwing activities.

COMBINED EXERCISE PATTERNS TO DEVELOP UPPER EXTREMITY FUNCTION

The importance of isolated muscle strength for throwers and swimmers has been discussed earlier. However, sport specific training of the upper extremity musculature has not been addressed. The following combined exercise patterns can be used to functionally train the muscles of the upper extremity that are used during throwing and swimming. These exercises improve both the concentric and eccentric phases of muscle contraction in sport-specific patterns. They allow muscles to work in combination rather than in an isolated fashion.[3]

Use of rubber tubing provides an inexpensive and efficient means to train muscles of the upper extremity concentrically and eccentrically. The internal and external rotators of the shoulder can be strengthened at varying levels of abduction. Initially strengthening of the shoulder rotators is performed with the arm at the side in 0 to 30 degrees of abduction. As the athlete improves and symptoms subside, exercise for the shoulder rotators can be progressed to higher levels of abduction, which is more functional for the athlete. Also diagonal exercise patterns can be performed to mimic the throwing motion (Fig. 19-15) and the pull-through and recovery phases of swimming (Fig. 19-16).

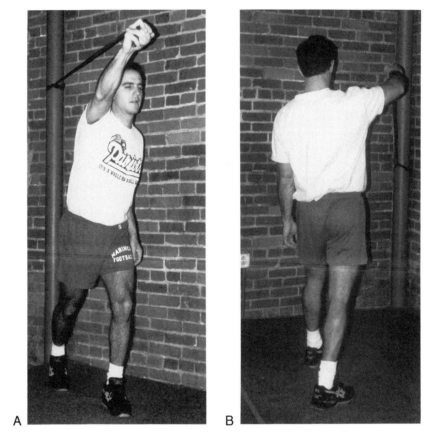

A   B

Fig. 19-15. Diagonal exercise patterns against rubber tubing can be performed to mimic the throwing motion. The exercise should be performed to strengthen the muscles that are involved in the acceleration **(A)** and deceleration **(B)** phases of throwing.

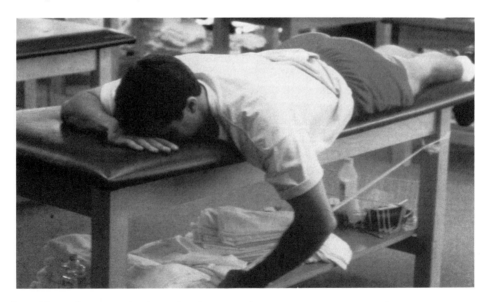

Fig. 19-16. Rubber tubing can also be utilized to provide resistance to exercises that mimic the pull-through and recovery phases of swimming.

The Inertial Impulse Exercise System (Engineering Marketing Associates, Newman, GA) has been shown to increase eccentric torque and is an excellent way to begin eccentric training for muscles of the upper extremity[1] (Fig. 19-17). This device allows resistance to move horizontally on rollers on a fixed platform. Many functional exercises the upper extremity can be performed on the Inertial Impulse Exerciser.

Exercises on this system that are important for throwing include internal and external rotation and extension of the shoulder. To load the internal rotators eccentrically, the athlete's shoulder is placed in external rotation with the arm at the side of the body (Fig. 19-18A). The athlete begins the motion by concentrically contracting the internal rotators to cause the resistance to move along the horizontal platform. Once the weight carriage passes the center of the platform, the internal rotators are loaded eccentrically to decelerate motion of the weight carriage along the platform (Fig.

19-18B). The internal rotators continue to contract eccentrically as the shoulder rotates back to the starting position of external rotation, where the sequence is initiated again. Over time this exercise can be progressed to 90 degrees of abduction, which loads the internal rotators in a manner similar to cocking and acceleration (Fig. 19-19).

The Inertial Impulse Exerciser can also be used to improve function of the external rotators. External rotation on the Inertial Impulse Exerciser is performed in a manner similar to the exercise for the internal rotators except that the direction of the movement is reversed. This is accomplished by having the athlete turn around to face the machine. The athlete begins with the shoulder internally rotated (Fig. 19-20). The external rotators contract concentrically to initiate movement of the weight carriage on the platform. As with the exercise for the internal rotators, as soon as the weight carriage passes the center of the platform, the external rotators contract eccentrically to decelerate movement of the weight carriage. This exercise can be progressed to 90 degrees of abduction as tolerated by the athlete (Fig. 19-21).

Many other functional activities for the upper extremity can be simulated with the Inertial Impulse Exerciser. For example, it can be used to simulate the deceleration phase of throwing and the forehand and backhand strokes of tennis. Its use allows the athlete to train concentrically and eccentrically in sport-specific patterns.

The Plyoball and Plyoback (Functionally Integrated Technologies, Watsonville, CA), which is a weighted ball system, is an excellent tool to incorporate in the reconditioning and return to sport program for throwing athletes. Initially the Plyoball is used with the assistance of an athletic trainer or physical therapist. As improvement occurs, the athlete can be progressed to the Plyoback device. The weight of the balls ranges from 0.91 to 5.4 kg. However, we have found that the circumference of the heavier balls is too large to catch and toss with one hand. If more weight is indicated for activities involving the use of one hand, we attach a cuff weight around the wrist. Exercises with the Plyoball are started with the arm at the side of the body. As the athlete improves, these exercises can be progressed at 90 degrees of shoulder abduction to mimic the throwing motion more closely.

The Plyoball can be used to train the internal and

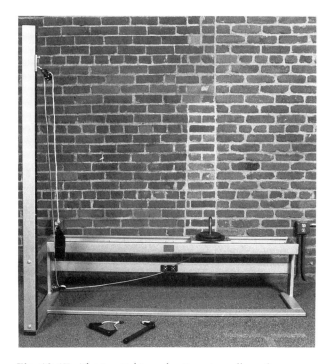

Fig. 19-17. The Inertial Impulse Exerciser allows for eccentric training of the muscles of the upper extremity. This device allows resistance to move horizontally on rollers. Once the weight carriage passes the center of the platform, the muscle is loaded eccentrically to catch the weight.

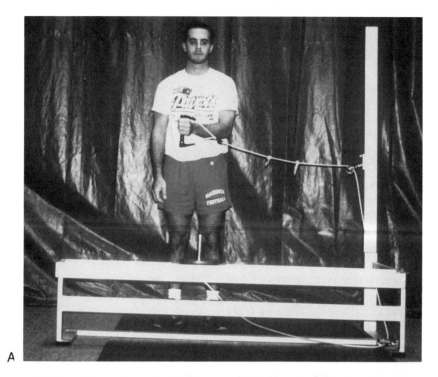

A

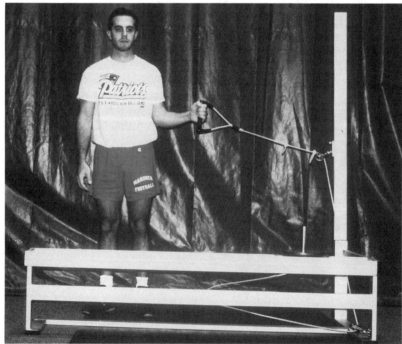

B

Fig. 19-18. The Inertial Impulse Exerciser can be used to strengthen the internal rotators. **(A)** The athlete begins motion by concentrically contracting the internal rotators to cause the resistance to move along the horizontal platform. **(B)** Once the weight carriage passes the center of the platform, the internal rotators are loaded eccentrically to decelerate motion of the weight carriage along the platform.

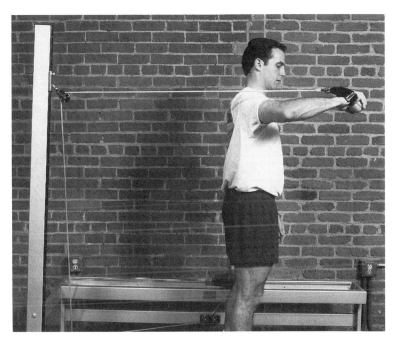

Fig. 19-19. As the athlete improves, training for the internal rotators on the Inertial Impulse Exerciser can be progressed to 90 degrees of abduction. This exercise loads the internal rotators in a manner similar to the late phase of cocking and acceleration.

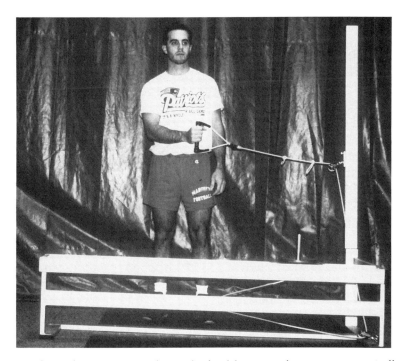

Fig. 19-20. The Inertial Impulse Exerciser can be used to load the external rotators concentrically and eccentrically. Initially this exercise is performed with the arm at the side.

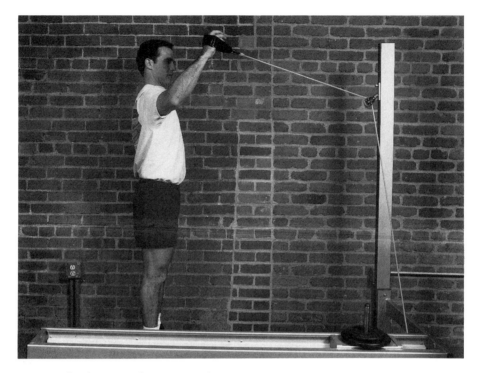

Fig. 19-21. Exercise for the external rotators on the Inertial Impulse Exerciser can be progressed to 90 degrees of abduction as tolerated by the athlete.

external rotators of the shoulder. To exercise the internal rotators the athlete should face the trainer or Plyoback device with the arm at the side and the shoulder externally rotated. The athlete throws the ball to the trainer or Plyoback device by internally rotating the shoulder (Fig. 19-22A). As the ball returns to the athlete, it is caught and decelerated through an eccentric contraction of the internal rotators (Fig. 19-22B). Initially the athlete performs this exercise with a 0.91-kg ball for the desired number of repetitions. As the athlete improves, the exercise can be progressed to use of heavier balls at greater degrees of external rotation and abduction of the shoulder.

The external rotators can also be trained with the Plyoball. To do so, the athlete stands with the back to a trainer or Plyoback device and the arm internally rotated at the side of the body. The elbow should be flexed to 90 degrees. To start the exercise, the athlete throws the ball backward by externally rotating the shoulder (Fig. 19-23A). As the ball returns to the athlete, it is caught and decelerated through an eccentric contraction of the external rotators (Fig. 19-23B). As the athlete becomes more skilled with this exercise and

can complete it without symptoms, higher degrees of shoulder abduction can be added (Fig. 19-24).

The Plyoball can also be used to train the deceleration and follow-through phase of throwing eccentrically. This exercise is performed with the assistance of an athletic trainer. The trainer, positioned behind the half-kneeling athlete, tosses the ball to the athlete. The athlete catches the ball with the arm in the position it would be in at ball release (Fig. 19-25). The athlete uses the posterior shoulder musculature to decelerate the arm to a position of shoulder adduction and internal rotation. This exercise mimics the muscle action of the upper extremity during the deceleration phase of throwing. The athlete follows the same path in reverse to return the ball to the athletic trainer.

The above exercises with the Plyoball can be used to train the upper extremity musculature specifically for overhead throwing. Wilk et al.[39] have described a variety of other exercises that make use of one- and two-handed tosses with the Plyoball. These exercises can be performed with or without trunk rotation to develop the entire kinetic chain including the trunk and legs.

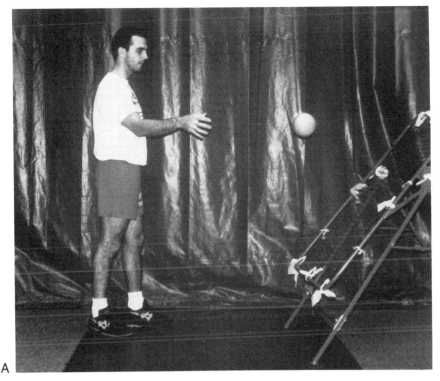

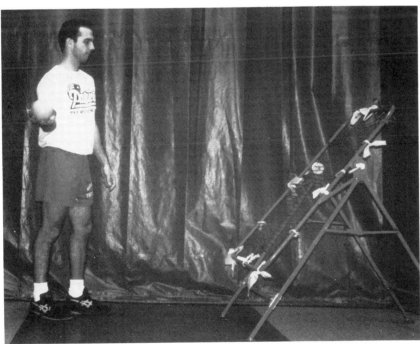

Fig. 19-22. The Plyoball and bounce back device can be used to train the internal rotators of the shoulder. **(A)** To start the exercise, the athlete throws the ball by internally rotating the shoulder. **(B)** As the ball returns to the athlete, it is caught and decelerated through eccentric contraction of the internal rotators. Initially this exercise is performed with the arm at the side. As the athlete improves, this exercise can be performed at greater degrees of external rotation and abduction of the shoulder.

317

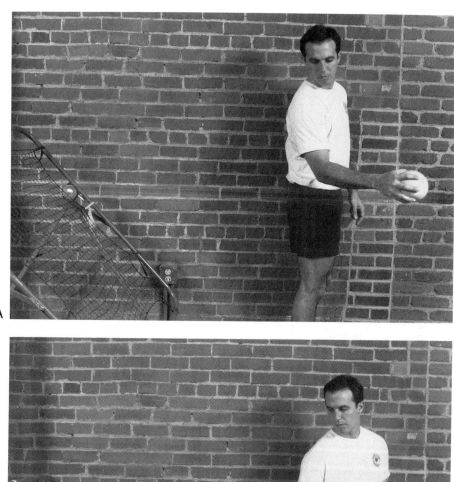

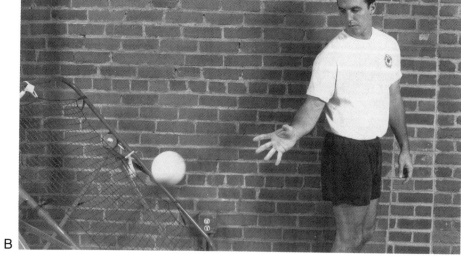

Fig. 19-23. The Plyoball and bounce back device can also be used to train the external rotators. **(A)** To begin the exercise, the athlete throws the ball backward by externally rotating the shoulder. **(B)** As the ball returns, the athlete catches and decelerates the ball through an eccentric contraction of the external rotators.

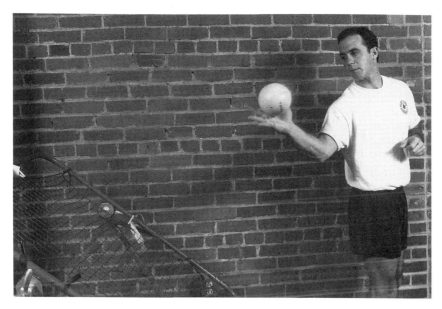

Fig. 19-24. As the athlete progresses and becomes more skilled, the Plyoball and bounce back device can be used to develop the external rotators with the shoulder at 90 degrees of abduction.

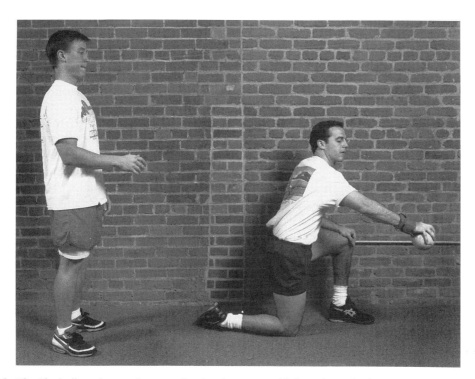

Fig. 19-25. The Plyoball can be used to train the deceleration and follow-through phase of throwing eccentrically. To perform this exercise the trainer is positioned behind the half-kneeling athlete and then tosses the ball to the athlete. The athlete catches the ball with the arm in the position that it would be in at ball release. This exercise mimics the muscle action of the upper extremity during the deceleration phase of throwing.

Many athletes such as throwers use the upper extremity as an open kinetic chain. Other athletes, however, use their upper extremity in a closed kinetic chain. These athletes move their body over the stationary upper extremity. Many events in gymnastics such as the floor exercise, vault, high bar, parallel bars, and pommel horse involve closed kinetic chain activities of the upper extremity. In swimming and rowing the athlete moves the body through a ROM over a stationary distal upper extremity. It is important to include closed-chain activities during the reconditioning and return to sport phase for these athletes.[35] The closed-chain activities should mimic the joint movement and muscle activity that is specific to the sport that the athlete participates in. As with open kinetic chain exercises, closed kinetic chain exercises should be added one at a time to monitor subjective complaints and objective changes of the athlete.

A low-level closed kinetic chain exercise that is often used clinically to strengthen the upper extremity is the "walking push-up." For this exercise, the athlete starts in the quadriped position and progresses to modified push-up, full push-up, and eventually to an inverted push-up. From the starting position the athlete walks with the arms in a side-to-side direction describing an arc of motion 2 to 6 feet in length. As the athlete progresses, other more challenging movement patterns can be begun with the hands such as circles, figure-of-eights, or cariocas in positions that involve increased weightbearing through the upper extremities.

Step-up exercises using the upper extremity are closed-chain exercises frequently used following successful completion of the "walking push-up." The upper extremity step-up is similar to the lower extremity step-up. The athlete starts in the quadriped position with both upper extremities on top of a small box or stool. The athlete begins the exercise by stepping with one hand at a time down off the elevated surface to the floor. The athlete then uses one hand at a time to step back up on the elevated surface (Fig. 19-26). The athlete may step down off the elevated surface utilizing side-to-side movement, which involves abduction and adduction of the upper extremity, or forward and backward, which involves flexion and extension of the upper extremity. It is recommended that an elevation of 2 inches or less be used initially. As the athlete improves, positions utilizing a modified push-up, full push-up or

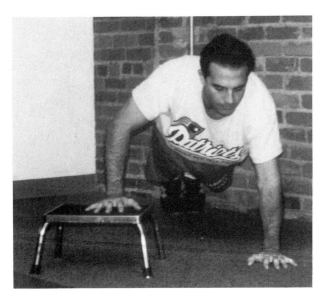

Fig. 19-26. Upper extremity step-up is a closed kinetic chain exercise that can be used to strengthen the upper extremity.

inverted push-up can be used. The height of the box or stool can be increased up to 8 inches.

The Fitter (Stack Enterprises, Alberta, Canada) can also be utilized for closed kinetic chain exercises for the upper extremity (Fig. 19-27A). The Fitter has a moveable platform and resistance is provided by elastic cords (Fig. 19-27B). The resistance of the platform to movement can be increased by increasing the number of elastic cords used. The athlete starts in a quadriped position and is aligned perpendicular to the Fitter. Initially this exercise should be performed with one cord attached for resistance. The athlete's hands are placed on top of the moveable platform. As the athlete horizontally abducts and adducts the shoulder, the moveable platform of the Fitter moves from side to side (Fig. 19-28A). The athlete can also be placed parallel to the Fitter so that flexion and extension of the shoulder causes the platform to move back and forth (Fig. 19-28B). By positioning the athlete at a 45-degree angle to the Fitter, diagonal patterns of the upper extremity can be performed (Fig. 19-28C). This exercise can be progressed by using different push-up positions described above and by adding resistance of additional cords.

A slide board can be used as another closed kinetic chain activity for the upper extremity. The athlete be-

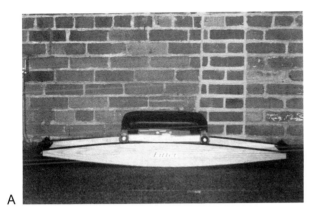
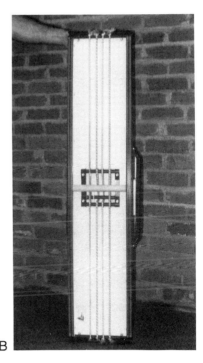

A   B

Fig. 19-27. The Fitter can be used to perform closed kinetic chain exercises for the upper extremity. **(A)** The Fitter has a movable platform. **(B)** Resistance is provided by elastic cords.

gins in the quadriped position with both upper extremities bearing weight on the slideboard. The hands should be covered with socks to minimize friction between the hand and the slideboard. The athlete begins by sliding the arms reciprocally forward and backward, which results in flexion and extension of the shoulder. The trainer or therapist needs to monitor the athlete closely to ensure that proper form is maintained throughout the exercise. If proper form is maintained, the athlete can be progressed to bilateral abduction and adduction exercises. The athlete uses the same position but now slides both arms simultaneously out to the side. The athlete slowly abducts and adducts the shoulders, trying to control position of the shoulder girdle. Each level is begun in the quadriped position and progressed to the push-up positions as described above.

The Stairmaster (Stairmaster Exercise Systems, Tulsa, OK) is a popular lower extremity closed kinetic chain exercise device that can be adapted for closed kinetic chain training of the upper extremity. The athlete begins in a quadriped position and places both

hands onto the foot pedals of the Stairmaster. The trainer or therapist should initially program the Stairmaster for a bodyweight of 5 to 10 lb with a step rate of 100 to 120 steps/min. The athlete should shift the body weight from side to side to depress the foot pedals in a reciprocal fashion (Fig. 19-29). This exercise can be used to improve muscular endurance of the upper extremity. As the athlete progresses, the body weight and rate of stepping programmed into the Stairmaster can be increased. The duration of exercise can be increased as tolerated by the athlete. Additionally the athlete can be progressed from the quadriped position to the push-up positions described above.

Reconditioning and return to sport for athletes involved in activities that utilize the upper extremity should include combined exercise patterns for the upper extremity. These combined exercise patterns should include open and closed kinetic chain exercises as described above. The exercise patterns should be specific to the sport that the individual participates in. Athletes involved in sporting activities that utilize the upper extremity in an open chain fashion should per-

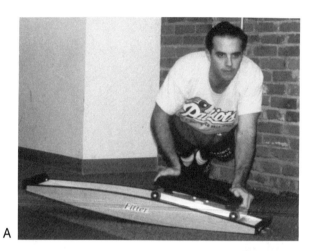

A

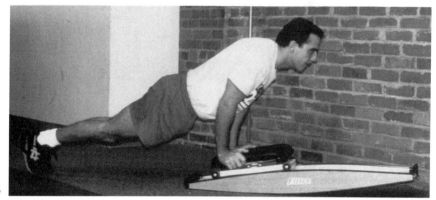

B

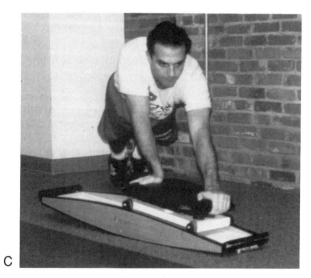

C

Fig. 19-28. The Profitter can be used to perform: **(A)** horizontal abduction and adduction of the shoulder; **(B)** flexion and extension of the shoulder; and **(C)** diagonal patterns for the upper extremity.

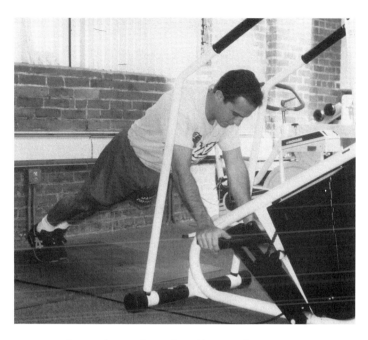

Fig. 19-29. The Stairmaster can be used to perform closed kinetic chain exercises for the upper extremity. When performing this exercise, the athlete should shift the body weight from side to side to depress the foot pedals in a reciprocal fashion. This exercise can be used to improve muscular endurance of the upper extremity.

form open kinetic chain exercises during the reconditioning and return to sport phase. Closed kinetic chain exercises should be used for those who make use of the upper extremity in a closed kinetic chain fashion while participating in their sport.

These combined exercise patterns should help prepare swimming and throwing athletes for competition by training the upper extremity in sports-specific patterns. They make use of concentric and eccentric contractions to prepare the athlete for the particular activity. They should be added one at a time to monitor subjective and objective changes properly. The athletic trainer needs to monitor the athlete closely to detect fatigue and substitute motion patterns. We generally have the athletes perform this functional training after they have completed a warm-up exercise program.

It should be remembered that in addition to these open and closed kinetic chain activities for the upper extremity, the entire kinetic chain including the trunk and lower extremities should be developed. The reconditioning and return to sport phase of the athlete's program is an important link between rehabilitation and successful return to full competition. The Specific Adaptation to Impose Demands (SAID) principal indicates that the later stages of rehabilitation should be specifically tailored to meet the individual needs of the athlete. When used properly these combined exercise patterns can successfully achieve sport-specific strength and function of muscles throughout the upper extremity.

USE OF WEIGHT-TRAINING AND WEIGHTLIFTING EXERCISES

Weight-training and weightlifting exercises that utilize free weights or machines, or both, have a secondary role in reconditioning and return to sport for throwers and swimmers. These exercises develop large muscles in nonfunctional patterns. Generally, reconditioning of these athletes should initially rely on specific exercises to improve isolated muscle function and should then progress to activities designed to improve muscle function in patterns that are functional for the athlete (the combined exercise patterns described above).

Weight-training and weightlifting exercises can be used to assist in development of muscle function for the upper extremity. Additionally, they can be used to develop the trunk and lower extremity, which is important to recondition the athlete fully for return to sports. They should not be relied upon to improve isolated muscle function of weak muscles, particularly that of the rotator cuff, nor should they be relied on to improve muscle performance in sport-specific functional patterns. Weight-training and weightlifting exercises should only be used as a supplement to the exercises and activities described above to improve isolated muscle function and muscle performance in sport-specific patterns.

It should also be noted that if these exercises are performed improperly they may contribute to further pain and injury. Caution should be used when lifting weights overhead to avoid impingement of the shoulder. To prevent impingement, weight training should be performed with the weights in front of the chest. This is important for weightlifting exercises such as the military press and latissimus pull-downs. Care should be taken to avoid undue stress on the anterior capsule and ligaments, which may contribute to development of anterior shoulder instability. Exercises such as the wide grip bench press should be avoided for those athletes who have anterior shoulder instability. For these athletes the bench press should be performed utilizing a narrow grip with the hands placed shoulder width apart. Weight-training and weightlifting exercises should be used cautiously when reconditioning throwers and swimmers. These exercises should be modified or discontinued if they contribute to an increase in the athlete's symptoms.

PROGRESSION FOR RETURN TO SPORT

Overhead Throwing Sports

Throwing may begin when the athlete is symptom-free and has recovered adequate ROM and the muscle function necessary for throwing. Return to throwing must be carefully monitored. Progression must be slow in order to ensure adequate time for the tissues to adapt to the stresses imposed upon them. Proper mechanics must also be emphasized. Initially this can be accomplished by slow and deliberate rehearsal of the throwing motion. Visual feedback can be given by use of mirrors or videotape to ensure use of correct technique. As the throwing motion is perfected, the speed and force of the throwing motion can be increased.

Several authors have outlined a progression for return to throwing for baseball players.[5,28,38] Generally, these programs make use of interval throwing with a progressive increase in intensity, frequency, and duration of throwing to allow the arm time to adapt to the stresses being imposed. Progression of the program is controlled by symptoms. The athlete should remain symptom-free during this progression. If symptoms develop, the program should be regressed to the pain-free level.

Initial emphasis is on the long toss program. Prior to beginning the throwing session, the athlete should warm up by stretching the arm as well as trunk and lower extremities. This should be followed by a period of short throws (30 to 45 feet) for several minutes. Once the athlete has properly warmed up, the interval throwing program, which consists of throws from 45 to 180 feet, may begin. Prior to increasing distance, the athlete should be able to complete 75 throws without pain[38] (Appendix 1). Once the athlete can complete 75 throws from 180 feet, return to the respective position in the field is appropriate.

Pitchers, however, will require further progression of the throwing program once they have completed the long toss program. Once the long toss program has been completed, pitchers may begin throwing fastballs at 50 percent effort from the mound. Over time they should progress to throwing at 75 percent and then to 100 percent effort. Once they can throw fastballs from the mound at 100 percent effort without symptoms they may progress to throwing more stressful pitches such as breaking balls and simulated game conditions[38] (Appendix 2).

While the throwing progression for baseball players has been well described, the progression for return to activity for athletes who perform similar overhead activities has been less well described. Generally, the return to sport for these athletes should consist of progression in sport-specific activity from a submaximal to maximal effort. The athlete should begin the progression using low-force, slow-speed, controlled motions. Over time the intensity, duration, and frequency of the effort should be progressed until they can perform their sport-specific skills with maximal force and speed. Prior to return to full participation, they should be exposed to game-simulated conditions.

Throughout this process, the athlete should be closely monitored to ensure correct technique and a symptom-free condition. Any technical faults should be closely investigated and corrected.

Return to Swimming

As with throwing, return to swimming should be a gradual process to allow time for the soft tissues to adapt to the stresses being imposed. Before return to swimming, the swimmer should demonstrate a full, pain-free ROM and normal strength. Additionally, the swimmer should be able to move through the arc of the swimming stroke against manual resistance without discomfort. Upon return to sport, the swimmer should swim a set amount of time rather than a set distance so that the speed of swimming is not an issue. Initial sessions in the pool should be limited to 10 to 15 minutes to determine the athlete's response. If the athlete responds favorably, the length of time and distance should be increased approximately 10% a week. Training for speed or sprints should be incorporated only after the swimmer has established baseline endurance in the water. Coaches and clinicians should carefully observe the swimmer to detect a "dropped elbow," which is the universal sign of fatigue in swimmers. Muscular fatigue of the dynamic stabilizers may result in secondary impingement, which can create further dysfunction for the swimmer.

More than 50 percent of swimmers have been reported to swim with shoulder pain.[32] The coach and swimmer need to understand clearly that the athlete should stop swimming on the initiation of pain or fatigue, as evidenced by "dropped elbow." Continued swimming through pain or fatigue will result in further irritation of the shoulder.

REFERENCES

1. Albert M: Eccentric Muscle Training in Sports and Orthopaedics. p. 63. Churchill Livingtone, New York, 1991
2. American Academy of Orthopaedic Surgeons: Joint Motion: Method of Measuring and Recording. Chicago, 1965
3. Arrigo C, Wilk K: Advanced strengthening exercises for the throwing athlete. Presented at the 11th Annual Injuries in Baseball Course, Birmingham, AL, January 21, 1993
4. Beach ML, Whitney SL, Dickoff-Hoffman SA: The correlation between shoulder flexibility, external/internal rotation, abduction/adduction strength and endurance ratios to shoulder pain in competitive swimmers. J Orthop Sports Phys Ther 16:262–268, 1992
5. Blackburn TA: The off-season program for the throwing arm. p. 2/7. In Zarins B, Andrews JR, Carson WG (eds): Injuries to the Throwing Arm. WB Saunders, Philadelphia, 1985
6. Blackburn TA, McLeod WD, White B, Wofford L: EMG analysis of posterior rotator cuff exercises. Athletic Training Spring:40–45, 1990
7. Counsilman JE: The Complete Book of Swimming. Athenum, New York, 1977
8. Cuillo JV, Stevens GG: The prevention and treatment of injuries to the shoulder in swimming. Sports Med 7:182–204, 1989
9. Fleisig GS, Dillman CJ, Andrews JR: Proper mechanics for baseball pitching. Clin Sports Med 1:151–170, 1989
9a. Glousman R, Jobe F, Tibone J et al: Dynamic electromyographic analysis of the throwing shoulder with instability. J Bone Joint Surg Am, 70:220–226, 1988
10. Greipp FJ: Swimmer's shoulder: the influence of flexibility and weight training. Phys Sports Med 13:92–105, 1985
11. Harryman DT, Sidles JA, Clark JM et al: Translation of the humeral head on the glenoid with passive glenohumeral motion. J Bone Joint Surg [Am] 72A:1334–1343, 1990
12. Irrgang JJ, Whitney SL, Harner CD: Nonoperative treatment of rotator cuff injuries in throwing athletes. J Sport Rehabil 1:197–222, 1992
13. Jobe FW, Moynes DR: Delineation of diagnostic criteria and a rehabilitation program for rotator cuff injuries. Am J Sports Med 10:336–339, 1982
14. Jobe FW, Tibone JP, Moynes D: An EMG analysis of the shoulder in throwing and pitching: a preliminary report. Am J Sports Med 11:3–5, 1983
15. Jobe FW, Moynes DR, Tibone JE et al: An EMG analysis of the shoulder in throwing and pitching: a second report. Am J Sports Med 12:218–220, 1984
16. Kamkar A: Electromyographic analysis of serratus anterior muscle exercises. University of Pittsburgh Masters Thesis, 1992
17. Kamkar A, Irrgang JJ, Whitney SL: Nonoperative management of secondary shoulder impingement syndrome. J Orthop Sports Phys Ther 17:212–224, 1993
18. Kendall FP, McCreary EK: Muscle Testing and Function. Williams & Wilkins, Baltimore, 1983
19. Kibler B: Role of the scapula in the overhead throwing motion. Contemp Orthop 22:525–532, 1991
20. Kisner C, Colby LA: Therapeutic exercise foundations and techniques. FA Davis, Philadelphia, 1990
21. Lucas DB: Biomechanics of the shoulder joint. Arch Surg 107:425–432, 1973

22. McLeod WD: The pitching mechanism. In Zarins B, Andrews JR, Carson WG (eds): Injuries to the Throwing Arm. WB Saunders, Philadelphia, 1985

23. McLeod WD, Andrews JR: Mechanisms of shoulder injuries. Phys Ther 66:1901–1904, 1985

24. Maglischo EW: Swimming Faster. p. 1. Mayfield Publishing, Mountain View, CA, 1982

25. Moseley JB, Jobe FW, Pine M et al: EMG analysis of the scapular muscles during a shoulder rehabilitation program. Am J Sports Med 20:128–134, 1992

26. Moynes DR: Electromyography and motion analysis of the upper extremity in sports. Phys Ther 66:1905–1911, 1986

27. Nuber GH, Jobe FW, Perry J, Antonelii D: Fine wire electromyography analysis of muscles of the shoulder during swimming. Am J Sports Med 14:7–11, 1986

28. Pappas AM, Zawacki RM, Sullivan TJ: Biomechanics of baseball pitching: a preliminary report. Am J Sports Med 13:216–222, 1985

29. Penny JN, Smith C: The prevention and treatment of swimmer's shoulder. Can J Appl Sports Sci 5:195–202, 1980

30. Perry J: Anatomy and biomechanics of the shoulder in throwing, swimming, gymnastics and tennis. Clin Sports Med 2:379–390, 1983

31. Pink M, Perry J, Browne A: The normal shoulder during freestyle swimming: an electromyographic and cinematographic analysis of twelve muscles. Am J Sports Med 19:569–576, 1991

32. Richardson AR: The biomechanics of swimming: the shoulder and knee. Clinics Sports Med 5:103–113, 1986

33. Richardson AR, Jobe FW, Collins HR: The shoulder in competitive swimming. Am J Sports Med 8:159–163, 1980

34. Smith FL, Brunolli J: Shoulder kinesthesia after anterior glenohumeral joint dislocation. Phys Ther 69:106–112, 1989

35. Stone J, Lueken J, Partin N et al: Closed kinetic chain rehabilitation for the glenohumeral joint. J Athletic Training 28:34–37, 1993

36. Townsend H, Jobe FW, Pink M, Perry J: Electromyographic analysis of the glenohumeral muscles during a baseball rehabilitation program. Am J Sports Med 19:264–272, 1991

37. Werner SL, Fleisig GS, Dillman CJ, Andrews JR: Biomechanics of the elbow during baseball pitching. J Orthop Sports Phys Ther 17:274–278, 1993

38. Wilk KE, Arrigo C, Andrews JR: Rehabilitation of the elbow in the throwing athlete. J Orthop Sports Phys Ther 17:305–317, 1993

39. Wilk KE, Voight ML, Keirns MA et al: Stretch-shortening drills for the upper extremities: theory and clinical application. J Orthop Sports Phys Ther 17:225–239, 1993

40. Worrell TW, Corey BJ, York SL, Santies-Taban J: An analysis of supraspinatus EMG activity and shoulder isometric force development. Med Sci Sports Exerc 24:744–748, 1992

Appendix 1

Return to Throwing: Long Toss Program[a]

45-ft Phase

Step 1
- A. Warm-up throwing
- B. 45 ft (25 throws)
- C. Rest 15 minutes
- D. Warm-up throwing
- E. 45 ft (25 throws)

Step 2
- A. Warm-up throwing
- B. 45 ft (25 throws)
- C. Rest 10 minutes
- D. Warm-up throwing
- E. 45 ft (25 throws)
- F. Rest 10 minutes
- G. Warm-up throwing
- H. 45 ft (25 throws)

60-ft Phase

Step 3
- A. Warm-up throwing
- B. 60 ft (25 throws)
- C. Rest 15 minutes
- D. Warm-up throwing
- E. 60 ft (25 throws)

Step 4
- A. Warm-up throwing
- B. 60 ft (25 throws)
- C. Rest 10 minutes
- D. Warm-up throwing
- E. 60 ft (25 throws)
- F. Rest 10 minutes

- G. Warm-up throwing
- H. 60 ft (25 throws)

90-ft Phase

Step 5
- A. Warm-up throwing
- B. 90 ft (25 throws)
- C. Rest 15 minutes
- D. Warm-up throwing
- E. 90 ft (25 throws)

Step 6
- A. Warm-up throwing
- B. 90 ft (25 throws)
- C. Rest 10 minutes
- D. Warm-up throwing
- E. 90 ft (25 throws)
- F. Rest 10 minutes
- G. Warm-up throwing
- H. 90 ft (25 throws)

120-ft Phase

Step 7
- A. Warm-up throwing
- B. 120 ft (25 throws)
- C. Rest 15 minutes
- D. Warm-up throwing
- E. 120 ft (25 throws)

Step 8
- A. Warm-up throwing
- B. 120 ft (25 throws)
- C. Rest 10 minutes
- D. Warm-up throwing
- E. 120 ft (25 throws)
- F. Rest 10 minutes
- G. Warm-up throwing
- H. 120 ft (25 throws)

[a] Interval throwing program allows the athlete to progress in throwing from 45 to 180 feet.

(Adapted from Wilk et al.,[38] with permission.).

327

150-ft Phase

Step 9
  A. Warm-up throwing
  B. 150 ft (25 throws)
  C. Rest 15 minutes
  D. Warm-up throwing
  E. 150 ft (25 throws)

Step 10
  A. Warm-up throwing
  B. 150 ft (25 throws)
  C. Rest 10 minutes
  D. Warm-up throwing
  E. 150 ft (25 throws)
  F. Rest 10 minutes
  G. Warm-up throwing
  H. 150 ft (25 throws)

180-ft Phase

Step 11
  A. Warm-up throwing
  B. 180 ft (25 throws)
  C. Rest 15 minutes
  D. Warm-up throwing
  E. 180 ft (25 throws)

Step 12
  A. Warm-up throwing
  B. 180 ft (25 throws)
  C. Rest 10 minutes
  D. Warm-up throwing
  E. 180 ft (25 throws)
  F. Rest 10 minutes
  G. Warm-up throwing
  H. 180 ft (25 throws)

Step 13
  A. Warm-up throwing
  B. 180 ft (25 throws)
  C. Rest 10 minutes
  D. Warm-up throwing
  E. 180 ft (25 throws)
  F. Rest 10 minutes
  G. Warm-up throwing
  H. 180 ft (25 throws)

Step 14
  A. Begin throwing off the mound or return to respective position

Appendix 2

Internal Throwing Program for Pitchers[a]

Stage One: Fastball Only

Step 1: Interval throwing
15 throws off mound 50%

Step 2: Interval throwing
30 throws off mound 50%

Step 3: Interval throwing
45 throws off mound 50%

Step 4: Interval throwing
60 throws off mound 50%

Step 5: Interval throwing
30 throws off mound 75%

Step 6: 30 throws off mound 75%
45 throws off mound 50%

Step 7: 45 throws off mound 75%
15 throws off mound 50%

Step 8: 60 throws off mound 75%

Stage Two: Fastball Only

Step 9: 45 throws off mound 75%
15 throws in batting practice

Step 10: 45 throws off mound 75%
30 throws in batting practice

Step 11: 45 throws off mound 75%
45 throws in batting practice

Stage Three

Step 12: 30 throws off mound 75% warm-up
15 throws off mound 50% breaking balls
45 to 60 throws in batting practice (fastball only)

Step 13: 30 throws off mound 75%
30 breaking balls 75%
30 throws in batting practice

Step 14: 30 throws off mound 75%
60 to 90 throws in batting practice 25% breaking balls

Step 15: Simulated game: progressively by 15 throws per workout

---

[a] Pitchers are progressed from throwing fast balls at 50% effort from the mount to throwing breaking balls in game-simulated conditions.

(Adapted from Wilk et al.,[38] with permission.).

20

Sports Injuries of the Upper Extremity in Children and Adolescents

LYLE J. MICHELI
EDWARD S. FORMAN

INTRODUCTION

With the current trend toward physical fitness (and sports medicine) that is sweeping throughout the world, people of all ages are becoming involved with organized sports. Children and adolescents, including 25 to 30 percent of adolescents who participate in organized high school sports, are no exception.[28] Unlike their adult counterparts, children and adolescents require specific consideration of their injuries because they are skeletally immature and have open growth plates. Longitudinal growth is manifested through the epiphysis; injury to the epiphysis carries the potential for rapid healing as well as growth disturbances. Growth plate injuries may be classified as acute or chronic. Acute injuries have been described by Salter and Harris[44] and also by Ogden.[36] Overuse injuries from repetitive microtrauma, previously seen primarily in adult recreational athletes, are now being seen with increased frequency in children and adolescents.

GROWTH PLATE INJURIES

A thorough understanding of the normal epiphyseal anatomy is imperative to understanding and treating potential epiphyseal plate injuries. The epiphyseal plate is a cartilaginous disk through which skeletal growth occurs between the epiphysis and the metaphysis.[39,44] The two types of epiphyses are pressure epiphyses and traction epiphyses, or apophyses. Pressure epiphyses are located at the ends of long bones; they provide longitudinal growth of the bone and also are subjected to pressures transmitted through the joints into which they enter.[44] A traction epiphysis is the site of origin or insertion of major muscles or muscle groups and is therefore subjected to traction rather than pressure. Traction epiphyses are nonarticular and contribute neither to joint formation nor longitudinal growth of long bones.[44] The epiphysis is rarely fractured without involving the growth plate, and injuries involving the growth plate account for about one-third of all skeletal fractures in children. Injuries to the epiphyseal plate may potentially lead to growth problems, with angular deformity, limb length discrepancy, joint surface incongruity, and or cessation of growth. Growth disturbances are caused by one of the following etiologies: (1) avascular necrosis of the plate, (2) crushing or infection of the plate, (3) formation of a callus bridge between the bony epiphysis and the metaphysis; (4) nonunion, or (5) hyperemia producing local overgrowth.[39]

In the prepubescent child, fractures through bone are much more common than are epiphyseal fractures. In the adolescent, however, and particularly during growth spurts, the epiphyseal plate spanning the joint may be weaker than the ligaments. Adolescents tend to sustain epiphyseal plate injuries, whereas the prepubescent child or skeletally mature individual would sustain a tendinous or ligamentous injury. In addition, the epiphyseal plate is not as strong as the fibrous joint capsule, and therefore traumatic dislocations of joints are less common and epiphyseal separations more common in these joints.

The three main types of epiphyseal injuries sustained by children and adolescents are (1) separation of the epiphysis, (2) fractures that cross the epiphysis or have a component that transverses the epiphysis, and (3) crush injuries.[12] The etiology is one of the following mechanisms: shearing, avulsion, splitting, or crushing.[44]

The epiphyseal plate is composed of four distinct cell layers: (1) resting cells, (2) proliferating cells, (3) hypertrophying cells, and (4) endochondral ossification cells. The resting cell zone lies just proximal to the epiphysis and is composed of compact cartilaginous cells. The resting cells act as a reservoir for future growing cartilage cells and are nourished by vessels through the epiphysis.[20] The zone of proliferating cells is identified by the appearance of microscopic mitotic figures. In the zone of hypertrophying cells the cells begin to arrange in vertical columns as they hypertrophy and then eventually degenerate. Epiphyseal fractures in children and adolescents most commonly occur through the zone of hypertrophied cells, the weakest part of the epiphyseal plate. The fourth zone, that of endochondral ossification, is adjacent to the metaphyseal region of bone. The appearance of osteoblasts, the replacement of dying cartilage cells by trabeculae of bone, and the outgrowth of capillaries from the metaphysis characterize this bone.[12]

Anatomically, the zone of hypertrophied cells is felt to be the weak link in the growth plate. However, because of its metaphyseal and epiphyseal vasculature, separation of the growth plate through this zone does not interfere with the blood supply to the cartilage cells in the zone of endochondral ossification or the future cartilage cells in the zone of proliferating cells.

Salter-Harris Classification

Salter and Harris classified epiphyseal plate fractures based on the mechanism of injury and the relationship of the fracture line to the growing cells of the epiphyseal plate[44] (Fig. 20-1).

Type I

The radiographs are commonly negative and the diagnosis is made on clinical suspicion. Type I injuries are usually a result of a shearing or torsion force, or, in the case of an apophyseal fracture, an avulsion force. Healing in type I fractures usually occurs with 3 weeks and complications are rare. It is important to note that even with type I fractures, which usually have an excellent prognosis, it is difficult to distinguish between a type I and a type V injury in which the epiphyseal plate is crushed, which has a poor prognosis. Type V fractures are usually caused by an axial loading force and are best distinguished from type I fractures by the history of the injury.

Type II

Type II fractures are produced by a lateral displacing force that ruptures the periosteum on one side and leaves it intact on the side with the metaphyseal fragment. Reduction of this type of fracture is carried out with relative ease, and overreduction is prevented by the intact periosteal sleeve.

Type III

Type III fractures are seen in partially closed growth plates and therefore growth disturbances are not usu-

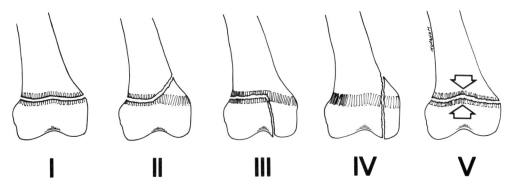

Fig. 20-1. The Salter-Harris classification of physeal fractures. (From Micheli,[26] with permission.)

ally a problem. These fractures are intra-articular and require anatomic reduction to prevent malarticulation.

Type IV

Type IV fractures must be anatomically reduced, usually by open reduction and internal fixation in order to preserve a smooth joint surface and to close the fracture gap; such treatment will prevent nonunion and cell-to-cell apposition of the growth plate, ensuring that growth is not disturbed.[39]

Type V

Type V fractures, as stated earlier, are usually caused by axial loading forces and are usually crush-type injuries. A potential consequence of this type of fracture is that all or part of the plate may be affected.

All injuries to the epiphyseal plate should be followed for at least 6 months and potentially for up to a year or more to rule out the possibility of any growth disturbance.

OVERUSE INJURIES

In recent years, with the growing popularity of organized sports among children and adolescents, an increased number of injuries have been demonstrated in this population. In addition to the expected acute traumatic injuries in children and adolescents, new types of injury are occurring. These overuse injuries have a common mechanism of injury: repetitive microtrauma. Microtrauma results from chronic repetitive insult to the local tissues and is the major etiologic factor in overuse injuries. In the past, these injuries were thought to have reflected a breakdown of the "aged" tissues of the often inadequately trained or maintained adult athlete or "weekend warrior." The growing involvement of children and adolescents participating in organized sports has been paralleled by an increased number of overuse injuries. Organized sports or fitness for children have resulted in a whole new genre of injuries that have rarely occurred in the free play situation.[27]

The number of children and adolescents presenting to the Division of Sports Medicine Clinic at Boston's Children's Hospital with overuse injuries has increased significantly.[25] This has led to the development of a simple check list of risk factors, which is helpful in determining the etiology of a given overuse injury and is useful as a first step in determining ways of preventing the occurrence or recurrence of other overuse injuries in the young athlete.

Growth in children and adolescents occurs in disproportionate fashions. The lower extremities grow before the upper extremities, and bone growth precedes ligament, muscle, soft tissue, and tendon growth. A sudden increase in growth, commonly seen in children and adolescents, compounded with their increased involvement in organized sports, has placed this population at risk of overuse injuries. Listed below are specific risk factors that have been documented for overuse injuries.[25,27,35]

1. Training error
2. Muscle-tendon imbalance
3. Anatomic malalignment
4. Footwear/playing surface
5. Associated disease state
6. Growth

Training error is the most frequently encountered etiology (e.g., when a child or adolescent who plays pick-up basketball or ice hockey for an hour a day, three to four times a week, is sent away to a sport-intensive summer camp with training for 6 to 8 hours a day).

Muscle-tendon imbalance can involve strength, flexibility, or bulk. Growth leads to a decrease in flexibility and is also associated with increased strength. This increased strength, however, may predispose toward muscle and tendon imbalances about the joints. For example, a child or adolescent athlete in repetitive overhead throwing sports or specific swimming strokes such as the backstroke or the breaststroke and develops capsular contractures about the shoulder that demonstrate a loose anterior capsule and a tight posterior capsule. Resistance to this imbalance may result in an impingement syndrome or even anterior subluxation of the shoulder. Muscle-tendon imbalance may thus be summarized as part of a four-part equation[35]:

1. Growth decreases flexibility
2. Strength increases with growth
3. Increases in strength may not be uniform, additionally contributing to imbalances about the joints.
4. Overstress of particular muscle-tendon units can cause subtle neurovascular injury

Anatomic malalignment, footwear, and playing surface may also be factors in the occurrence of overuse injuries. These factors predominantly deal with the lower extremity and the spine and therefore are only noted for completeness in this chapter.

PHYSICAL EXAMINATION

When examining a young athlete, the examiner must consider the differences between skeletally mature and skeletally immature bones. Young bones have greater elasticity, whereas older bones become stiff and brittle with age. This principle makes the skeletally immature epiphysis susceptible to forms of stress different from those observed in skeletally mature epiphyses. Because of the increased elasticity of young bones, remodeling of potentially permanent deformities of bone may be corrected. This property of bone is due to a strong periosteum, which often remains partially intact. This allows for remodeling of angular deformities, but it cannot correct rotational deformities.

SPECIFIC UPPER EXTREMITY INJURIES

Included in this review are upper extremity bony, cartilaginous, ligamentous, and tendinous injuries sustained by children and adolescent athletes. Child and adolescent athletes may sustain unique injuries to the upper extremity that are age-specific and that may be predicted by the biomechanical patterns of the athlete's sport and age. Upper extremity fractures and dislocations from macrotrauma may occur commonly as sports-specific injuries in football, wrestling, and hockey.[16] Overuse injuries from microtrauma may occur in sports requiring repetitive overhead activities such as swimming, tennis, and baseball.

As with any injury, the most important factor in treating injured children and adolescent athletes is to make the correct diagnosis. To do this, a thorough history must be taken and a careful physical examination performed of the entire athlete, concentrating on the injured extremity and adjacent structures, must be done. In addition, comparison with the contralateral extremity is imperative. Radiographs of the injured extremity, including the joint above and below the injured area,

are necessary in the evaluation process. Also, radiographs of the controlateral side should be obtained for comparison views whenever a question exists about a bony or cartilaginous defect (or both). In patients with acute epiphyseal trauma, the radiographs may appear normal, but the clinical examination may demonstrate a Salter-Harris I fracture. Radiographs should be repeated in 10 to 14 days to demonstrate periosteal reaction at the fracture site. When examining a skeletally immature athlete, the presence of open epiphyseal plates requires consideration of multiple factors as potential causes of clinical instability or deformity.

Clavicle

The clavicle is the most commonly fractured bone in the shoulder girdle. This fracture is usually a result of direct trauma and is usually seen in athletes participating in contact sports like football and hockey. Clavile fractures ordinarily occur in the middle one-third of the bone and generally progress to complete union. Open reduction and internal fixation is rare in the treatment of clavicular fractures in children and adolescents since primary union is the norm. On occasion, a physeal separation of the distal clavicle may occur, simulating an acromioclavicular (AC) separation.

Acromioclavicular Joint

Although uncommon, AC joint separations can occur in children and adolescents. In children and adolescents, grades I and II acromioclavicular sprains are more common than are grade III sprains. Management of grades I and II AC sprains is similar to that of skeletally mature patients, with symptomatic treatment, initial immobilization, and a sling and swathe for support. Grade III AC sprains have been treated successfully nonoperatively,[48] but the treatment remains controversial.[32,40,41,49]

Shoulder

Injuries to the shoulder have been found to account for as many as 44.6 percent of all upper extremity injures.[2] Injuries of the shoulder include fractures (Little League shoulder), impingement syndrome, rotator cuff injuries, instabilities, and neuromuscular injuries.

In 1966, Adams[1] studied Little League baseball pitchers in California and first described an overuse Salter

I fracture of the proximal humerus resulting from repetitive overhand throwing; he termed this injury *Little League shoulder*. Radiographs usually demonstrate a widening of the proximal humeral epiphyseal plate. Treatment for this type of fracture is relative rest, with the athlete avoiding throwing for 4 to 6 weeks. Physical therapy is instituted to restore strength and range of motion (ROM). In our experience, this fracture occurs in relatively tight individuals.

Subacromial shoulder pain with motion may result from impingement of the rotator cuff on the coracoacromial ligament or acromium. Rotator cuff tears are rare in children and adolescents, but impingement with tendinitis has been well described, most frequently in young competitive swimmers.[10,13,19,50] In 1972, Neer[29] described the pathoanatomy of shoulder impingement, and in 1983, Jobe and Jobe[18] suggested that impingement was caused by repetitive microtrauma. This injury is most commonly seen in individuals who participate in overhead activities such as swimming and tennis. Treatment is similar to that of most other overuse injuries: modification of activity, relative rest, nonsteroidal anti-inflammatory drugs (NSAIDs), physical therapy, internal and external rotator strengthening, and ice massage.

The supraspinatus tendon and the long head of the biceps are in close proximity and may often confuse the examining physician: does the patient have a rotator cuff derangement, a biceps tendinitis, or a biceps tendon subluxation? In 1973, O'Donohue[34] described subluxation of the biceps tendon in the athlete. This entity has been seen in young athletes but is rare. Shoulder instability is commonly seen in the adolescent athlete. Although anterior subluxations and dislocations are most common, improved radiographic skill and technique have made the diagnosis of posterior subluxations, once thought to be a very rare entity, more common.[16] In addition, many recent studies have demonstrated that patients with posterior glenohumeral instability tend to respond to conservative rehabilitation strengthening of the posterior shoulder musculature with a better prognosis for successful nonoperative treatment than anterior instability.[14,46,47,52] Neer[30] has described multidirectional instability in the shoulder and states that it can be involuntary. Prior to puberty, bilateral "physiologic" painful glenohumeral subluxation may be seen in young athletes. This condition is commonly seen in young athletes with generalized laxity. Strengthening exercises

of both the glenohumeral and scapulothoracic joints can allay symptoms. Recurrence can be seen, however, as training is resumed. Surgery should be avoided in these cases with multiaxial instability (Fig. 20-2).

When treating children and adolescent athletes with shoulder instability, radiographs should be obtained to rule out associated bony abnormality. Labral avulsions, Hill-Sachs lesions, and reverse Hill-Sachs lesions can be seen. Unidirectional glenohumeral joint instability, whether anterior or posterior, may improve with conservative treatment. Exercises to strengthen the shoulder and stretch any detected contracture can be combined with activity modification. These patients may demonstrate an associated rotator cuff impingement with shoulder instability.[51]

If recurrent subluxations or dislocations occur despite a well-supervised rehabilitation program, surgical repair may be required. If surgical repair is considered, the physician must consider the patient's open epiphyseal plates and the patient's compliance with postoperative rehabilitation. The physician may postpone surgical repair until physical and emotional maturity has been attained. For patients with anterior laxity, a standard anterior capsuloraphy should achieve a 95 percent success rate.[3,6,14,15,31,37,42,46,50] For patients with posterior laxity, a posterior capsuloraphy is usually satisfactory. Preoperative computed tomography (CT) scan should be attained to rule out glenoid insufficiency, in which case posterior osteotomy or bone may be necessary.

Long Thoracic Nerve Palsy

Long thoracic nerve palsy with scapular winging is a rare entity observed in young athletes.[22] It has been seen in young athletes who bench press, young throwers, and patients using crutches who support their body weight with the crutches. To test for scapular winging and long thoracic nerve function, the patient should push on the wall with the arm forward and abducted and the elbow extended. These injuries are usually transient and are treated expectantly.

Elbow

Overuse injuries of the elbow are most commonly seen in children and adolescents involved in sports that require overhead activities such as throwing. The elbow has been found to be the most frequent area of

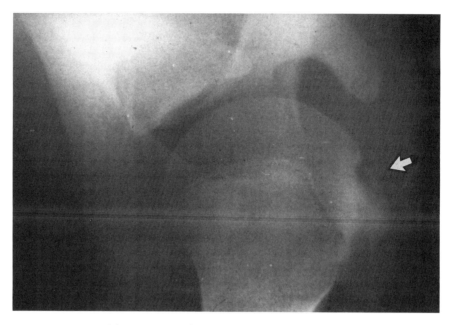

Fig. 20-2. Repetitive anterior subluxation in a 14-year-old baseball pitcher resulting in an osteochondral injury of the anterior humerus (*arrow*).

complaint in children and adolescent baseball players.[11]

The type of injuries depends on the athlete's age and bony development. A knowledge of the anatomy of the elbow and the appearance and fusion of the secondary ossification centers of the elbow is imperative to understand the young athlete's elbow (Tables 20-1 and 20-2). In addition to clinical examination, radiographs of the contralateral elbow are necessary to rule out the presence of a possible fracture or avulsion of the patient's ossification center.

Pappas[37] reviewed injury patterns at the elbow in the young athlete and related them to stage of development. The three stages of development (childhood, adolescent, and young adult) are associated with differ-

ent characteristic physical and hormonal changes. Childhood terminates with the appearance of all secondary centers of ossification; adolescence terminates with fusion of all secondary centers of ossification to their respective long bones; and young adulthood demonstrates the completion of all bone growth and the attainment of final muscular development.

In 1966, Adams[1] described elbow pain with associated pathologic changes in young throwers, particularly pitchers, and labeled this entity *Little League elbow.* These changes included osteochondral changes in the capitellum, fragmentation of the medial epicondyle, and premature proximal physeal closure of the radius. Subsequent investigations have suggested that

Table 20-1. Age of Appearance for Secondary Ossification Centers: Elbow

	Boys	Girls
Capitellum	1–2 months	1–6 months
Radial head	3–6 years	3–6 years
Medial epicondyle	5–7 years	3–6 years
Trochlea	8–10 years	7–9 years
Olecranon	8–10 years	8–10 years
Lateral epicondyle	12 years	11 years

(Modified from Ogden,[36] with permission.)

Table 20-2. Age of Fusion for Secondary Ossification Centers: Elbow

	Boys (Years)	Girls (Years)
Capitellum	14.5	13
Radial head	16	14
Medial epicondyle	17	14
Trochlea	13	11.5
Olecranon	16	14
Lateral epicondyle	15	12.5

(Modified from Pappas,[37] with permission.)

these changes are due to repetitive compression of the radius against the capitellum laterally and traction of the epicondyle medially due to a valgus strain at the elbow during the overhead delivery of the ball.

Pappas[37] has established six factors to be considered when evaluating musculoskeletal problems about the elbow:

1. Musculoskeletal development of the elbow
2. Biomechanical demands of throwing
3. Throwing pattern and variety of pitches thrown
4. Frequency of throwing
5. Genetic history of the individual
6. Other individual considerations

When examining the musculoskeletal development of the elbow in children and adolescents, it is important for the physician to know the ages at appearance, ossification, and fusion of the secondary ossification centers within the elbow. Radiographs should also be obtained of both the affected elbow and the contralateral elbow to observe any potential variations in appearance of the ossification centers that could suggest possible abnormal development. Variations seen in size, density, or radiographic appearance and the presence of loose bodies within the elbow joint are commonly associated with osteochondrosis. Repetitive trauma to the elbow joint, usually from throwing, may lead to avascular necrosis of a susceptible epiphyseal plate and may manifest as chronic elbow pain.

Pappas[37] has divided the throwing mechanism into three general phases of motion: the cocking phase, the acceleration phase, and the follow-through phase. During the late cocking phase, distraction forces are produced medially, compressive forces are applied laterally, and translational forces exist across the joint between the humerus and the olecranon. The acceleration phase acts to neutralize the forces the joint, and the follow-through phase creates increased forces posteriorly. These posterior forces are created by contraction of the triceps mechanism and compressive and shear forces across the radiocapitellar articulation, which are caused by rapid pronation of the forearm.

Repetitive trauma to the athlete's elbow commonly seen in overuse or increased frequency of pitching has been found to be a significant factor in predicting the frequency of elbow problems.[1] With this information, Little League organizations have established rules that limit the number of innings a player may pitch, thereby hopefully lowering the number of pitches thrown and decreasing the amount of repetitive microtrauma to the elbow sustained by the athlete.

Clinical features of Little League elbow can be said to occur in different anatomic regions of the elbow. In the medial elbow, the medial epicondyle (the site of origin for the flexor tendons of the forearm), the ligaments stabilizing structures between the humerus and the ulna, and the ulnar nerve within the ulnar groove are the most vulnerable anatomic structures. The medial epicondyle is an extra-articular structure. It is important to remember this when evaluating an elbow radiograph for a possible anterior fat pad sign because such a sign may not be present. It is also important to note that since the epicondyle is extra-articular, it is uncommon for irreversible changes to occur and affect joint function. Conservative treatment is recommended, with a period of relative rest. Steroid injections or NSAIDs are not recommended (Fig. 20-3).

As the athlete matures and enters the adolescent phase of growth, physical strength increases and bones

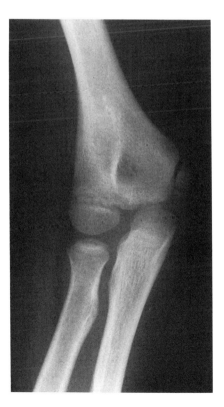

Fig. 20-3. Medial epicondylitis in a young baseball pitcher with fragmentation of the epicondyle.

are beginning to fuse. At this stage in development the throwing athlete may sustain an increase in valgus stress to the elbow along with a sudden contraction of the flexor mechanism that may potentially lead to a medial epicondyle avulsion fracture; such a fracture would require open reduction and internal fixation. As the athlete continues to develop and the ossification centers continue to fuse, a more common occurrence is for a small fragment to be avulsed rather than the entire medial epicondyle. Occasionally, these fragments may become painful and asymptomatic within the flexor mechanism and may require surgical excision. Failure of the medial epicondyle to fuse or nonunion of the avulsed epicondyle has been reported to occur in adolescent baseball pitchers secondary to chronic stress to the medial epicondyle. As the athlete matures and enters the young adult phase, the ossification centers have fused. Injuries at this stage of development are more commonly muscular avulsion from bone rather than bony fractures.

Another important anatomic concern of the medial elbow is that of the ulnar nerve. The ulnar nerve courses around the medial epicondyle in the ulnar groove and then distally into the forearm and hand. Repetitive stress on the medial side of the elbow may stretch the ulnar nerve and lead to inflammation of the nerve and possibly even neurologic changes in the function of the nerve. If signs and symptoms persist, an electromyelogram with nerve conduction velocity study (EMG with NCV) may be performed to evaluate the condition of the nerve. If the EMG with NCV studies are abnormal and the athlete still has neurologic complaints, an ulnar nerve transposition may be proposed.

The lateral condyle is different from the medial epicondyle in that the capitellum and radial head are usually well along with their ossification process by the time the athlete is in grade school. As the athlete matures during the adolescent growth period, repetitive forces on the ossifying capitellum and radial head may result in damage to the articular surface of the elbow joint, leading to eventual joint incongruency and possibly even avascular necrosis. Articular changes associated with subchondral avascular necrosis that are seen following the age of 10 years are considered symptomatic of osteochondritis dissecans.[4,11] Avascular necrosis may weaken the subchondral bone, may lead to secondary articular depression, and may cause changes in the joint surface. This may eventually lead to deformation of the capitellum, which may cause an alteration in the normal mechanics of the radiocapitellar joint and possible loose body formation (Fig. 20-4). If cessation of the offending activity (such as throwing a ball, swimming, or playing tennis) does not occur, additional changes to the radiocapitellar joint may occur, including restriction of joint motion, progressive joint surface degeneration, and formation of osteochondral fragments. The initial treatment for avascular necrosis of the capitellum is rest and cessation of the offending activities. If radiographs or magnetic resonance imaging demonstrate compromise of the joint, then surgical intervention should be considered with removal of the loose osteochondral fragments and either drilling of the subchondral bone to stimulate repair and or subchondral bone grafting.

The posterior elbow has its greatest involvement in the follow-through phase of throwing. In the skeletally immature adolescent athlete near complete ossification with persistent pain, two factors have been described by Pappas as possible causes.[37] The first is the formation of an avulsion fragment, which results in loose osteocartilaginous symptoms at the triceps insertion, and the second is the lack of fusion between the olecranon and its secondary ossification center. As the athlete matures and the ossification centers close, other causes of elbow pain may be seen: a forceful contraction of the triceps tendon, which may avulse off the olecranon and require surgical repair, or the formation of heterotopic bone at the tip of the olecranon, which may limit joint motion and may require surgical resection.

A relatively rare cause of elbow pain in the young athlete is radial head or proximal radial physeal injury. Although radial head fractures usually result from acute macrotrauma, injury may also result from repetitive valgus forces that are generated with elbow motion such as throwing. When an athlete presents with a history of repetitive throwing, pain with palpation over the radial head, loss of full extension and supination or active ROM, and positive radiographic fat pad sign, the physician should always suspect a radial head or neck fracture. Often, nondisplaced fractures may not be appreciated radiographically and the physician needs to use the clinical examination, history of the injury, and bone scan to determine if a fracture exists. Treatment for a nondisplaced radial head or neck fracture is sling immobilization until the patient is asymptomatic and then active ROM exercises.

Elbow joint dislocations are not uncommon in chil-

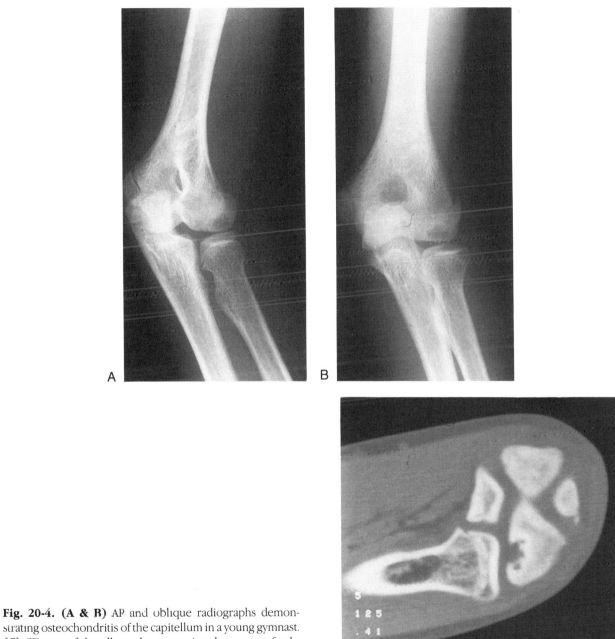

Fig. 20-4. (A & B) AP and oblique radiographs demonstrating osteochondritis of the capitellum in a young gymnast. **(C)** CT scan of the elbow demonstrating the extent of subchondral injury of the capitellum.

dren and adolescent athletes. They are usually seen in athletes who participate in contact sports like football and wrestling, in which the elbow joint may constantly undergo many different distracting forces, or high-load noncontact sports like gymnastics. Prompt recognition of such injuries are extremely important and early reduction should be performed. In addition, careful review of the prereduction and the postreduction radiographs is necessary to rule out any possible associated fracture. Early protected ROM is the preferred method of treatment along with repeat radiographs to evaluate the joint and observe any possible complications such as heterotopic ossification (Fig. 20-5).

One additional entity seen in the elbow of children and adolescent athletes is that of olecranon apophysitis. As described earlier, an apophysis is a traction epiphysis at the site of origin or insertion of major muscle groups, such as that seen with the attachment of the triceps tendon to the olecranon. Abnormal stresses, increased forces, musculotendinous imbalance, and rapid bony growth have all been identified as potential causes of chronic overuse or microtraumatic injuries. Conservative treatment is preferred for these injuries.

Hand and Wrist

As athletic participation has increased among children and adolescents so have the number of hand and wrist injuries, including certain sports-specific injuries.

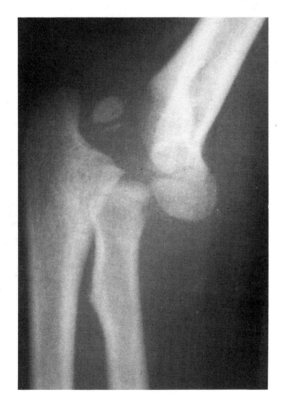

Fig. 20-5. Lateral radiograph of an elbow dislocation in a young athlete. Note the fractured medial epicondyle trapped in the joint.

Epiphyseal fractures of the distal radius and ulna are common injuries in children and adolescents. A thorough clinical examination needs to be performed to differentiate pain in the distal radius and ulna from pain in the proximal carpal row. The distal radial growth plate produces 75 to 80 percent of the entire growth potential of the radius, and the distal ulnar growth plate produces 40 percent of the growth potential for the entire ulna.[23] Acute fractures of the distal radius or distal ulna, or both, are usually caused when an athlete falls onto a hyperextended hand and wrist.[17,40,41] Wagner and Lyne[50] have reported that although it was thought that distal radius and ulnar epiphyseal fractures required a large force to cause a fracture, epiphyseal fractures at the distal radius or ulna, or both, may occur with loads of as little as 55 percent of the child or adolescent's body weight. Treatment of these types of fractures is best performed by a closed reduction with either a local hematoma block or general anesthesia, and then application of a cast for immobilization. It is important to note that because of the significant growth potential at the epiphyseal plates, the physician should not attempt multiple reductions, as this may increase the potential for growth plate injury.

Carpometacarpal (CMC) dislocations are rare in children and adolescents. The forces necessary to cause a carpometacarpal dislocation usually produce a fracture instead of a dislocation. However, if a dislocation occurs, it is most commonly seen in the adolescent age group. The most commonly injured CMC joint is that of the thumb. This injury is usually caused by an axial loading force on the thumb that produces a Salter III fracture, which would be equivalent to a Bennett's fracture in a skeletally mature individual. Treatment is similar to that of the adult, taking special care to obtain as complete an anatomic reduction as possible.

Although carpal bone fractures are less common in children and adolescents, scaphoid fracture is the next most common wrist fracture seen in this population. The most common site of fracture is through the distal third. These fractures also usually result from a fall on an outstretched hand. As with adults, children and adolescents commonly present with tenderness is the anatomic snuff box and decreased range of motion at the wrist. Often the initial radiographs are negative. If a high clinical level of suspicion exists, then the athlete should be placed in a short arm thumb spica and repeat radiographs should be obtained in 2 to 3 weeks. If the fracture is diagnosed late, with an apparent nonunion, then treatment is similar to that of the adult with a nonunion: immobilization for 8 to 12 weeks, possible bone grafting with or without internal fixation, and then repeat immobilization after surgery. If diagnosed at the time of injury, scaphoid fractures in the skeletally immature usually heal primarily with immobilization.[9,24,36]

The most common dislocation in the child's hand is dorsal dislocation of the thumb metacarpophalangeal (MP) joint.[41] MP dislocations of the index finger are the most common finger dislocation. The mechanism for these is hyperextension. Treatment depends on whether or not the volar plate is entrapped. If the volar plate is not entrapped, closed reduction is usually very successful. If the volar plate is entrapped or avulsed, or both, surgical repair is often required. Immobilization of the thumb should last for 3 to 4 weeks in a cast.[5,7,38,43] For the fingers, splinting in flexion for 10 days with immediate mobilization is recommended.[45]

The other common injury in the thumb MCP joint is avulsion of the ulnar collateral ligament from the proximal phalanx, commonly known as either a gamekeeper's or skier's thumb. A major function of the thumb is that of apposition or pinch between the thumb and the other fingers. A radially deviating force applied to the thumb of a young child may have a different outcome from that of an adolescent, and even that of an adult. In the young child, a Salter II fracture of the proximal first metacarpal may result. In the older child and adolescent a Salter III or IV fracture may occur, and in the skeletally mature athlete, an ulnar collateral ligament avulsion may occur. It is important to note that if a child or adolescent, or even an adult, presents with pain and tenderness over the ulnar collateral aspect of the thumb MCP and a history of radial deviation is known or suspected, radiographs should be obtained and carefully reviewed before the joint is stressed. If an undisplaced fracture exists, stressing the joint may displace the fracture. If the radiograph demonstrates a displaced fracture, either in a child or in an adult, open reduction is recommended to restore the anatomic alignment of the joint surface. If the radiographs are negative but the clinical examination demonstrates laxity and no end point with radial stress of the MCP joint, then open reduction and internal fixation of the ulnar collateral ligament is recommended.

Whether open reduction with internal fixation is performed or not, cast immobilization of the thumb is recommended.

Injuries to the interphalangeal joints are common; the *jammed finger* is seen in adolescents and in adults. This type of injury is the result of an axial loading force on the finger. It usually occurs when the distal interphalangeal joint is hyperflexed, the proximal interphalangeal joint is hyperextended, and an axial compression force is applied to the fingertip. The proximal interphalangeal joint is most commonly injured when this occurs. If the force is strong enough, the joint may dislocate, with the middle phalanx displacing dorsally on the proximal phalanx. Reduction of these injuries is usually done on site by either the player or the coach by applying distal traction to the digit and reducing the dislocation. Initial treatment after reduction should be to buddy tape the finger to an adjacent finger, and then seek medical attention to rule out fracture. A jamming injury at the distal interphalangeal joint may result in a *mallet finger*. This injury results from a torn terminal extensor tendon avulsion or a displaced Salter III fracture of the distal epiphysis. Treatment of this type of injury is reduction followed by immobilization in extension for 6 to 8 weeks, with full motion at the proximal interphalangeal joints. If closed reduction is not successful, open reduction or pinning may be necessary.

Tendinous injuries do occur in children and adolescents but they are rare. The most common closed flexor tendon injury that occurs in adolescents is that of an avulsed flexor tendon, most commonly occurring to the ring finger. This injury results when a hyperextension force to the distal interphalangeal joint is applied with a concomitant contraction of the flexor digitorum profundus tendon. It is commonly seen in contact sports when an athlete's finger gets caught on an opposing player's jersey and is forcibly hyperextended while flexing the flexor digitorum profundus. This injury has been called *jersey finger*. It is often diagnosed late. The avulsed tendon retracts, making treatment potentially more difficult. The tendon may retract just distal to the A4 pulley, often with a bony fragment; it may retract to the level of the proximal interphalangeal joint; or it may retract all the way into the palm, making for a potentially more extensive repair process.[45]

If the diagnosis is made within the first 3 weeks, the tendon usually may be reattached despite the extent

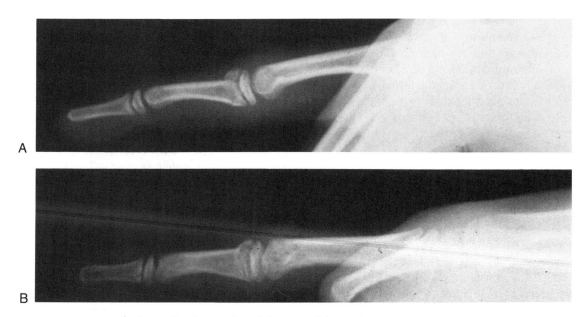

Fig. 20-6. (A & B) Salter II physeal fracture of the middle phalanx in a young athlete.

of the retraction. However, after the 3-week mark, the potential for performing primary repair of the tendon is significantly decreased because of adhesion. Therefore, if flexor function is to be restored, a free tendon graft must be done. Free tendon grafts have been reported to have good results in adolescents and young adults.[45]

Middle and proximal phalanx fractures are the most common hand fractures in children.[8] A significant majority of middle phalanx fractures are Salter II fractures of the proximal physis, caused by forced rotation and angulation.[38,45] Salter III fractures are more often seen in the proximal phalanx than in the middle phalanx. The reason for the difference in fracture pattern between the middle and proximal phalanx has been attributed to the fact that the collateral ligaments at the proximal interphalangeal joint insert on the epiphysis of the middle phalanx.[33]

Digital fractures are the most common physeal injuries encountered in sports (Fig. 20-6). Many differences exist between adult hand fractures and those of children and adolescents. The child and adolescent hand has the potential for remodeling, seen especially if the fracture occurs near the epiphysis and is within the plane of motion. Volar angulation in a child and adolescent finger fracture may be up to 30 degrees, whereas angulation greater than 25 degrees in an adult would potentially cause a disability to the patient when the finger is used.[41] The one condition that cannot be left to correct on its own is a rotational deformity, which must be corrected with either closed reduction or, if this procedure is unsuccessful, open reduction, each with possible fixation. Conservative treatment of most finger fractures in the child and adolescent population may be used, with only 10 percent requiring open reduction and internal fixation.[21] Nondisplaced phalanx fractures may be buddy taped to an adjacent finger and early ROM exercises begun after the initial pain from the injury subsides.

Distal tuft fractures of fingers occur in children and adolescents and in adults. They are often associated with axial forces on the distal tip of the finger or with compression injuries to the distal tip of the fingers. Nearly 50 percent of these fractures are open fractures with damage to the nail bed.[43] Treatment for simple closed tuft fractures is with a molded dorsal splint for 10 to 14 days in hyperextension. If the nail bed is involved, it should be repaired and the fracture immobilized in a dorsal splint.

CONCLUSIONS

At this time when athletic participation is on the rise, participation in organized sports has dramatically increased, especially among children and adolescents.

With this increase in participation has come increased potential for acute traumatic injuries of the upper extremity as well as new types of overuse injuries not previously seen in children and adolescents.

REFERENCES

1. Adams JE: Little League shoulder osteochondrosis of the proximal humeral epiphysis in boy baseball pitchers. Calif Med Assoc J 105:22–25, 1966

2. Andrish JT: Upper extremity injuries in the skeletally immature athlete. In Nicholas JA, Hershman EB (eds): The Upper Extremity in Sports Medicine. CV Mosby, St. Louis, 1990

3. Aronen JG, Regan K: Decreasing the incidence of recurrence of first time anterior shoulder dislocations with rehabilitation. Am J Sports Med 12:283–291, 1984

4. Brown R, Blazina ME, Kerlan RK et al: Osteochondritis of the capitellum. J Sports Med 2:27–46, 1974

5. Burton RI, Eaton RG: Common hand injuries in the athlete. Orthop Clin North Am 4:809–838, 1973

6. Cofield RH, Kavenagh BF, Frassica FJ: Anterior shoulder instability. p. 210. In: American Academy of Orthopaedic Surgeons, Instructional Course Lectures. Vol. 34. CV Mosby, St Louis, 1985

7. Dobyns JH, Sim FH, Linscheid RL: Sports stress syndromes of the hand and wrist. Am J Sports Med 6:236–254, 1978

8. Garcia-Moral CA: Injuries to the hand and wrist. p. 155. Sullivan JA, Grana WA (eds): The Pediatric Athlete. American Academy of Orthopaedic Surgeons, Park Ridge, IL, 1990

9. Greene MH, Hadied AM, LaMont RL: Scaphoid fractures in children. J Hand Surg 9A:536–541, 1984

10. Greipp JF: Swimmer's shoulder: the influence of flexibility and weight training. Phys Sports Med 13(8):92–105, 1985

11. Guggenheim JJ Jr, Stanley RF, Woods GW, Tullos HS: Little League survey: the Houston study. Am J Sports Med 4:189–200, 1976

12. Harris WR: Epiphyseal injuries. p. 206. In: American Academy of Orthopaedic Surgeons, Instructional Course Lectures. Vol. 15. CV Mosby, St. Louis, 1958

13. Hawkins RJ, Kennedy JC: Impingement syndrome in athletes. Am J Sports Med 8:151–158, 1980

14. Hovelius L: Anterior dislocation of the shoulder in teenagers and young adults. Five year prognosis. J Bone Joint Surg [Am] 69A:393–399, 1987

15. Hovelius L, Eriksson K, Fredin H et al: Recurrences after initial dislocation of the shoulder: results of a prospective study of treatment. J Bone Joint Surg [Am] 65A:343–349, 1983

16. Ireland ML, Andrews JR: Shoulder and elbow injuries in the young athlete. Clin Sports Med 7:473–494, 1988

17. Jacobs RA, Keller EL: Skateboard accidents. Pediatrics 59:939–942, 1977

18. Jobe FW, Jobe CM: Painful athletic injuries in the shoulder. Clin Orthop 173:117–124, 1983

19. Kennedy JC, Hawkins RJ, Krissoff WB: Orthopaedic manifestations of swimming. Am J Sports Med 6:1305–1322, 1978

20. Larson RL: Epiphyseal injuries in the adolescent athlete. Orthop Clin North Am 4:839–851, 1973

21. Leonard MH, Dubravcik P: Management of fractured fingers in the child. Clin Orthop 73:160–168, 1970

22. Makin JG, Brown WF, Ebers GC: C7 radiculopathy: importance of scapular winging in clinical diagnosis. J Neurol Neurosurg Psychiatry 49:640–644, 1986

23. Markiewitz AD, Andrish JT: Hand and wrist injuries in the preadolescent and adolescent athlete. Clin Sports Med 11:203–225, 1992

24. McCae FC, Baugher WH, Kurland DN et al: Hand and wrist injuries in the athlete. Am J Sports Med 7:275–286, 1979

25. Micheli LJ: Overuse injuries in children's sports: the growth factor. Orthop Clin North Am 14:337–360, 1983

26. Micheli LJ: Musculoskeletal trauma in children. p. 195. In Green M, Haggerty RJ (eds): Ambulatory Pediatrics. Vol. 3. WB Saunders, Philadelphia, 1984

27. Micheli LJ: Overuse injuries in children. p. 1103. In Lovell WW, Winter RB (eds): Pediatric Orthopaedics. 2nd Ed. Vol. 2. JB Lippincott, Philadelphia, 1986

28. Nelson MA: In Friedman SB (ed): Comprehensive Adolescent Health Care. Quality Medical Publishing, St Louis, 1992

29. Neer CS II: Anterior acromioplasty for the chronic impingement syndrome in the shoulder. J Bone Joint Surg [Am] 54A:41–50, 1972

30. Neer CS: Involuntary inferior and multidirectional instability of the shoulder is not rare. p. 232. In: American Academy of Orthopaedic Surgeons, Instructional Course Lectures. Vol. 34. CV Mosby, St Louis, 1985

31. Nielson AB, Nielson K: The modified Bristow procedure for recurrent anterior dislocation of the shoulder. Acta Orthop Scand 53:229–232, 1982

32. Niemien S, Aho AS: Anterior dislocation of the acromioclavicular joint. Ann Chir Gynaecol 73:21–24, 1984

33. O'Brien ET: Fractures of the hand and wrist region. p. 229. In Rockwood CA, Wilkins KE, King RE (eds): Fractures in Children. JB Lippincott, Philadelphia, 1984

34. O'Donohue DH: Subluxating biceps tendon in the athlete. J Sports Med Phys Fitness 1:20–29, 1973

35. O'Neill DB, Micheli LJ: Overuse injuries in the young athlete. Clin Sports Med 7:473–494, 1988

36. Ogden JA: Skeletal Injury in the Child. Lea & Febiger, Philadelphia, 1982

37. Pappas AM: Elbow problems associated with baseball during childhood and adolescence. Clin Orthop 164:30–41, 1982

38. Posner MA: Hand injuries. p. 495. In Nicholas JA, Hershman EB (eds): The Upper Extremity in Sports Medicine. CV Mosby, St Louis, 1990

39. Rang M: Children's Fractures. JB Lippincott, Philadelphia, 1974

40. Rockwood CA, Green DP, Bucholz RW: Fractures in Adults. Vol. 1. JB Lippincott, Philadelphia, 1991

41. Rockwood CA, Green DP, King RE: Fractures in Children. Vol. 3. JB Lippincott, Philadelphia, 1991

42. Rowe CR, Zarins B, Ciullo JV: Recurrent anterior dislocation of the shoulder after surgical repair. Apparent causes of failure and treatment. J Bone Joint Surg 66A(2):159–168, 1984

43. Ruby LK: Common hand injuries in the athlete. Clin Sports Med 2:609–629, 1983

44. Salter RB, Harris WR: Injuries involving the epiphyseal plate. J Bone Joint Surg [Am] 45A:587–622, 1963

45. Simmons BP, Lovallo JL: Hand and wrist injuries in children. Clin Sports Med 7:495–512, 1985

46. Simonet WT, Cofield RH: Prognosis in anterior shoulder dislocations. Am J Sports Med 12:19–24, 1984

47. Samilson RC, Prieto V: Posterior dislocation of the shoulder in athletes. Clin Sports Med 2:369–378, 1983

48. Taft TN, Wilson FC, Ogelsby JW: Dislocation of the acromioclavicular joint. J Bone Joint Surg [Am] 69A:1045–1051, 1987

49. Tibone JE: Shoulder problems of adolescents. Clin Sports Med 2:423–426, 1983

50. Wagner KT Jr., Lyne ED: Adolescent traumatic dislocations of the shoulder with open epiphyses. J Pediatr Orthop 3:61–62, 1983

51. Warner JJP, Micheli LJ, Arslanian LE et al: Patterns of flexibility, laxity, and strength in normal shoulders and shoulders with instability and impingement. Am J Sports Med 18:366–375, 1990

52. Warren RF: Subluxation of the shoulder in athletes. Clin Sports Med 2:339–354, 1983

Index